Health Inequalities in Japan: An Empirical Study of Older People

MODERNITY AND IDENTITY IN ASIA SERIES

Modernity and Identity in Asia Series

Globalization, Culture and Inequality in Asia
Timothy S. Scrase, Todd Miles, Joseph Holden and Scott Baum

Looking for Money: Capitalism and Modernity
in an Orang Asli Village
Alberto Gomes

Governance and Democracy in Asia
Takashi Inoguchi and Matthew Carlson

Liberalism: Its Achievements and Failures
Kazuo Seiyama

Health Inequalities in Japan: An Empirical Study of Older People
Katsunori Kondo

JAPANESE SOCIETY SERIES

General Editor: Yoshio Sugimoto

Lives of Young Koreans in Japan
Yasunori Fukuoka

Globalization and Social Change in Contemporary Japan
J.S. Eades, Tom Gill and Harumi Befu

Coming Out in Japan: The Story of Satoru and Ryuta
Satoru Ito and Ryuta Yanase

Japan and Its Others:
Globalization, Difference and the Critique of Modernity
John Clammer

Hegemony of Homogeneity:
An Anthropological Analysis of Nihonjinron
Harumi Befu

Foreign Migrants in Contemporary Japan
Hiroshi Komai

A Social History of Science and Technology in
Contemporary Japan, Volume 1
Shigeru Nakayama

Farewell to Nippon: Japanese Lifestyle Migrants in Australia
Machiko Sato

The Peripheral Centre:
Essays on Japanese History and Civilization
Johann P. Arnason

A Genealogy of 'Japanese' Self-images
Eiji Oguma

Class Structure in Contemporary Japan
Kenji Hashimoto

An Ecological View of History
Tadao Umesao

Nationalism and Gender
Chizuko Ueno

Native Anthropology: The Japanese Challenge
to Western Academic Hegemony
Takami Kuwayama

Youth Deviance in Japan: Class Reproduction of Non-Conformity
Robert Stuart Yoder

Japanese Companies: Theories and Realities
Masami Nomura and Yoshihiko Kamii

From Salvation to Spirituality:
Popular Religious Movements in Modern Japan
Susumu Shimazono

The 'Big Bang' in Japanese Higher Education: The 2004 Reforms and the Dynamics of Change
J.S. Eades, Roger Goodman and Yumiko Hada

Japanese Politics: An Introduction
Takashi Inoguchi

A Social History of Science and Technology in Contemporary Japan, Volume 2
Shigeru Nakayama

Gender and Japanese Management
Kimiko Kimoto

Philosophy of Agricultural Science: A Japanese Perspective
Osamu Soda

A Social History of Science and Technology in Contemporary Japan, Volume 3
Shigeru Nakayama and Kunio Goto

Japan's Underclass: Day Laborers and the Homeless
Hideo Aoki

A Social History of Science and Technology in Contemporary Japan, Volume 4
Shigeru Nakayama and Hitoshi Yoshioka

Scams and Sweeteners: A Sociology of Fraud
Masahiro Ogino

Toyota's Assembly Line: A View from the Factory Floor
Ryoji Ihara

Village Life in Modern Japan: An Environmental Perspective
Akira Furukawa

Social Welfare in Japan: Principles and Applications
Kojun Furukawa

Japan's Whaling: The Politics of Culture in Historical Perspective
Hiroyuki Watanabe

Escape from Work: Freelancing Youth and the Challenge to Corporate Japan
Reiko Kosugi

Gender Gymnastics: Performing and Consuming Japan's Takarazuka Revue
Leonie R. Stickland

Poverty and Social Welfare in Japan
Masami Iwata and Akihiko Nishizawa

Japan's Whaling: The Politics of Culture in Historical Perspective
Hiroyuki Watanabe

Health and Social Disparity in Japan: Japan and Beyond
Norito Kawakami, Yasuki Kobayashi and Hideki Hashimoto

The Modern Family in Japan: Its Rise and Fall
Chizuko Ueno

Widows of Japan: An Anthropological Perspective
Deborah McDowell Aoki

Social Stratification and Inequality Series

Inequality amid Affluence: Social Stratification in Japan
Junsuke Hara and Kazuo Seiyama

Intentional Social Change: A Rational Choice Theory
Yoshimichi Sato

Constructing Civil Society in Japan:
Voices of Environmental Movements
Koichi Hasegawa

Deciphering Stratification and Inequality: Japan and Beyond
Yoshimichi Sato

Social Justice in Japan: Concepts, Theories and Paradigms
Ken-ichi Ohbuchi

Gender and Career in Japan
Atsuko Suzuki

Status and Stratification: Cultural Forms in East and Southeast Asia
Mutsuhiko Shima

Globalization, Minorities and Civil Society:
Perspectives from Asian and Western Cities
Koichi Hasegawa and Naoki Yoshihara

Fluidity of Place: Globalization and the Transformation of Urban Space
Naoki Yoshihara

Advanced Social Research Series

A Sociology of Happiness
Kenji Kosaka

Frontiers of Social Research: Japan and beyond
Akira Furukawa

A Quest for Alternative Sociology
Kenji Kosaka and Masahiro Ogino

MODERNITY AND IDENTITY IN ASIA SERIES

Health Inequalities in Japan: An Empirical Study of Older People

edited by

Katsunori Kondo

foreword by

Ichiro Kawachi

TRANS PACIFIC PRESS

First published in Japanese in 2007 by Igaku Shoin as *Kenshō kenkō kakusa shakai: Kaigo yobō ni muketa shakai-ekigakuteki daikibo chōsa.*

This English edition first published in 2010 by
Trans Pacific Press, PO Box 164, Balwyn North, Victoria 3104, Australia
Telephone: +61-3-9859-1112 Fax: +61-3-9859-4110
Email: tpp.mail@gmail.com
Web: http://www.transpacificpress.com

Designed and set by Digital Environs, Melbourne. www.digitalenvirons.com
Figures set by the authors.

Printed by BPA Print Group, Burwood, Victoria, Australia.

Distributors

Australia and New Zealand
DA Information Services/Central Book Services
648 Whitehorse Road
Mitcham, Victoria 3132
Australia
Telephone: +61-3-9210-7777
Fax: + 61-3-9210-7788
Email: books@dadirect.com
Web: www.dadirect.com

USA and Canada
International Specialized Book Services (ISBS)
920 NE 58th Avenue, Suite 300
Portland, Oregon 97213-3786
USA
Telephone: 1-800-944-6190
Fax: 1-503-280-8832
Email: orders@isbs.com
Web: http://www.isbs.com

Asia and the Pacific
Kinokuniya Company Ltd.

Head office:
3-7-10 Shimomeguro
Meguro-ku
Tokyo 153-8504
Japan
Telephone: +81-3-6910-0531
Fax: +81-3-6420-1362
Email: bkimp@kinokuniya.co.jp
Web: www.kinokuniya.co.jp

Asia-Pacific office:
Kinokuniya Book Stores of Singapore Pte., Ltd.
391B Orchard Road #13-06/07/08
Ngee Ann City Tower B
Singapore 238874
Telephone: +65-6276-5558
Fax: +65-6276-5570
Email: SSO@kinokuniya.co.jp

ISBN 978-1-920901-71-4 (Hardback)

National Library of Australia Cataloguing-in-Publication entry

Title:	Health inequalities in Japan: an empirical study of older people / editor, Katsunori Kondo.
ISBN:	9781920901714 (hbk.)
Notes:	Includes bibliographical references and index.
Subjects:	Older people – Japan – Health and hygiene. Older people – Medical care – Japan. Health – Social aspects – Japan. Preventive health services for older people – Japan.
Dewey Number:	362.60952

Contents

Figures

Tables

Boxes

Contributors

Katsunori Kondo
Professor, Faculty of Social Welfare
Director, Center for Well-being and Society
Nihon Fukushi University

Hideki Endo
Associate Professor, Faculty of Economics
Nihon Fukushi University

Hiroshi Hirai
Chief Researcher, Center for Well-being and Society
Nihon Fukushi University

Yukinobu Ichida
Visiting Researcher, Center for Well-being and Society
Nihon Fukushi University

Etsuko Kato
Associate Professor, Faculty of Social Welfare
Nihon Fukushi University

Ichiro Kawachi
Professor and Chair, Department of Society, Human Development, and Health
Harvard School of Public Health

Ryozo Matsuda
Professor, Faculty of Social Sciences
Ritsumeikan University

Chiyoe Murata
Assistant Professor, Department of Community Health and Preventive Medicine
Hamamatsu University School of Medicine

Miyo Nakade
Associate Professor, Faculty of Human Wellness
Tokaigakuen University

Yoshitaka Saito
Associate professor, Department of Health & Welfare Management
Bunri University

Yumika Shirase
Researcher, Department of Empirical Social Security Research,
National Institute of Population and Social Security Research

Kei Suemori
Associate Professor, Faculty of Social Welfare
Nihon Fukushi University

Tokunori Takeda
Professor, Division of Occupational Therapy, Faculty of Rehabilitation
Seijoh University

Kiyoko Yoshii
Associate Professor, Faculty of Social Welfare
Nihon Fukushi University

Goshu Yoshikawa
Research Fellow, Graduate School of Global Environmental Studies
Kyoto University

Translators
Ross Mouer: Chapters 1–3
Fumiko Tachibana: Chapter 4 and Appendix
Kikuko Onoda: Chapters 5–7, 11
Dougal Phillips: Chapters 8–10
Minako Sato: Chapters 12–15

Structural editor
Karl Smith

Foreword

The publication of the English translation of Professor Katsunori Kondō's book marks a watershed in the field of the social determinants of health. The findings of his landmark Aichi Gerontological Evaluation Study (AGES) are significant for three reasons. First, Japan leads the world in the rapid pace of population aging. Owing to a combination of increasing life-spans and a declining fertility rate, Japan leads the world in having the highest proportion of individuals older than 65 years of age in the population, currently over 1 in 5 individuals. Japan's profile offers a glimpse of the future for other countries which are following close on the heels of Japan's demographic transition. As Japanese society grapples with the challenges of an aging population, the rest of the world has much to learn from both the country's successes and failures. On the positive side of Japan's achievement is the much-touted fact that the Japanese are the longest-living individuals on the planet, with an average life expectancy *at age 65* of more than 22 years for women – in other words, the average 65 year old Japanese woman can expect to live for another two decades. On the negative side, Japanese society is heading for a crisis brought on by population decline, falling worker-to-retiree ratios, rising costs of social security payments and – unless something is done – an eventual decline in living standards.

One of the major planks of Japanese health policy to meet the needs of an aging population has been to improve access to long-term care. The revised Long-Term Care Insurance Law, introduced by the Japanese government in April 2006, is part of this effort. Whether the new policy has been successful is still debatable, and this book provides a critique of that policy. Using impeccable epidemiological logic, Professor Kondō's analysis points out that the current screening procedures to determine eligibility for long-term care are able to correctly identify less than 0.2 percent of older individuals who eventually end up needing long-term care. That is an important lesson for other countries grappling with policies to meet the needs of an aging population.

In contrast to the high risk screening approach adopted by Japanese government, Professor Kondō's analysis points the way to a more sustainable approach to prevent long-term care dependency, based upon core principles of population-based prevention. His prescription is based upon life-long investment in factors that promote "healthy aging". What is remarkable about Professor Kondō's far-reaching analysis is that his prescription consists of not just the usual advice dispensed to individuals to avoid smoking, exercise regularly, and floss their teeth, but also broader investments at the community and societal level, including investing in education earlier in life, strengthening community bonds (the notion of "social capital"), reducing inequalities in the distribution of wealth and income, and assuring financial and occupational security. In other words, Professor Kondō's prescription is aimed not just at what individuals can do for themselves, but what communities and societies ought to be doing to assure the healthy aging of the population. For readers familiar with the World Health Organization's 2009 Commission on the Social Determinants of Health, Professor Kondō's radical message echoes the new direction in health promotion advocated by the WHO. It amounts to a call to re-direct the focus of our health care policies, backed by hard evidence.

A second reason for the significance of this book is that it represents the first time that the social determinants of health have been examined within Japanese society in such a comprehensive and in-depth manner. "The social determinants of health" refers to a broad set of factors including social class (education, income, occupational status), stress, social relations, and community social capital which are believed to influence the health of people over and above their lifestyle habits, genetic endowment, and access to health services. The field of social determinants represents a burgeoning area of research throughout the world. So far, however, the bulk of research has been carried out in western societies (primarily North America, Europe, Australasia), and the field is still nascent in Asian countries. The value of studying social determinants in non-western contexts is obvious. Quite apart from the need to replicate findings from the West in other cultural contexts, the emerging studies in Asia are beginning to paint a very different picture of the relationships between social determinants and health outcomes.

To give a simple example, marital status has attained near-canonical status in studies based in western populations as a fundamental determinant of health. As a broad generalization, married men and women tend to live longer than the never married, the widowed, the separated and divorced. The association between marriage and longevity is partly due to selection bias (i.e. healthy people are more successful in finding marriage partners). But there is now also sufficient evidence to convince most social scientists that the association is partly causal – that is, marriage promotes health through financial security,

Box 1: Japan as an Aged Society

Tokunori Takeda

Introduction

Japan is an aged society. The average life expectancy was 78.4 years for men and 85.3 years for women and the aging rate was 19 percent in 2003, both of which were among the highest in the world (Cabinet Office 2004). Japan's transition to an aged society has precipitated new problems posed by a growing number of older people who require long-term care due to immobility, dementia, depression and housebound behavior. The promotion of 'long-term care prevention' has thus become a real challenge for Japan in order to prevent older people from becoming invalid and those already receiving nursing care from deteriorating further.

This box will explain the changes in the aging rate and the average life expectancy underlying Japan's aged society. It will then outline the circumstances surrounding the establishment of the 'long-term care insurance' system to deal with the increasing number of people requiring nursing care.

Aging rate

The total population of Japan is projected to rise from 126.39 million in 2000 to 127.62 million in 2003, 127.77 million in 2007, then begin to shrink to around 125.40 million by 2015 (Cabinet Office 2004).

The aging rate (the ratio of the population aged 65 or older to the total population) is rising rapidly. Figure 0.1 shows changes in the aging rate (Cabinet Office 2007). It shows that Japan became an aging society when the aging rate reached 7 percent in 1970 and grew into an aged society within a period of 24 years when the aging rate hit 14 percent. It was an extremely short period in comparison with other countries. For example, France took 115 years to reach that stage, Sweden 85 years, the USA 75 years and the UK 45 years. Japan's aging rate reached 17.3 percent in 2000, 19 percent in 2003 and exceeded 20 percent in 2005, topping the world ahead of Italy's 19.7 percent. The aging rate is forecast to climb to 23.1 percent in 2010, 26.9 percent in 2015 and 29.2 percent in 2020 when one in three Japanese will be 65 years old or older (Cabinet Office 2007).

A characteristic of the impending expansion of an older population is an increasingly higher ratio of the late-stage older population (aged 75 or older) relative to the early-stage older population (aged 65–74) and to the total population. Figure 0.2 shows this trend (Cabinet Office 2004). The proportion of the late-stage older population was

Figure 0.1: World trends in aging rate

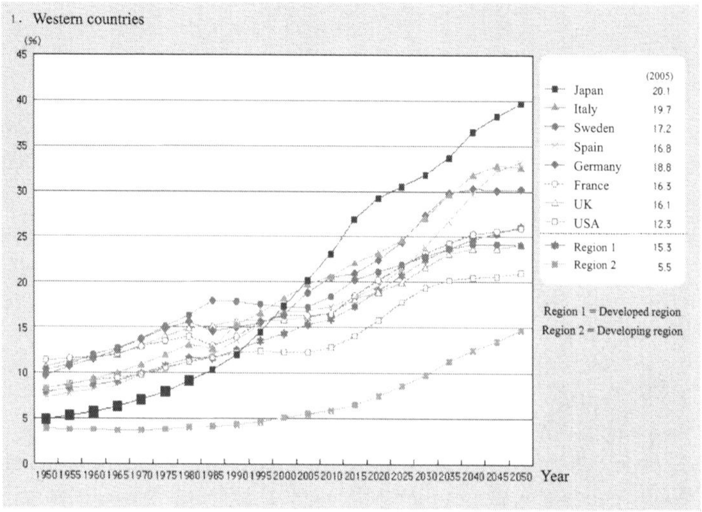

Source: Compiled from Cabinet Office, Heisei 19-nen-ban *kōrei shakai hakusho* (Annual report on the aging society 2007).

2.1 percent in 1970 when Japan became an aging society, a figure which had almost tripled by 1995 to 5.7 percent and nearly quadrupled by 2003 to 8.3 percent, within only 30 years or so. It is expected to increase to 13.1 percent by 2015.

Average life expectancy

Japan's average life expectancy is among the highest in the world for both men and women. According to data from the OECD, Japan's average life expectancy was 78.4 years for men and 85.3 years for women in 2003 while the average was 76.9 years and 82.9 years in Italy, 77.9 years and 82.4 years in Sweden, 75.8 years and 82.9 years in France, 76.2 years and 80.7 years in the UK, 74.5 years and 79.9 years in the USA and 73.4 years and 80.4 years in Korea (OECD 2005).

Figure 3 shows the future trend for average life expectancy in Japan (Cabinet Office 2007). The 2005 figures of 78.5 years for men and 85.5 years for women will increase to 80.2 years and 87.0 years by 2015 and 81.3 years and 88.1 years by 2025, after which women's life expectancy is projected to exceed 90 years. Japan is indeed a nation of longevity. However, this is not a product of any genetic characteristics peculiar to the Japanese. This is due to the rapid rise that Japan experienced after the postwar period (1945–1965) as shown in Figure 0.1.

Figure 0.2: Trends in aging rate and late-stage older population ratio

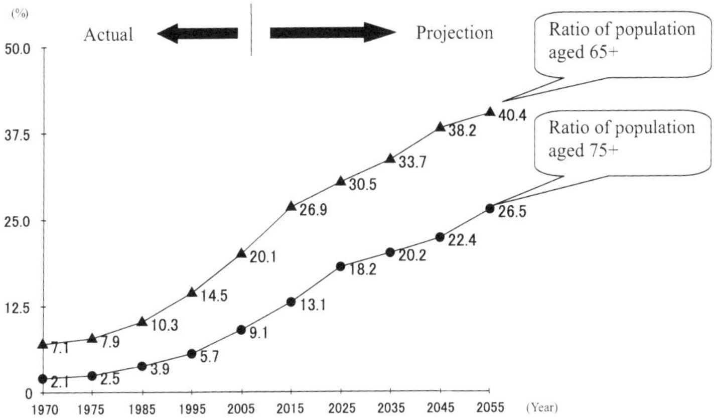

Source: Compiled from Cabinet Office, *Heisei 16-nen-ban kōrei shakai hakusho* (Annual report on the aging society 2004).

Furthermore, average life expectancy at the age of 65 was 18.02 years for men and 23.04 years for women in 2003 (Ministry of Health, Labour and Welfare 2008). Compared with 12.50 years for men and 15.34 years for women in 1970, the life expectancy has increased, especially for women. This means that people spend more years in their old age. The way they spend their old age is important not only for their QOL but also for long-term care prevention.

Healthy life expectancy

Healthy life expectancy proposed by the WHO in 2000 refers to 'the length of life lived in full health'. According to an international comparison of 2002 figures contained in its 2004 report (WHO 2004), Japan's healthy life expectancy was the longest in the world at 72.3 years for men and 77.7 years for women. Other high-ranking countries for men included Iceland at 72.1 years, Sweden at 71.9 years, Switzerland at 71.1 years and Australia at 70.9 years. It was 69.3 years in France, 69.1 years in the UK and 67.2 years in the USA.

High-ranking countries for women included San Marino at 75.9 years, Spain at 75.3 years, Switzerland at 75.3 years and Monaco at 75.2 years. It was 74.7 years in France, 72.1 years in the UK and 71.3 years in the USA.

Long-term care insurance system

When Japan's aging rate reached 7 percent in 1970, the number of older

Figure 0.3: Trends in average life expectancy in Japan

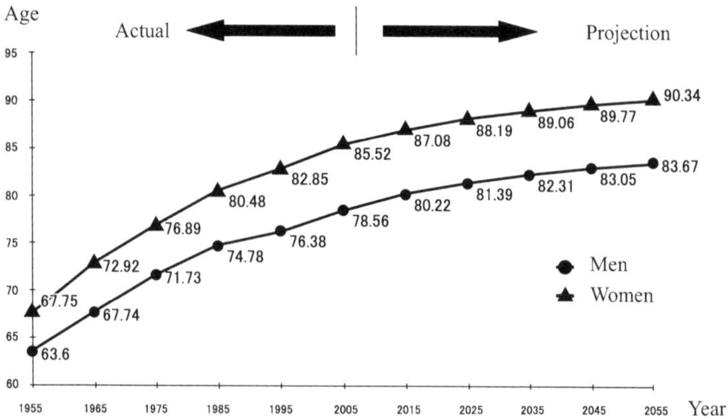

Source: Compiled from Cabinet Office, Heisei 19-nen-ban *kōrei shakai hakusho* (Annual report on the aging society 2007).

people who are bedridden, suffering from dementia and requiring long-term care began to increase. This gave rise to new social problems. First, their family members were also aging and unable to provide adequate nursing care at home. Second, they were requiring care for increasingly longer periods of time. Third, medical services and facilities were inappropriately using long-term hospitalization for nursing care (so-called social hospitalization). Last, the system at the time was vertically divided between medicine and welfare. Users could not freely choose the service they wanted and had to pay unequal amounts of co-payment at the point of service.

The government was pressed to resolve concerns about problems and establish mechanisms to distribute the cost burden of long-term care, which was expected to rise rapidly, among the entire nation equitably into the future. The Long-Term Care Insurance Law was passed in 1997 and the system was put into operation in April 2000.

Long-term care insurance covers those who are aged 65 or older (Category 1 Insured) and those aged from 40 to 64 (Category 2 Insured). These people become eligible to receive services if:

1. they require care and support for daily activities such as bathing, toilet and meals (persons requiring long-term care), or
2. they are in a frail state and require appropriate services to stop them from deteriorating to a long-term care status (long-term care risk). (Long-term Care Insurance, Ministry of Health, Labour and Welfare 2002)

Figure 0.4: Changes in the number of people certified for long-term care

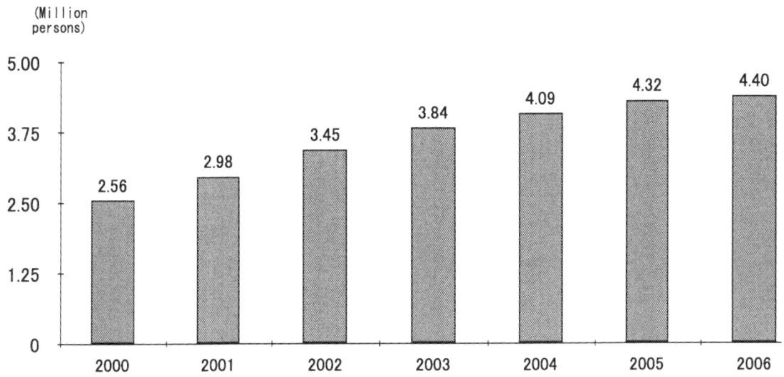

Compiled from Cabinet Office, *Heisei 18-nen-ban kōrei shakai hakusho* (Annual report on the aging society 2006).

Long-term care prevention

Figure 0.4 shows changes in the number of certified persons requiring long-term care since the introduction of the long-term care insurance system in April 2000. The total number increased from 2.56 million in 2000 to 4.32 million in 2005 and 4.40 million in 2006, an increase of 1.84 million. In five years from 2000, the number of persons requiring support (not yet requiring long-term care) more than doubled from 290,000 to 670,000. For this reason, the 2005 review of the system proposed shifting the emphasis to long-term care prevention and implementation of this change began in 2006.

Long-term care prevention is defined as 'preventing (delaying) the older person from falling into a state requiring long-term care as much as possible and preventing the older person in a state requiring long-term care from deteriorating further as much as possible' (Kaigo Yobo Manyuaru 2009). It does not only aim for the improvement of individual elements such as motor function and nutritional status of older people. Rather, it attempts to increase the living activities (activity level) and participation (role level) of individual older persons as per the International Classification of Functioning, Disability and Health (ICF, 2001) through the improvement of mental and physical functions and environmental factors and thereby support the endeavors for individual fulfillment and self realization in order to improve their quality of life (QOL). Long-term care prevention aspires to create a longevity society that is truly worth celebrating as well as to maximize healthy life expectancy for the nation.

the exchange of love and social support. Curiously, however, when the same studies are repeated in Japan, a different pattern emerges. In the Japan Collaborative Cohort study of over 94,000 men and women prospectively followed for 10 years, Ikeda and colleagues recently reported that widowed and divorced Japanese men were at 1.5–2.0 times the risk of dying during follow-up compared to married men. By contrast, however, widowed/divorced Japanese women were at no greater risk of mortality compared to married Japanese women (Ikeda et al. 2007 *BMC Public Health*; 7:73). Apparently, being married does not confer the same health protection to Japanese women as to women in the west! This finding is also echoed in Professor Kondō's AGES study (Chapter 10), where his team found that married Japanese women were more likely to report poor health than the never married, divorced, and widowed. Both of these findings contradict decades of studies conducted in western societies which suggest that health is better for the married than for those who were not married. What could explain this curious discrepancy? When researchers are confronted with a major contradiction in research results, they must conclude either that: a) one set of studies gave the wrong answer (for example because they were of poor quality), or b) the theory itself is incomplete. In this instance, both of the studies conducted in Japan were of high quality, and thus one is forced to conclude that the "canonical" relationship between marital status and health is not so canonical after all.

The intriguing discrepancy in the association of marriage and health between east and west suggests that the same social determinant (marital status) can influence health in different ways depending on the social context. In the case of Japanese society, it throws up the intriguing possibility that marriage does not serve the same functions as it does in the west. Whereas most western marriages are based upon shared lives between husband and wife, Japan has been referred to as a "homo-social" society in which men and women lead largely separate lives, at least during their working years. The typical Japanese "salaryman" leaves the house early in the morning (often before the kids are up), and returns home after everyone has gone to bed. The weekends are for dads to catch up on their sleep. By contrast, Japanese women's lives are centered on the children, friends, relatives, and neighbors. The result is that when a man retires from work, he is forcibly brought together with his wife for the first time in decades, often to share the typically restricted confines of a Japanese apartment. In contrast to many western couples who eagerly look forward to retirement as a period in life when they can go on road trips together in the family Winnebago, post-retirement life for many Japanese couples represents a period of heightened tension and stress. Indeed, many support groups have formed throughout Japan in recent years to provide counseling to distressed couples, and the demeaning term "*nuré-ochiba*" (wet, clinging leaves) was minted in the popular lexicon to describe the pitiful predicament of retired husbands who mope about the house with nothing to do. In short, there is a rich vein to be tapped in conducting cross-cultural research on the social determinants of health, and Professor Kondō offers many nuggets of insight throughout this book.

The third and final reason for citing the significance of this book is because it, for the first time, provides a snapshot of the emerging health inequalities in Japanese society. Japan has been long heralded as an egalitarian land of the broad middle class. That all changed with the asset bubble collapse in 1989, and the decade long economic slump ("the Lost Decade" – now extending to two decades) that followed. During the slow and excruciating path to economic recovery, Japanese society was radically reshaped from an egalitarian one – with lifelong employment and job security – to an American-style society consisting of "winners and losers". The Japanese have only recently woken up to the changed reality of their lives, and the news media are now constantly blaring about the emergence of a new "poverty class" as well as the sharp increase in wealth and health inequalities. The rising awareness of the concept of the "health gap society" (*kenkou kakusha shakai*) is due in no small part to the tireless efforts of Professor Kondō to raise consciousness about the issue in his academic research as well as his popular writings on the topic. The AGES study was, in fact, the first academic study to reveal that there was a seven-fold difference in the risk of depressive illness comparing the least well off Japanese to the most well off. The sheer magnitude of that inequality was a wake-up call, and the shock still reverberates throughout the Japanese public health community. Professor Kondō's study has laid down the benchmark against which all subsequent descriptions of health inequalities in Japan will be compared. His study also lays down an explicit challenge to all health policy makers in the country – will they continue to tolerate the widening health disparities that could eventually jeopardize the health achievements of the post-War years, or will they reverse the trend by investing in the broader social determinants of health? Now is the time to act.

Ichiro Kawachi
Professor of Social Epidemiology
Harvard University
January 2010

Preface

Japan boasts the world's healthiest population with the longest average lifespan. Few books in English, however, give a complete picture of Japan's older population. The aim of this book is to profile Japan's older population by using findings from a large-scale survey which targeted over 30,000 people. It paints a multi-faceted picture of Japan's older population from a variety of perspectives: depression; self-rated health; oral functions; malnutrition; history of falls; health-promoting activities; insomnia; hobbies; abuse; household make-up; participation in community organisations; social support; work; and social capital (which has been attracting attention across many fields in recent years). This book summarises the research findings on these factors and their relationship with socioeconomic factors such as income and educational attainment. It also presents results on the disparity between urban and rural regions. Readers interested in an overview would be well served by reading Chapter 15, which presents a summary of each chapter.

However, this book has three additional aims which draw upon the domestic and overseas research and policy trends I introduced in my book, 'The Health-Gap Society: What is harming our minds and health?' (*Kenkou kakusa shakai – nani ga kokoro to kenkou wo mushibamu no ka*) (Igaku-Shoin, 2005). These aims are detailed below.

Japan was once regarded as a relatively egalitarian country, one which came a close second to the countries of northern Europe. However, since the 1990s Japan has seen a dramatic widening of socioeconomic inequalities, such as the income gap indexed by the Gini coefficient. These inequalities would be expected to give rise to disparities in health. The first aim of this book, then, is to evaluate the degree to which health inequalities exist among Japan's older population. For instance, men in the lowest income group are 6.9 times more likely to be depressed than those in the highest income group (Chapter 2).

The second aim of this book is to highlight the necessity of reviewing the strategy behind healthy ageing and 'long-term care prevention' which seeks to prevent people from deteriorating to a point at which they require long-term care. In 2000, Japan saw the introduction of social insurance for long-term care. However, the fact that benefits increased beyond expectations led to a review of the long-term care insurance system in April 2006. This brought about greater emphasis on long-term care prevention in order to help keep costs under control. The long-term care prevention system targets older people who are vulnerable to the risks of their functions deteriorating to a state in which they require long-term care. This system, however, has not been functioning well. It has attempted to identify participants for long-term care prevention by screening people who attend health checkups. However, it has only been possible to identify a mere 0.14% of participants for home-based care programs despite the original estimate that such people accounted for approximately 5% of the elderly population.

This book clarifies the reasons for this. The lower a person's level of income, the more likely they will have multiple health problems (e.g. poor self-rated health) and the higher the risk that they will eventually require long-term care (long-term care risk). Further, it is also clear that people with a low level of education have a higher long-term care risk from factors such as depression or a history of falls. This is despite the fact that the education in question occurred some 50 years earlier. Despite this relationship, the fact is that the lower a person's socioeconomic status, the less likely they are to attend health checkups. In other words, the 'high risk' strategy by screening high risk individuals at health checkups and the interventions has its limitations after old age. This book aims to highlight the necessity of adopting a population strategy from an earlier age and an ecological perspective which focuses on the interaction of multiple factors.

The third aim is to demonstrate the importance of social epidemiological research. Current health policy and long-term home-based care prevention policy focus solely on health behaviours relating to nutrition, exercise, smoking and alcohol as risk factors. While these are important, the present book highlights the psychological and social factors which also relate to poor health in similar ways. In order to draft more effective policy on health and long-term care prevention in the future, it is imperative to conduct social epidemiological research which takes account of psychological and social factors. The World Health Organization (WHO) has released two editions of the book, *Social Determinants of Health: The Solid Facts* (1998, 2003). WHO then established the Commission on Social Determinants of Health (CSDH) in 2005. In their final report, they noted the importance of measuring health inequities and raising public awareness about the social determinants of health. It is my hope that, through this book, many people will discover the important role played by the social determinants of health and the significance of social epidemiology in highlighting such factors. I hope that social epidemiological research can progress to the next level.

It is desirable that empirical research such as that featured in this book be published in a peer reviewed journal. This is because the peer review process maintains the quality of research by only publishing research articles which can stand up to the critical eye of fellow researchers. The collection of articles published in this book have not been subjected to the formal peer review process (with the exception of Chapters 5, 9 & 11) since the cohesiveness of the whole was considered a greater priority. It is not our intention as authors, however, to publish research that, by obviating the peer review process, is of poor quality. Rather, in order to enhance the quality of the articles, during the process of drafting the articles and bringing them together in a book, we have had many opportunities for mutual criticism amongst the authors and at meetings of the Health Inequality Workgroup which have led to ongoing refinements.

Nevertheless, it has been my experience from past peer reviews that, while collaborators may engage in mutual critiques, the potential for blind spots remains. Accordingly, the manuscripts for each chapter were submitted for comment to researchers with an interest in the areas of social epidemiology and long-term care prevention, and were also submitted to editorial committee members of the *Japanese Journal of Public Health*. On condition of anonymity (with the exception of the editor), these reviewers ensured that: the basic data had been covered and nothing relevant had been inadvertently omitted; the limits of the research had been described; no blind spots existed; no claims had been exaggerated; and that the articles were well-structured, in addition to other editorial considerations. Only after completing the editing process by incorporating these comments did this book come into being. I would like to take this opportunity to express my thanks to all of the people who so kindly cooperated in improving the quality of this book including: Tadayuki Ahiko, Masao Ishizaki, Toshiyuki Ojima, Naoki Kondo, Hidehiro Sugisawa, Shigeru Soukejima, Toshio Takatorige, Akizumi Tsutsumi, Satoshi Toyokawa, Takeo Nakayama, Shigeki Nishida, Hideki Hashimoto, Kenji Hayashi and Yoshiharu Fukuda. I would also like to acknowledge the other collaborators who preferred to remain anonymous. However, it goes without saying that, as its editor, I assume all responsibility relating to the content of this book.

The present research was carried out as part of the Nihon Fukushi University 21 Century Center of Excellence Program "Asian COE toward new policy science for social well-being and development"

(2003–2007) with the support of a 2003–2005 Grant-In-Aid for Scientific Research (14310105) and a 2002–2006 Academic Frontier Project grant (Japanese Ministry of Education, Culture, Sports, Science and Technology (MEXT)). Publication of the English version of the book was supported by a Grant-in-Aid for Publication of Scientific Research Results (2009). On behalf of the Center for Well-being and Society (CWS) which was established with a Strategic Research Foundational Project grant for Private Universities (MEXT, 2009–2013) at Nihon Fukushi University, it gives us great pleasure to publish the research findings in English and hence make them available to researchers overseas. I would like to express my thanks for the many research subsidies.

I would also like to express my gratitude to all the people who participated in the study, to the long-term care insurance staff at the regional local governments, and the various other people who provided feedback at various conferences. Finally, I would also like to express my appreciation to Igaku-Shoin for their publication of the Japanese version of this book and to Trans Pacific Press for publication of the English version.

August 2010

Katsunori Kondō
Director,
Center for Well-being and Society,
Nihon Fukushi University

Chapter 1

Introducing a Survey on Health of Older People in Japan: AGES (Aichi Gerontological Evaluation Study) project

Katsunori Kondō

Introduction

Since becoming the most aged society in the world, attention in Japan has shifted to the issues involved in healthy aging and "nursing or long-term care prevention" (Koreisha Kaigo Kenkyukai 2003; Koreisha Rihabiriteeshon Kenkyukai 2004). "Nursing or long-term care prevention" means preventing frailty and disability for older people. The causes of frailty and disability among older people are not limited to the effects of strokes, hip fractures and other such ailments (Koreisha Rihabiriteeshon Kenkyukai 2004). Many older people lose the capacity to lead a normal or independent life style owing to an array of socio-psychological factors such as social isolation and depression, etc. In order to develop effective preventative policies, it is necessary to study the ways that such phenomena are distributed across the older population.

The study of how various socio-psychological factors affect health is being taken up by a new sub-discipline known as "social epidemiology". Social epidemiology is defined as the "branch of epidemiology that studies the social distribution and social determinants of health" (Berkman and Kawachi 2000). I have introduced the theoretical framework of this field and relevant empirical data in a recently published volume entitled 'The Health-Gap Society: What is harming our minds and our health?' [*Kenkou kakusa shakai – nani ga kokoro to kenkou o mushibamu no ka*] (Kondō 2005).

The view that Japan is an egalitarian society is firmly entrenched in the minds of many Japanese. It has often been the case that information such as income and educational background is not carefully reported in social surveys and the government has often been reluctant to release information on the socio-economic background of the

Figure 1.1: Social epidemiological model of relationship examined in this book

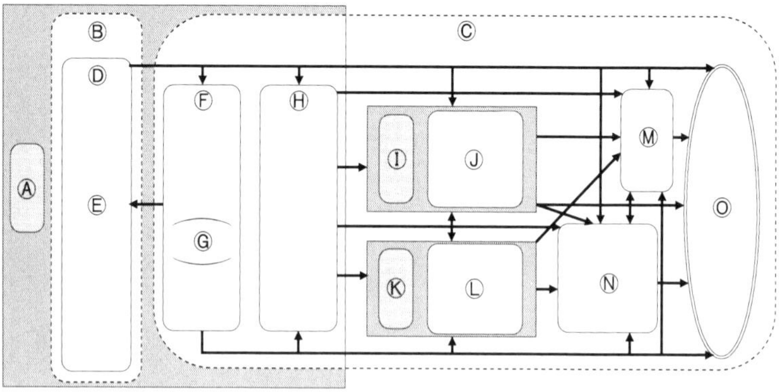

Legend:

Ⓐ Social factors.

Ⓑ Community-level factors.

Ⓒ Individual-level factors.

Ⓓ Characteristics of community-level factors.

Ⓔ (Semi-)urban, rural. ②–⑬
Social capital. ⑭

Ⓕ Socio-economic status.

Ⓖ Income. ②–⑬
Years of education. ②–⑬
Employment status. ⑬

Ⓗ Household composition, marital status, marital satisfaction. ⑩
Participation in community organizations. ⑪
Giving/receiving social support. ⑫

Ⓘ Psychological factors.

Ⓙ Stress management ability. ⑥

Ⓚ Living conditions.

Ⓛ Hobby activities. ⑦
Housebound behavior. ⑧
Abuse. ⑨

Ⓜ Self-rated health & depression. ②

Ⓝ Lifestyle choices & falls. ③
Dental, oral & nutritional statuses. ④
Insomnia. ⑤

Ⓞ Healthy life expectancy.

Note: the numbers in circles denote chapter numbers.

citizens from whom it gathers data. Reflecting that proclivity perhaps, we do not have any empirical research focused on how differential health outcomes might be related to the socio-economic situation in which individuals find themselves. There is an insufficient accumulation of good descriptive social epidemiological reports that assess the extent to which health outcomes are unequally distributed across the population. This volume was conceived as a means of beginning to fill that lacuna.

Aims and hypotheses

This volume reports on the findings from a large survey of older Japanese, looking at some of the basic tabulations and providing a socio-epidemiological analysis. First, it considers the physical, mental and social realities that define old age in Japan. Second, it examines the main factors shaping those realities. Third, it analyses how these various factors might be correlated. Fourth, based on the findings that emerge, it seeks to comment on the geographic spread of health outcomes. The final aim is to show the importance of social epidemiology in helping health professionals gain a better understanding of health outcomes, healthy aging, preventative care and the social determinants of health.

Figure 1.1 provides a theoretical framework that shows how the social determinants of health affect the health of the aged. The right side of the diagram shows a number of psychological factors (such as the self-rating of health or the sense of coherence [see Antonovsky 1987]). The diagram shows how those factors and life-style choices (such as hobbies and housebound behavior [see Box 12]) impact health directly and indirectly through influences of daily habits (such as smoking, the consumption of alcohol, or regular exercise). Major dependent variables in this book are self-rated health and depression. The self-rated health at a given point in time has been shown to be a good predictor of mortality by many longitudinal cohort data (Idler 1997) (see Box 6). The occurrence of depression has also been shown to be correlated with morbidity and other measures of health. The findings presented in this volume suggest relationships between healthy aging or longevity and a variety of factors. Social factors include spatial location (positioning in an urban or rural environment) and access to various forms of social capital as well as individual characteristics (including socio-economic status and interpersonal support networks). The following chapters examine the extent to which the correlations shown in Figure 1.1 realistically portray the situation in Japan's aged population.

The chapters are aligned so that the discussion progresses from the variables and the relationships to the right in Figure 1.1 to those on the left. They start with a consideration of self-rated health and depression.

The AGES project

The data presented in this volume is from a study organized at the Nihon Fukushi University (Nihon Fukushi Daigaku). Data were produced from a project known as the Aichi Gerontological Evaluation Study (AGES).

The aim of the AGES project was to evaluate policies and services provided under long-term care insurance. The project has three data sets: one on independent aged persons, one on persons with disability and requiring care services under long-term insurance, and one on family carers. The first of those data sets provides the basis for the analyses found in this volume. The data set consisted of information on those who are covered by long-term care insurance but who were not receiving any benefits because they are functionally independent. Information was collected on their lifestyles and social /psychological characteristics. The project was conducted with ethical clearance from the University's Research Ethics Committee (Kenkyu Rinri Shinsa Iinkai).

An overview of the AGES project is provided in Box 2. Five features of the project stand out. First, the sample of aged Japanese included over 30,000 individuals. Second, the researchers who joined the project came from a range of disciplines. The result was an interdisciplinary approach in line with the way social epidemiology has developed. In order to better develop preventative policies, third was the focus on factors that help maintain a healthy life or delay the loss of such life (either through death or functional decline). Fourth is the follow-up on cohorts so that a longitudinal data set could be created. Fifth is the inclusion of information on social capital and other community level factors.

The sample

The present analysis is based on a sample of persons aged 65 or older who are registered in a municipality which provides long-term care insurance. We excluded those who have a disability and those certified

Box 2: What is the AGES Project?

Katsunori Kondō

"AGES" is an acronym for the Aichi Gerontological Evaluation Study.

The project aims to provide empirical data that might serve as a basis for developing policies for aged care. The study began with a survey of aged persons in two municipalities in Aichi Prefecture, initially funded by a research grant from the (then) Ministry of Health and Welfare. The survey was aimed at (i) aged persons requiring care, with the survey to be filled in by the care manager for each person, (ii) family members who were carers, and (iii) older people who were independent and had not yet been certified as eligible to receive benefits from long-term care insurance.

The data used for the analysis in this volume comes from 32,891 individuals who were drawn in 2003 from category (iii) and were living in fifteen municipalities across three prefectures. In 2004 data was gathered from a further three municipalities in two prefectures. In 2006 ten municipalities in three prefectures assisted in administering a follow up survey.

The survey was constructed and the responses were analyzed by a wide range of persons interested in social epidemiology. The research team drew together persons with expertise in areas such as public health, epidemiology, nutrition, the sociology of the family, psychology, gerontology, social welfare, social policy, economics, regional planning and geography.

The AGES project has had financial support since 2002 from the Fund to Promote Frontier Research (Gakujutsu Furonteia Suishin Jigyo), which is overseen by the Mombu Kagaku Sho (Ministry of Education, Culture, Sports, Science and Technology). Those funds were augmented from 2003 by an injection from the 21st Century Center of Excellence Program by the Mombu Kagaku Sho as a part of a project known as "Asian Perspectives on the Formation of a Science of Policy for the Development of a Welfare Society" of Nihon Fukushi University. In 2002–2004 the project proceeded under Grant No.14310105 from the Mombu Kagaku Sho, and then extended from 2006 by Grant No.18390200. In this manner the project was able to develop as a cohort research project. The project received further recognition from the Ministry with funding for 2009–2013 to establish the Center for Well-being and Society (CWS) at Nihon Fukushi University. With that funding the Center plans to launch a panel survey in 2010.

Based on findings from the survey of persons needing care and the survey of family members who provide care, research on aging in Japan has moved ahead. Such research will throw light on the maltreatment of aged persons and help us to understand better the burden felt by those having to care for older people.

An overview of that research and a list of papers undertaken as part of the AGES project can be found in Katō and Kondō (2008).

as eligible to receive benefits from long-term care insurance because older people with a disability find it too difficult to respond to our self-administered survey. The sample consisted of 59,622 individuals living in 15 municipalities. In the second half of the 2003 fiscal year (October 2003–March 2004) a survey was mailed to all in the sample. The self-administered survey was returned by 32,891 persons for a 55.2% response rate. Tables 1.1 and 1.2 show the value of N and the rate of return by prefecture, by the insurer and by the type of region. In principle, each municipality performs the role of insurer independently, but 4 municipalities organized one insurer body. There are therefore 12 insurer bodies for 15 municipalities. A comparison of those who returned the survey and those who did not is provided in Box 20. In general the response rate was lowest among those aged over 80, women and those with low incomes.

The questionnaire and the main variables

A copy of the questionnaire is appended to this volume. It extends over 16 A-4 pages and covers the following areas:

i. life style factors, including a history of past medical examinations, time spent walking, smoking habits, and the consumption of alcohol;
ii. psychological factors that included the ability to deal with stress (sense of coherence, Antonovsky 1987), and the sense of well-being (using the Philadelphia Geriatric Center's morale scale, Lawton 1975);
iii. social factors such as social supports, social networks, level of income, years of formal education, and social capital; and
iv. health indicators such as self-rated health (see Box 6) and the Geriatric Depression Scale (see Box 7) (Yesavage, Brink, Rose *et al.* 1982).

For socio-economic background, the equivalent income (see Box 3) and years of formal education (see Box 5) were used. Since the major-

Table 1.1: The distribution and return of surveys by the twelve long-term care insurers, by type of region covered

	Number of questionaires distributed				**Number of questionaires returned**	
	Questionaire subsections					
Insurer	**Dementia**	**Family and maltreatment**	**Oral health and nutrition**	**Total**	**Total number (N)**	**%**
Urban						
A-1	1,667	1,667	1,666	5,000	2,772	55.4
A-2	1,667	1,667	1,666	5,000	2,471	49.4
A-3	1,767	1,766	1,766	5,299	2,693	50.8
Subtotal	5,101	5,100	5,098	15,299	7,936	51.9
Semi-urban						
A-4	1,667	1,667	1,666	5,000	2,655	53.1
A-5	1,281	1,281	1,281	3,843	2,132	55.5
Subtotal	2,948	2,948	2,947	8,843	4,787	54.1
Rural-agricultural						
A-6	1,538	1,538	1,537	4,613	1,980	42.9
A-7	1,873	1,873	1,873	5,619	2,566	45.7
B-1	8,800	8,800	8,800	8,800	5,244	59.6
B-2	2,432	2,432	2,432	2,432	1,681	69.1
B-3	3,017	3,017	3,017	3,017	2,265	75.1
C-1	2,000	1,999	1,999	5,998	3,177	53.0
C-2	1,667	1,667	1,667	5,001	3,255	65.1
Subtotal	21,327	21,326	21,325	35,480	20,168	56.8
Total	29,376	29,374	29,370	59,622	32,891	55.2

Notes.
1. The upper case alphabetic letters in column 1 indicate the three prefectures from which the insurers were drawn.
2. The random sample was drawn for A-1. A-2, A-4 and C-2. Insurer A-2 was a unified insurer that provided coverage for aged persons in four municipalities.

ity of persons in the sample would be retired from the labor force, information on occupational status was not obtained

As for income, each respondent was asked to place themselves into one of fourteen income brackets based on the entire pre-tax income for their respective household. The income brackets ranged from under 500,000 to over 10 million yen. (US$1 = 90–120 Japanese yen). Box 3 explains how the equivalent income value was then calculated by the researchers using the mid-point for each income bracket (with 250,000 yen being the value assigned to those in the lowest category and 10.5 million yen assigned to those in the top bracket. As for the level of education, respondents were asked to indicate the number of years of formal education they had completed, with the multiple choice

Table 1.2: Numbers of questionnaire distributed/returned and response rate by prefecture

	Subsection of questionnaire											
	Dementia			Family and abuse			Oral health and nutrition			Total		
Prefectures	**Distributed**	**Returned**	**Response rate**	**Distributed**	**Returned**	**Response rate**	**Distributed**	**Returned**	**Response rate**	**Distributed (a)**	**Returned (b)**	**Response rate (b/a)**
A	11,460	5,667	49.5%	11,459	5,887	51.4%	11,455	5,715	49.9%	34,374	17,269	50.2%
B	14,249	9,190	64.5%	14,249	9,190	64.5%	14,249	9,190	64.5%	14,249	9,190	64.5%
C	3,667	2,123	57.9%	3,666	2,180	59.5%	3,666	2,129	58.1%	10,999	6,432	58.5%
Total	29,376	16,980	57.8%	29,374	17,257	58.7%	29,370	17,034	58.0%	59,622	32,891	55.2%

Note: Only in Prefecture B was the questionaire sent with all three subsections.

answers ranging from '6 or fewer' up through '13 or more'. As for the education level of the older population in Japan, see Box 5.

Three different versions of the questionnaire were prepared: One version included a sub-section on dementia related questions. Another version included a sub-section on family and society, and the third version included a sub-section on oral hygiene and nutrition. Eighty to ninety percent of the questions were the same in all three versions. The different versions were randomly sent out from each insuring body as indicated in Table 1.1. The person responsible for the three insurers in Prefecture B decided to send out the surveys to everyone in those municipalities in a format that included all three sub-sections. Because the sub-sections did not go to everyone in the other prefectures, the number of cases in the analyses involving sub-section material were fewer than 32,891. Moreover, as is standard practice, cases with missing values were also missing from the relevant tabulations.

Regional variation and other patterns

In order to determine whether geographical positioning was a significant factor, the twelve insuring bodies were classified into three groups; urban, semi-urban, and rural, according to population density on inhabitable land as shown in Figure 1.2 and Tables 1.1, 1.3 and 1.4: urban with a population density over 1500 persons per square kilometer, semi-urban with densities between 1000 and 1500 persons, and rural agricultural-type regions with densities below 1000 persons per square kilometer. The outcome was that three insurers were urban types, two were semi-urban types, and seven were of the rural-agricultural type. To ascertain how well the twelve insurers represented the other insuring bodies (i.e. municipalities), data from the research was compared with data from the Japanese Bureau of Statistics (Somu Sho Tokei Kyoku 2004). The results are shown in Figure 1.2 and Table 1.3.

If we look at the population density on inhabitable land as an index showing the extent to which a community is urbanized, we can also see that the densities recorded for the urban and semi-urban communities in our study place those municipalities in the top quartile, and that the rural-agricultural communities in our survey had densities above the median density. Likewise, when we look at the per capita pre-tax income, we can see that the per capita income for the urban and semi-urban communities surveyed in the AGES research project placed those communities in the top quartile of all communities in Japan. It placed the rural-agricultural communities in our study above the median income. In other words, the communities studied were not

Figure 1.2: Type of region – population density on inhabitable land and rate of involvement in primary industry

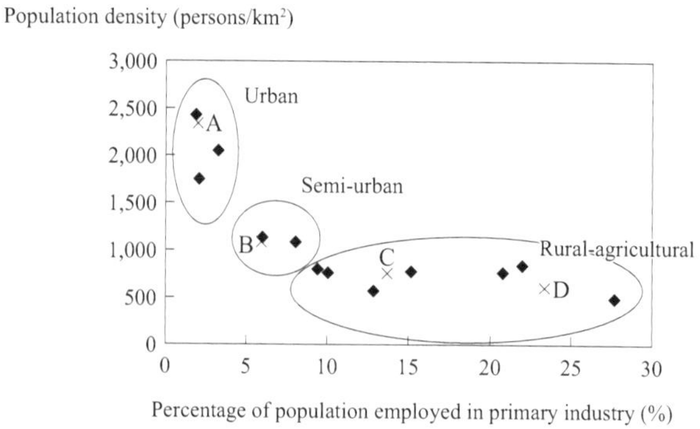

Four similar cities in other prefectures are represented by alphabetic letters:
A = Takasaki City (Gunma Prefecture)
B = Izumo City (Shimane Prefecture)
C = Toba City (Mie Prefecture)
D = Obuse Town (Nagano Prefecture)

◆ = the 12 insurers
× = shows similarly situated municipalities in other prefectures for reference

representative of all communities in Japan, and the urban bias needs to be acknowledged.

Some key demographic variables and the twelve insuring bodies

Looking at age, it is clear that the average age of the samples rises as we move from the more densely populated cities through the towns to the rural agricultural regions where the average is the highest. Age also correlates negatively with level of income and years of formal education completed. The gap in income levels of regions is particularly noticeable. More than 50 percent of those in the rural agricultural-type municipalities had an income below 2 million yen, whereas the figure was only 40 percent in the urban regions, a difference of 10 percentage points. Even more noticeable was the difference in the percentage of older persons with an income below 1 million yen. Although not shown in Table 1.4, levels of income and years of education vary inversely with age for reasons explained in Boxes 4 and 5). Even when we control for gender and age, the same city-size variable correlates with income and years of education (Table 1.4).

Table 1.3: Comparing the three types of regions in AGES with municipality data for all of Japan

	Urban regions (3 insurers)	Semi-urban regions (2 insurers)	Rural-agricultural regions (7 insurers)	Total in study	Quantile values for all municipalities in Japan		
					25%	50%	75%
Number of surveys returned	7,936	4,787	20,168	32,891			
Measures of urbaness							
Population density (Persons/km^2)	2,092.60	1,109.00	738.2	1,326.80	1,005.50	486.7	277
Per-capita pre-tax income (1 million yen)	3.71	3.55	3.19	3.57	3.34	3.09	2.85
Measures of ruralness							
Percentage of labor force in primary industry	3.1	6.9	16.9	7.3	23.7	13.4	5.5
Percentage of aged population	13.3	18.8	22.7	16.3	28.4	23.5	18.2

Source for national data: Ministry of Internal Affairs and Communications, Statistics Bureau (2004)

Table 1.4: Number of respondents by gender, age and level of education for each type of region

	Urban regions (n = 7,936)			Semi-urban regions (n = 4,787)			Rural-agricultural regions (n = 20,168)			All regions (n = 32,891)	
	N	%	%*	N	%	%*	N	%	%*	N	%
Gender											
Males	3,784	50.8	–	2,104	46.9	–	8,104	43.5	–	13,992	45.8
Females	3,663	49.2	–	2,386	53.1	–	10,511	56.5	–	16,560	54.2
Age groups											
65–69	2,744	37.5	37.2	1,538	34.9	34.9	5,154	28.4	28.5	9,436	31.6
70–74	2,203	30.1	30	1,272	28.9	28.9	5,390	29.7	29.8	8,865	29.7
75–79	1,453	19.9	19.9	918	20.9	20.9	4,120	22.7	22.7	6,492	21.7
80–84	625	8.6	8.7	448	10.2	10.2	2,368	13.1	13	3,441	11.5
85–	301	4.2	4.2	226	5.1	5.2	1,100	6.1	6.1	1,627	5.4
Number of years of education											
<6	329	4.4	5	204	4.5	4.8	1,049	5.6	5	1,582	5.1
6–9	3,987	53.5	53.9	2,510	55.8	55.7	10,637	56.6	56	17,134	55.7
10–12	2,347	31.5	31.3	1,351	30	30.1	5,664	30.2	30.9	9,362	30.5
13+	792	10.6	9.9	434	9.6	9.4	1,430	7.6	8	2,656	8.6
Equivalent income (10 thousand yen)											
< 100	695	10.8	11.7	445	12	12.7	3,159	22	21.6	4,299	17.6
101–200	1,887	29.3	28.6	1,081	29.1	27.9	4,647	32.4	32.2	7,615	31.1
201–300	1,889	29.3	28.8	1,024	27.5	27.2	3,264	22.8	23	6,177	25.2
300–400	1,188	18.5	18.5	696	18.7	18.6	2,003	14	14.2	3,887	15.9
≥ 400	780	12.1	12.4	473	12.7	13.6	1,256	8.8	9	2,509	10.2

Notes.

1: To obtain comparability, the percentages were recalculated for age group with weightings to correct for gender and age differences. These percentages are provided in the columns marked '%*'.

2: Household income was calculated as equivalent value by dividing total household income by the square root of the number of household members.

3: N = the number of cases (i.e., aged persons) actually tabulated in the analysis.

Box 3: Equivalent Income

Hiroshi Hirai

Along with years of education and occupation, income is generally considered to be an indicator of socio-economic status. Income is conceived in a number of ways that include household income, per capita household income, and equivalent income. The relevant measure of household income for the AGES project was equivalent income – a figure derived when household income is divided by the square root of the number of persons living in the household. That measure was chosen for the reasons given below.

A single-person household and a multi-person household, each with an income of 4 million yen, experience rather different financial realities. One approach that takes into account such differences is to calculate the per person income of each household, an approach which results in the average income per person. However, the cost of running a household does not increase by as much as twice or three times when the number of household members doubles or triples. In other words, as family or household size increases, economies of scale come into play. If a household increases, say, from one to two persons, or from two to four persons, it generally does not buy a second stove or double the floor space required for living.

The notion of 'equivalent income' is one that factors in household size while also taking into account economies of scale. To calculate equivalent income for the AGES, we sought to divide household income by an index that set the equivalent number of household members as the actual number of household members taken to the power of 0.5. The aim was to represent the actual number of household members in a way that would reflect the cost elasticity of having each additional household member. The power used (also known as the "equivalence elasticity") for this exercise was 0.5. An equivalence elasticity of 0.5 has been used in studies of the older population in ten countries in Europe and North America as one means of judging socio-economic status. In Japan it has been used by the Ministry of Health, Labour and Welfare in its white papers and by the national government's Bureau of Statistics.

Box 4: The Distribution of Income

Hideki Endō

Since around 1990 it has become clear that older people in Japan do not necessarily have low levels of income (*e.g.*, Takayama 1994). At the same time, it has also become clear that great income disparities exist among them. This box will consider briefly what the government's official statistics tell us about the incomes of older people in Japan.

The various major surveys conducted by the government do not define income in a consistent manner. We adopt gross income as the definition of income that is similar to the one (pre-tax total household income) used in the AGES project. Gross income includes remuneration from gainful employment, interest and dividends. It also includes cash payments from public pensions and other benefits.

Figure 1.3 shows the average gross household income and gross equivalent income by the age bracket of the household head. In this book the household head is the person nominated by the household as its spokesperson without regard to that person's income or age. Households headed by someone in their fifties had an average gross household income of 7.396 million yen, the highest average among households bracketed by the age of the household head. The average gross household income of all other households, save those headed by a person aged under 29, is higher

Figure 1.3: The average gross household income and the average gross equivalent income by the age of the household head (2005)

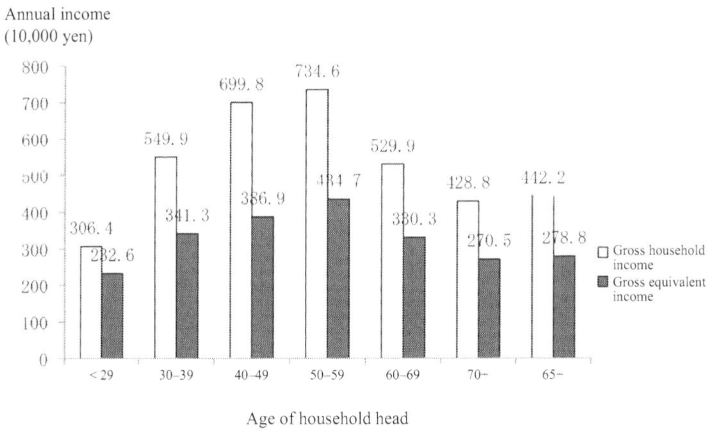

Source: Ministry of Health, Labour and Welfare (2008), from Figure 2.3.1.

Figure 1.4: Distribution of income (gross equivalent value) by the age of the household head (2005)

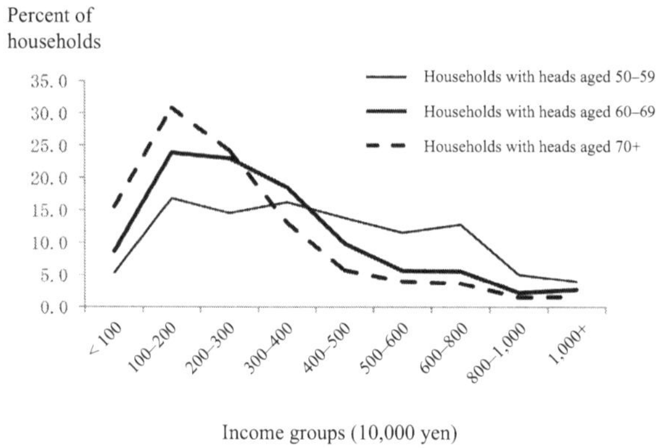

Source: Ministry of Health, Labour and Welfare (2008), from Figure 2.3.2.

than that of households headed by someone aged over 65 (which stood at 4.422 million yen).

Persons aged over 65 have an income distribution that is different to that of those aged below 65. Figure 1.4 shows how gross equivalent income is distributed for households categorised into three groups according to the age of the household head (50–59, 60–69, and 70+). Households headed by someone in their fifties are spread fairly evenly over a range of 1 million to 8 million yen. As the age of the household head increases, the distribution becomes increasingly skewed to the lower income brackets. Reflecting this reality, the Gini coefficient for households headed by someone aged over 55 is around 0.37, whereas for households with younger heads (not shown in Figure 1.4) the range of the Gini coefficient is between 0.25 and 0.33.

Two factors explain this. One is the system of mandatory retirement that many firms impose when their employees reach a certain age (OECD 2004: 16–17). The other influence is the system of public pensions. Although revisions to the Law Concerning the Stabilization of Employment of Older Persons called for firms to implement a mandatory retirement age of 65 or above or to provide alternative employment opportunities for all of their employees aged 60–64 who desire to continue working, the retirement age at some firms remains between 60 and 64 and no alternatives are yet available. As for the public pension, the qualifying age has been raised to 65. However, in 2005 some pensions could still be accessed from the age of 60, e.g., Rōrei Kōsei Nenkin (Old-age Employees' Pension), although, this is scheduled to be raised in stages.

Both the retirement age and the pension system encourage employees to retire in their sixties, and effect a direct change in their income situations. Moreover, some pensions are paid according to a formula whereby a sliding scale is applied so that the amount of pension one receives varies inversely with other income they might receive. In this way, the Japanese Pension system tends to encourage older people to change their employment status from full-time regular employment to various forms of casual employment.

Old age is thus characterized by a withdrawal from permanent employment and a reduction in the hours worked. The outcome is typically a huge drop in income. At the same time, however, the financial and fixed assets of older people remain at levels which are much higher than those of younger people, and their liabilities are correspondingly less. Accordingly, when considering the overall financial situation of older people, the fluidity of their assets needs to be considered alongside their incomes. More specifically, it is important to recognize that 60 percent of their assets are in real estate: land, houses and buildings (which are difficult to convert to liquid assets). One source of disparity in disposable income within each age cohort, however, is the difference in home ownership, with some having to pay rent and others not having to do so. A number of statistical surveys suggest that approximately 80 percent of those aged over 65 live in a home that they own. Data from the 2005 Population Census can be retabulated to show that for urbanized cities 74.3 percent of households with a member aged 65 or older are in premises owned by the family, whereas for semi-urbanized municipalities the figure rises to 86.0 percent. The figure is highest for households in rural agricultural municipalities at 91.5 percent. For those in the AGES data, the figure is still higher at 94.2 percent. At least three reasons come to mind when explaining that finding. First, the average personal income levels in the twelve areas selected for the AGES project are in the upper half of the top quartile of all incomes in Japan. Second, because those non-responders were more prevalent among lower income groups, respondents tend to be in higher income groups than non-responders. Third, 61.3 percent of respondents came from rural agricultural municipalities where we know that home ownership is highest.

Readers seeking more details concerning the retirement system, pensions and how they relate to the labor force participation of Japan's older people are referred to the OECD (2004) report mentioned above. For more information on the situations of income and assets of Japan's older people, readers may consult Ministry of Health, Labour and Welfare (2008).

Box 5: Changes in the System of School Education

Yumiko Shirase

AGES used income and years of formal education as its indicators of socio-economic status (SES). As Dore (1997: 35–50) has observed, some of Japan's leaders came to attach a great deal of importance to the role of education as one of the drivers of economic growth as the country began its move to modernize during the Meiji period. When we look at the data produced by the AGES research, we find that the level of education is inversely related to age, evidence that education became more widely available with changes to the system of education that was established during the occupation following World War II. For this reason it is worth briefly reviewing the changes that were experienced by many Japanese aged over 65.

In 1872 steps were taken to introduce a modern system of education, and all children were to attend primary school when they turned six. The number of years that children attended primary school varied from one region to another. In 1900 the Ministry of Education issued the Primary School Edict which stipulated that all ordinary primary schools were to offer four years of instruction. That became six years in 1907. At the same time, compulsory education was extended from four to six years. In 1910 over 98 percent of all appropriately aged children were in primary school.

Figure 1.5: The prewar system of education in Japan (circa 1920)

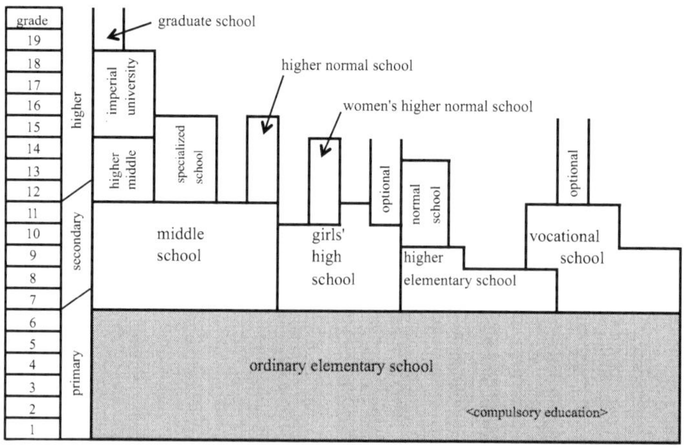

Source: Ministry of Education (1972), p. 338.

Table 1.5: A cross tabulation by age and the years of education received among participants in the AGES research project

Age in 2003 years	Year in which respondent was born	Years of formal education (%)			
		Up to 5 years	6–9 years	10–12 years	13+
65–69	1934–1938	1.1	53.0	34.3	11.7
70–74	1929–1933	3.1	57.7	31.2	8.0
75–79	1924–1928	5.7	54.9	31.9	7.5
80–84	1919–1923	12.5	58.6	23.0	6.0
85+	–1918	20.8	55.5	17.6	6.1

Hence, those who returned the AGES questionnaire should have received at least six years of compulsory education.

A look at the AGES data (as shown in Table 1.5), however, reveals that 12.5 percent of those aged 80–84 (*i.e.*, those born between 1919 and 1923) received less than the six years of compulsory education, compared to 20 percent of those aged over 85 who had not received such an education. This prompts us to ask why our data diverged from the official view. One answer is that respondents reported on the number of years they actually attended and not the number of years they were officially enrolled. Those who lived in urban slums and girls in rural agricultural villages often had to work to augment family income and absented themselves from school, a fact picked up in social surveys conducted in the 1920s. In those days absenteeism was not seen as a serious problem, and the government was not proactive in devising policies to encourage attendance.

While the primary school system was rather straightforward, the approach to developing middle school and senior high schools was more complex (see Figure 1.6). The outcome reflected the varied demands for graduates that could be slotted into a rapidly developing and changing economy in which different technologies were being introduced. What emerged was a system with multiple avenues for advancement. In that sense it was a very flexible system. The secondary system embraced normal schools (*shihan gakko*), vocational schools (*jitsugyo gakko*), various optional courses (*hoshuka*) and other types of schools with various curricula and years of study. Accordingly, among those aged 70 and over (i.e., those born before 1933) there were some respondents who had 13 or more years of education without having attended a university.

Figure 1.6: Comparison of the education levels of adults in three countries: Japan (1950), USA (1950) and England (1951)

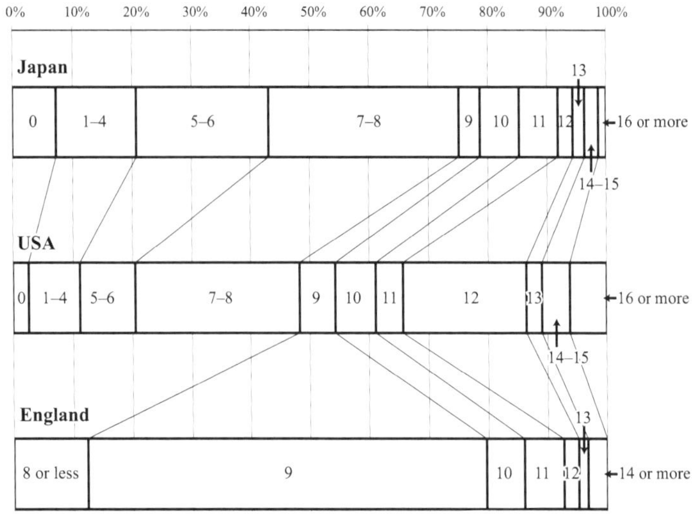

Accumulated percentage showing those who had completed various levels of education (years of formal education completed)

Source: Ministry of Education (1959), p. 5.

At the beginning of the 1950s the educational level of the generation coming into the work force was not necessarily high by international standards. In 1950 about 20 percent of Japanese aged 25 or more (i.e., those born before 1925) would have had ten or more years of education, a figure on par with that found in England, but considerably below the figure of 45 percent found in the USA. In England, about two thirds of that age cohort had completed the 9 years of compulsory education whereas only 32 percent had received 7–8 years of education.

The system that was in place in the 1920s continued with only minor changes until the end of the Second World War. The present system, as shown in Figure 1.7, was established in 1947 when compulsory education was set at nine years – with six in primary school and another three in junior high school. Beyond those compulsory years were a further three in senior high school. About 30 percent of the participants in the AGES project who were aged 65–70 (i.e., born between 1934 and 1938) received their education through the new system, and 10 percent had gone to university. Accordingly, as Figure 1.8 shows, that cohort had a higher level of education than those who preceded them. With

Figure 1.7: The postwar system of education in Japan (circa 1949)

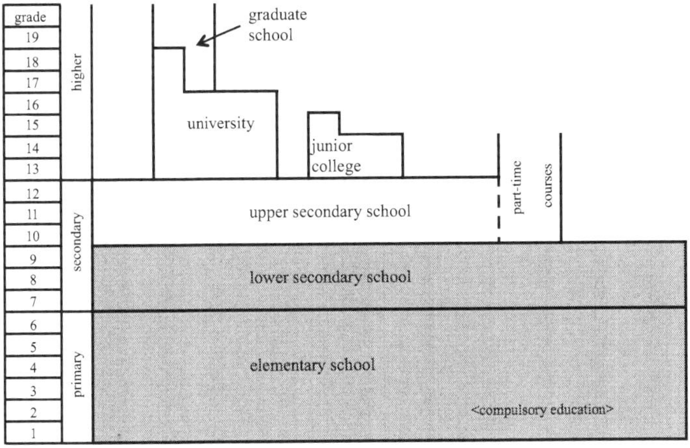

Source: Ministry of Education (1972), p. 336.

Figure 1.8: Percentage of corresponding age groups attending a secondary school or enrolled in a tertiary institution (1900–1960)

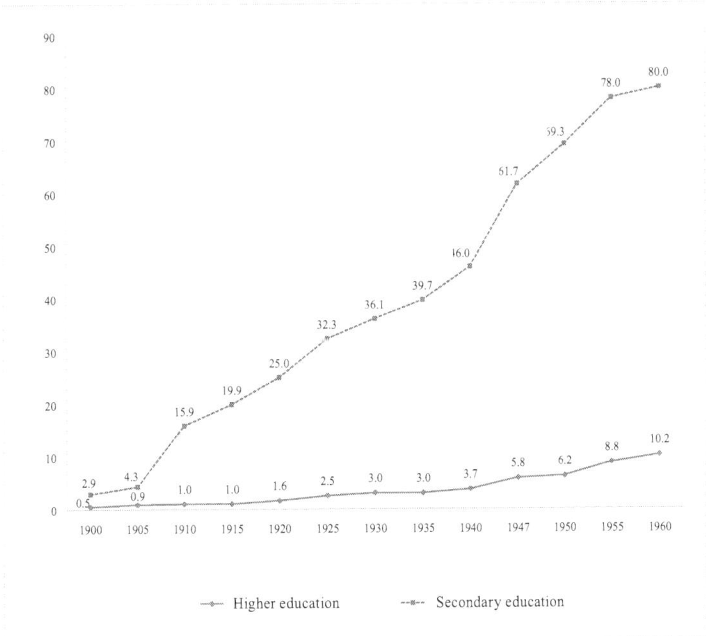

Source: Ministry of Education (1963), p. 181.

the new system of education in place, we can speculate as to the extent to which the life chances of those with fewer than six years of formal education would have been restricted in postwar Japan.

Chapter 2

Self-rated Health Status and Depression

Kiyoko Yoshii

Overview

This chapter looks at the correlation between socio-economic status (SES) and two measures of health: self-rated health status and depression. (2) The relationship between SES and health has been frequently researched in many countries (Lynch and Kaplan 2000). Nevertheless, compared to those who are younger, older people have received less attention when it comes to the relationship between SES and health indices, a point made both by Grundy and Holt (2001) and by Dalstra, Kunst and Mackenbach et al. (2006). House, Lepkowski and Kinney et al. (1994), Ross and Wu (1996) and Berkman and Gurland (1998) suggest several explanations for the relationship between SES and health indices among older persons.

One view is that the correlations between the two phenomena weaken within age cohorts as they progress into their later years. Persons with low SES are not as likely to live to old age. At the same time, those who do are exceptionally strong already, more than offsetting what disadvantage there might have been for others who also had low incomes. The result is a weakening of the correlation between income and health. Another consideration could be that the influence initially brought to bear by differences in education also diminishes over time and that SES is less dependent on income after retirement (Dalstra, Kunst, Mackenbach et al. 2006).

Another view, however, is that the effects of living in a poor physical and social environment and unhealthy habits are cumulative and serve only to reinforce the correlations between SES and health outcomes later in life (Ross and Wu 1996).

Other research reveals that the relationship between SES and health varies between countries and even among regions in the same country (Kimura, Gotō, Tsunoda et al. 2003; von dem Knesebeck, Lüschen, Cockerham et al. 2003; Nakaya and Dorling 2005). The review by Kimura et al. (2003) of nine other research projects using cross-societal data led to the conclusion that the correlation varies across the countries in which research has been conducted (USA, England, Finland, China and Japan) as well as across regions in each country. In their study of the relationship of SES and health, van dem Knesebeck et al. (2003) found that the health disparity was greater in Germany than in the United States. In another study of the relationship in Japan and the United Kingdom, Nakaya et al. (2005) found that there was a negative correlation between income levels and the incidence of death in all age groups in the United Kingdom, but that in Japan there was a negative correlation only among the working-age group, whereas the correlation disappeared among the older population.

In recent years researchers have begun to focus on differential health outcomes resulting from regional differences in socio-economic profiles (Macintyre and Ellaway 2000; Roberts 1998). In Japan, Tanaka, Mori and Shigemura et al. (2002) and Nohara, Onoda and Okayama (2003) have examined regional variations in death rates and suicide. Their work, however, has left a number of questions unanswered.

In this research two measure of health are employed. One is self-rated health status (a subjective self-assessment of health). The other is depression. Values for the first variable were derived by asking respondents to indicate how they felt on a Likert scale ranging from a category of 'excellent' to a category of 'poor' (see Box 6). The appraisal goes beyond an assessment of mental well-being and attempts to capture an indication of each person's physical well-being by requesting information about medical examinations and other assessments made by their doctors. The goal is to obtain a comprehensive view of the respondent's overall well-being with regard to their health (Sugisawa and Sugisawa 1998). A range of longitudinal research has shown that self-rated health correlates well with the death rate (Kaplan, Barell and Lusky 1988; Idler, Kasl and Lemke 1990; and Fujita and Hatano 1990) and physical deterioration (Stuck, Walthert, Nicolaus et al. 1999).

Depression has also been shown to correlate well with death (Ganguly, Dodge and Mulsant 2002), physical deterioration (Stuck, Walthert, Nikolaus et al. 1999) and dementia (Jorm 2000). The two subjective appraisals mentioned above cannot be seen as being a perfect fit with, or a replacement for, proper medical diagnoses. However, in view of the research introduced here, we think such assessments can play a useful role in the large-scale research that is necessary to develop policies that limit the need for aged care by extending the number of years that aged citizens enjoy good health.

The survey includes questions about the ability to perform various daily tasks, hospital visits, and any treatment that had been received. The first of the questions is put to respondents who have not yet been designated as needing care and who are still living independently. Because a high percentage of aged persons visit the hospital from time-to-time for one ailment or another, such visits were not seen by the research team for this project as a very sensitive indicator; accordingly, these are not used in the analysis presented in this chapter.

Comparative studies on the prevalence of depression suggests that it is extremely high in the USA, Ukraine, and Australia. They are followed by Canada, Europe (including Lebanon) and Mexico. China (including Hong Kong), Taiwan and Nigeria report much lower prevalences. The prevalence in Japan appears to be below the levels recorded in Europe and the United States, and is comparable with that found in countries such as China.

With the preceding discussion in mind, this chapter is written with two aims. One is to clarify the relationship between (i) socio-economic status (years of education completed and income) and (ii) self-rated health status and depression. The second is to provide a picture of variation among regions in terms of indices measuring health and the extent to which health outcomes for older people vary by the degrees of urbanization (i.e., by contrasting the situation in urban, semi-urban and rural-agricultural communities). In this regard, we will also consider the extent to which regional differences in health are explained by socio-economic variables.

Method

Subjects

Our sample of 32,891 individuals was drawn randomly from the 15 municipalities that yielded data for the AGES project in 2003 (see Table 1.1). The sample was drawn from residents who were aged over 65 and who had not been recognized as needing care.

Health as a variable

Two measures of health were used. One was a self-rated health status based on the four-point scale outlined in Box 6. The other was the fifteen-question depression test GDS (see Box 7) that was developed as a means of screening older persons for depression (see Sheikh and Yesavage 1986 and Yesavage, Brink, Rose et al. 2004). The screening score ranges from 0–15, with persons scoring 0–4 being seen as being 'not depressed', those scoring 5–9 being seen as having 'mild depression', and those scoring 10 or more being seen as having 'moderate to severe depression'.

Other variables

The socio-economic variables were (i) years of education (see Box 5) and (ii) the level of equivalent household income (see Box 3). The two variables have been revealed as effective SES indices in all countries where similar studies have been conducted in Europe and North America (Dalstra, Kunst, Mackenbach et al. 2006). The demographic variables were age and gender. In addition, residential location was recorded as 'urban', 'semi-urban' and 'rural-agricultural'.

Analysis

Because the measure for health and socio-economic status correlate strongly with age, it is necessary to control for variations in age when looking at other correlations. Bivariate analysis was conducted using SPSS to look at models of linear regression.

Findings

Frequency distribution for two health variables

Approximately 70 percent of the respondents answered that they were well, with 7.3 percent answering 'excellent' and 62.9 percent answering 'good'. The remaining 30 percent answered 'fair' (24.3 percent) or 'poor' (5.7 percent). On the GDS measurement, 8.1 percent scored 10 or more points and would be classified as 'moderate to severe depression', with another 25.0 percent scoring between 5 and 9 points and being designated as 'mild depression'.

Correlation of socio-economic indices and health

The correlations between SES and the health variables are shown in Table 2.1. To assist in understanding those relationships, Figure 2.1 shows the relationship between income and depression. Table 2.1 shows that those with lower levels of education are much more likely to have poor health and depression. The same relationship holds for income, with lower income also associated with negative outcomes.

Table 2.1: The effect of level of education and income on health indices

	Number in the sample by gender		Self-rated health (% respondents claiming to be 'excellent' or 'good')				The prevalence of depression using GDS (% respondents with scores of 10 or more)			
	Males	Females	Males	p-value	Females	p-value	Males	p-value	Females	p-value
Years of education										
<6	414	1,073	44.5	***	36.1	***	17.4	***	12.8	***
6–9	7,515	9,087	31.7		30.8		9.7		9.2	
10–12	4,041	5,185	26.3		25.1		4.9		5.7	
13+	1,815	813	24.2		24.1		5.4		5.3	
Level of equivalent income per annum (1 million yen)										
<1	1,603	2,438	40.0	***	34.8	***	15.8	***	15.0	***
1–2	3,898	3,458	30.7		29.7		9.8		7.7	
2–3	3,296	2,680	26.9		25.9		5.5		6.0	
3–4	2,068	1,731	24.6		22.7		4.2		3.7	
4+	1,239	1,201	21.0		21.2		2.3		3.7	

Notes.

The figures are adjusted by age with a general linear model.

***: $p = 0.001$

Figure 2.1: Level of equivalent income and the prevalence of depression

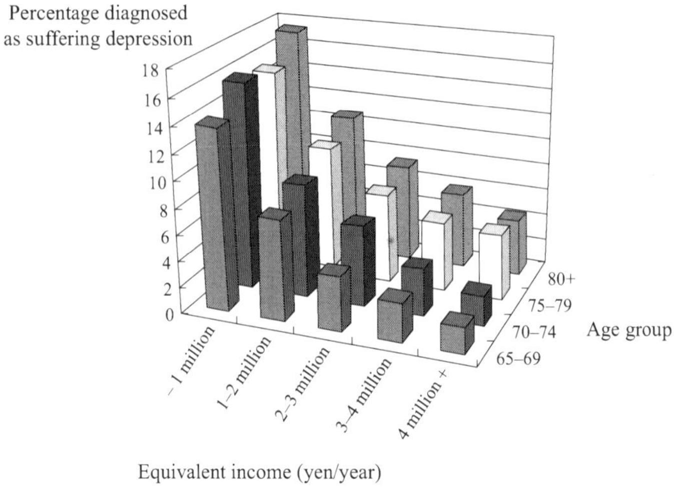

As Table 2.1 shows, these distributions yield a probability value (p) that is less than 0.001.

When these findings are evaluated, it is important to consider the relative interaction of income and education. There is thus a need to isolate their independent influence. When that is done and the two measures of health are analyzed separately as dependent variables (*mokuteki hensu*), education and income always result in correlations at significant levels.

Variation in health by type of region

The frequency distribution by age varies considerably from one type of region to another. Accordingly, we looked at health outcomes for each type by controlling for age. The range for feeling unhealthy or very unhealthy ranged from 26.9 percent to 36.9 percent; the percentage of individuals judged to be suffering from depression ranged from 6.8 to 12.0 percent. These are significant differences.

The scatter plot diagram in Figure 2.2 shows how these differences manifest themselves with regard to depression, income and type of municipality. The unit of analysis is the insuring body (as shown in Table 1.1 there were 12 insurers covering 15 municipalities). The horizontal axis showing income is scaled as an index where '100' represents the national average (Asahi Shimbun Sha 2004). Three

Figure 2.2: Income and the prevalence of depression by insurer

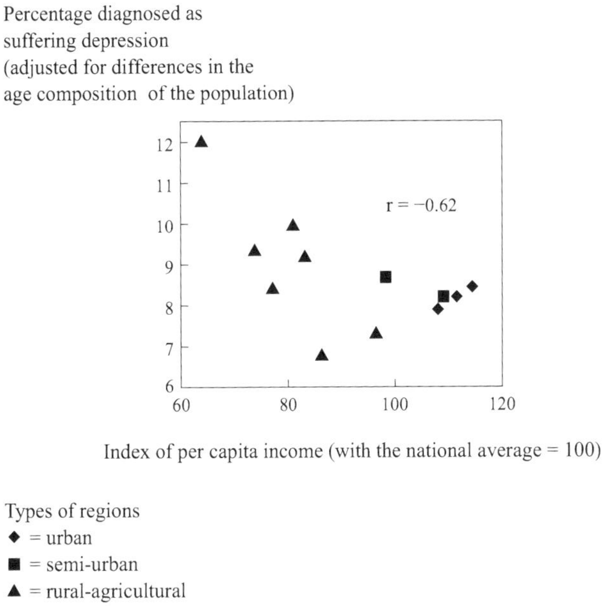

facets of the diagram in Figure 2.1 stand out. First, urban and semi-urban regions are characterized by high per capita incomes; rural-agricultural regions by low per capita incomes. Second, the regression lines would yield a negative correlation with r = -0.62. In other words, depression is more prevalent in the rural-agricultural regions where income levels are lower. Third, the correlation is even stronger when only the seven rural-agricultural regions are considered. Among those regions, the variation in income and in the incidence of depression is considerable, whereas the urban and semi-urban regions are bunched together in a concentrated area in Figure 2.2. In this regard it is important to note that the two rural-agricultural regions with the highest incomes also had an incidence of depression below that recorded in any of the more urbanized locales.

The data in Tables 2.2 and 2.3 provide a closer look at the situation. For men, the two tables show that health deteriorates as we move from urban to rural locations whereas, in line with the findings in Figure 2.1, the incidence of depression increases. For women, however, that relationship holds for depression, but not for self-rated health status. These differences were significant at the level of $p<0.001$ even when

Box 6: Self-rated Health

Chiyoe Murata

The notion of assessing one's own health or recording 'subjective feelings of physical well-being' (*shukanteki kenkokan*) used in the AGES research represents a concept expressed variously in English as 'self-rated health', 'self-assessed health', 'self ratings of health', and 'self-reported health'. Subjective assessments of an individual's health refer to the way that individuals feel about their own health. Such assessments were introduced in the United States in the late 1950s. Because such measures allow respondents to rate their own health by answering questions on their own, they have become a convenient means through which health information can be collected. This is especially so when large-scale surveys are conducted (see Sugisawa and Sugisawa 1995).

At first glance, self-rated health does not seem to be highly reliable. However, many longitudinal cohort studies have shown that self-assessments at one point in time have been good predictors of death or physical decline at a later stage in life. For example, respondents who have answered questionnaires by indicating that their health was poor or very poor on the average have ended up dying sooner than those who had answered the same question more positively. This was true even when the data was statistically controlled for age, blood pressure and a range of ailments.

In practical terms, some surveys use a five-point scale, ranging from 'excellent' through 'good', 'fair' and 'poor' to 'very poor'. Others use a three-point collapsed scale with options such as 'good', 'average' and 'poor'. The terms used and the way the questions are asked may vary from one survey to another. For the AGES data, the question was: 'How do you rate your health?' A four-point scale was used: 'excellent', 'good', 'fair' and 'poor'. Another question posed the inquiry differently: 'Compared to other persons of a similar age, how is your health?' Or, 'Compared to one year ago, how is your health today?'

What do these self-ratings represent? First, they are a proxy for a proper medically confirmed diagnosis, and it must be noted that such assessments do not always align with the clinical diagnosis of a doctor. However, many reports indicate that the self-appraisal of individuals correlates with the occurrence of death or levels of physical decline at a later date more highly than does the doctor's diagnosis (Sugisawa and Sugisawa 1995; Kaplan, Goldberg and Everson 1996; Idler and Benyamini 1997). Another perspective forwarded by Murata, Kondō and Tamakoshi (2006) is that subjective self-assessments also incorporate a holistic consideration of other important factors such as a person's mental outlook, their income and the surroundings or situation in which they find themselves.

the data were controlled for age. The relationship of income and education to scores on measures of health were analyzed separately by gender for each type of region. With only one exception (level of education for women in semi-urban regions), variation was significant at the level of $p < 0.001$. Generally, the variation by type of region was lower for women than for men.

Discussion

At the outset two goals were set for this chapter. First, we found for both men and women that the incidence of poor health and depression was inversely correlated with each measure of socio-economic status (SES) and that the correlations were significant. Moreover, it became clear that the incidence of poor health outcomes became increasingly pronounced as the measures of SES approached the lower end of the two scales. Consistent with the findings of Koskinen and Martelin (1994) elsewhere, we too found that the correlation was weaker for women than for men. The AGES data reveal that among those with depression, the number of men in the lowest income group (with per capita equivalent household incomes below ¥1 million) was 6.9 times the number from the highest income group (with equivalent incomes above ¥4 million). For women the figure was 4.1 times. As shown in Table 2.1, for those in the lowest groups in terms of the two measures of SES, the incidence of poor health outcomes was about 5 percent higher for men than for women. There seems to be a tendency for poor health to have a cumulative effect, particularly among men in the lowest SES groupings.

Second, the data showed that there were significant differences in health outcomes among the different types of regions. It is clear that better health outcomes were recorded for locales with higher levels of income. At the same time, that the health outcomes were not as good in semi-urban and rural-agricultural types of regions could not be fully explained simply by reference to their different levels of SES.

Other research has sought to compare the respective levels of health in urban and rural communities. Verheji (1996), however, found that the results of those studies were inconclusive. Some of them (Tang, Wang, Meng et al. 1999; Senior and Higgs 2000; and Levin

Table 2.2: Self-rated health levels by level of education, income and regional type: Age-adjusted percentage of respondents who indicated they were 'excellent' or 'good'

	Males				Females			
	Urban	Semi-urban	Rural-agricultural	p-value[a]	Urban	Semi-urban	Rural-agricultural	p-value[a]
Number in sample	3,621	2,012	7,716		3,513	2,264	9,974	
Overall average percentage	26.1	29.1	31.4	***	28	29.8	29.3	n.s.
Years of education								
<6	39.6	52.1	45.3		39.7	32.3	35.9	
6–9	27.7	31.1	33.6		29.1	31.1	31.3	
10–12	21.4	25	29.2		22.9	26.7	25.5	
13+	23.2	24.8	24.5		19.2	22.6	26.5	
p-value[b]	***	***	***		***	n.s.	***	
Equivalent annual income (million yen)								
<1	35.3	37.3	41.6		32.8	33	35.7	
1–2	26.9	31.7	32.2		29.8	32.9	29	
2–3	25	29	27.3		25.8	28.4	25.1	
3–4	23.7	25.3	24.8		23.1	23.4	22.2	
4+	18.5	20.1	22.9		17.3	20.4	23.5	
p-value[b]	***	**	***		***	**	***	

Notes.
a: Test of differences between the three area types.
b: Test of differences within each area type between socio-economic categories. All calculations are age-adusted.
**: p = 0.01; ***: p = 0.001; n.s.: not significant.

Table 2.3: Self-rated health by years of education, income and regional type: Age-adjusted percentage of respondents who indicated they experienced 'mild depression' or 'moderate to severe depression'

	Males				Females			
	Urban	Semi-urban	Rural-agricultural	p-value[a]	Urban	Semi-urban	Rural-agricultural	p-value[a]
Number in sample	3,321	1,818	6,431		2,929	1,879	7,685	
Overall average percentage	29.2	30	34.3	***	30.5	34.5	34.4	***
Years of education								
<6	43.5	52.3	58.2		42.2	45.2	46.7	
6–9	33.4	33.5	39		31.7	38.4	37.5	
10–12	22.7	24.5	27.7		25.5	26.6	28.1	
13+	23.5	24.2	24.5		24.8	21.7	28.1	
p-value[b]	***	***	***		***	***	***	
Equivalent annual income (million yen)								
<1	45.8	48.3	50.9		42.8	46.4	44.8	
1–2	34.7	33.9	38.1		35.8	41.1	35.3	
2–3	26.6	30.2	28.2		25.9	32.1	28.1	
3–4	20.3	22.3	21.8		20.8	20.4	23.2	
4+	17.4	12.1	19.3		17.3	19.1	24.2	
p-value[b]	***	***	***		***	***	***	

Notes.
a: Test of differences between the three area types.
b: Test of differences within each area type between socio-economic categories. All calculations are age-adusted.
**: p = 0.01; ***: p = 0.001; n.s.: not significant.

and Leyland 2005) found that suicide, overall mortality rates and the occurrence of disabilities were more pronounced in agricultural villages and towns than in urban settings. Others (Levin and Leyland 2004; Barnett, Roderick, Martin et al. 2001) found considerable variation even within areas with high concentrations of agricultural activity, while agricultural communities in closer proximity to urban nodes or centers did much better than those at some distance from such concentrations. In this way it is easy to see how the different studies might be generating countervailing or inconsistent findings. One issue here is the way in which locales are classified as 'urban' or 'rural'. Another difficulty is in the way 'health outcomes' are defined. There is a further challenge in trying to assess how historical and other factors give a distribution of the population a socio-political context, a concern which emerges from the great variation found in income levels among various rural communities (which often have different economic beginnings).

Others have applied multiple regression analyses to the same data, controlling for age, the number of ailments, self-rated health status, marital status and the extent to which one is able to perform a range of daily tasks independently (Murata, Kondō, Hirai et al. 2008). No matter how the data are analyzed, however, those with lower education and those in more rural locales are found to have a higher incidence of depression. When education and income are compared, the level of income comes out as the variable that is most strongly linked to depression.

The findings introduced above indicate how differences in health outcomes tend to stay with an age cohort into old age. Earlier research has found that physical dexterity also deteriorates more rapidly among older people with lower levels of SES (Grundy and Glaser 2000). Although the situation of the poor members of society is frequently mentioned in discussions of social welfare, there is a need to pay more attention to how to maintain good health among them and thus prevent the need for care. At the same time, it is important to be cognizant of the fact that older people are at a stage in life where it is difficult for them to alter their lives in terms of the two most important variables affecting their well-being: educational background and income. As explained in Chapter 1 (see Figure 1.1), the mechanisms that influence health outcomes in a society are multifaceted. Various factors come into play, including the physical environment, daily habits and lifestyle practices, psychological stress, the ability to deal with such stress, and participation in social networks and activities. In a very real sense, investigations into these and other factors in terms of any health

Box 7: GDS (Geriatric Depression Scale)
Kiyoko Yoshii

'Depression' is one of the more important mental health problems. It is desirable to diagnose depression based on a clinical interview conducted by a psychiatrist. However, it is unrealistic to interview all subjects in an epidemiological study to find out the proportion of depressive people among the general public. Various questionnaires for assessing depression have therefore been developed. The questionnaires ask survey subjects to answer a set of questions and detect signs of depression based on the score. Geriatric Depression Scale (GDS) is one of these questionnaires, developed specifically to measure depression in older people. It was recommended as a self-reported evaluation instrument in *Guidelines on Depression in Older People: Practising the Evidence* prepared under the auspices of the World Psychiatric Association Sections of Old Age Psychiatry and Affective Disorders.

It originally had 30 items, but a 15-item version was later developed (equivalent to items 6 and 12–24 under Question 3 in the family abuse version of the survey: Appendix 2). It is widely used in Japan and overseas since it has been tested for sensitivity (abnormal subjects are considered positive) and specificity (normal subjects are considered negative) and the yes/no response method is easier for older people to use. Scores range from 0 to 15. Scores from 0 to 4 are classified as 'not depressed', scores from 5 to 9 as 'mild depression' and scores 10 and over as 'moderate to severe depression'.

determining mechanisms are an important first step forward toward developing proper strategies for intervention. As for the health differences between regions, in addition to the variation in SES indices, we can mention climate and geographical features, local health practices, cultural proclivities, traffic conditions, the nature of social relationships at the local level, and the provision of medical facilities and services. To prevent or postpone the need for aged care it is necessary to investigate the relations of those kinds of factors to health outcomes so that policies and strategies can be introduced that are appropriate to the specific needs of each community.

Conclusions

Two overall conclusions emerge. First, the measures of SES were found to be negatively correlated to the health outcomes at significant levels. The prevalence of depression among those with incomes below ¥1 million was 4.1–6.9 times that of those with incomes above ¥4 million. Second, as for the inter-municipal variations, the percentage of those feeling very unwell or somewhat unwell ranged from 26.9 to 36.9 percent. For the percentage of those designated as 'depressed', the range was from 6.8 to 12.0 percent. Both findings mean that inter-municipal variations deserve further consideration. Moreover, the analysis also revealed that the locale-by-locale variations cannot be explained simply by the variations in SES.

Chapter 3

Life-Style Choices and Falls

Ryōzō Matsuda

Introduction

The discussion in this chapter focuses on the relationship between socio-economic status (SES) and (i) life style choices related to one's health and (ii) one's history of falls. Steptoe and Marmot (2002), Kondō (2004), Bartley (2004) and Wilkinson (2000) argue that the habits formed in the course of day-to-day living affect health outcomes within a socio-economic context – which marks one's access to social resources – and psychologically charged situations in which individuals find themselves.

Research in several Western European countries by Lantz, House, Lepkowski et al. (1998), Jarvis and Wardle (1999), Varo, Martinez-Gonzáles, de Irala-Estevez et al. (2003) and Wardle, Farrell, Hillsdon et al. (1999) revealed that the prevalence of unhealthy habits – such as smoking, lack of exercise, being overweight and consuming junk food – varies inversely with level of education and occupational status, with unskilled laborers and manual workers being more likely to develop such habits. However, Kim, Symons and Popkin (2004) found the reverse to be true in China, with unhealthy habits being positively correlated with SES. Clearly, then, the relationship between SES and health vary from one country to another just as social institutions, culture and economic structures differ from one society to another.

This chapter will examine the AGES data for 2925 men and 5206 women across three types of region providing information on (i) the extent of smoking, (ii) the level of exercise, (iii) the consumption of alcohol, and (iv) whether respondents had had a health check. It considers how that information is related to SES. The numbers that appear in each analysis vary according to the number of missing values for any given variable. The chapter will also consider the extent to which the prevalence of falling is related to SES.

Falls are a major source of disabilities among older people (Shakai Hoshō Shingikai Kaigo Hoken Bukai 2004). Fewer falls means less need for rehabilitation and care by others (Suzuki 2003). For older people falls can mean a loss of mobility and even death. According to one Cabinet survey, about 70 percent of older Japanese who experienced a fall end up with some kind of injury, with about 5 percent breaking bones (Cabinet Office 2004). Estimates suggest that about 20 percent of accidental deaths occurring among Japan's population aged over 65 result from falls, and that falls are a more common source of deaths than traffic accidents (Ministry of Health, Labour and Welfare, Statistics and Information Dept. 2003). Experts overseas attach huge importance to safeguarding against falls as central to any policy designed to improve health outcomes for older people. One's history of previous falls is an important precursor when it comes to predicting the likelihood of falling. It is one of ten items in Mose's risk assessment scale for falls (Suzuki 2003). According to the guidelines of the American Geriatric Society et al. (2001), depression (which correlates with SES) is linked with the likelihood of falling. We can also imagine how the cost of erecting fall-resistant residential accommodation might relate to indices of SES such as income.

Method

AGES data for 12,925 men and 16,206 women contained information on the: (i) extent of smoking, (ii) level of exercise, (iii) consumption of alcohol, (iv) utilization of health check-ups, and (v) history of previous falls. The analysis looked at some of the relationships among (i) health-related habits, (ii) socio-economic status, (iii) falls, (iv) years of education, (v) equivalent household income, (vi) subjective assessments of physical well-being, (vii) the occurrence of depression (as recorded on the GDS depression scale), and (viii) the overall feelings of happiness (as recorded on the moral scale developed by the Philadelphia Geriatric Center [PGC]). For each analysis the data was adjusted to correct for differences in the age profiles of each sub-sample. The statistics were produced by using SPSS. When disaggregating the data by type of region (classified according to population density), attention was paid to how regions varied in terms of SES and unhealthy habits. Missing values for some variables meant that the number of cases varied from the analysis of one relationship to another.

A multi-faceted index was conceived as a means of measuring the extent to which individuals engaged in unhealthy practices. The data was manipulated so it would yield a number of binary variables as developed by the Ministry of Health, Labour and Welfare. First, with regard to smoking, respondents were asked if they ever smoked. Only those who answered that they were currently smoking were deemed to have an 'unhealthy habit'. Second, as for the consumption of alcohol, those consuming 30 grams or more each day were judged to have an unhealthy habit. Here 30 grams was judged to be the equivalent of 750 ml of beer, 90 ml of whiskey or 270 ml of sake. The third question concerned exercise: 'How many minutes do you walk on an average day?' Those who answered less than 30 minutes were seen as having an 'unhealthy habit'. The fourth question asked was about having had a physical examination: 'Have you ever had a health check-up?'[1] Those who had never had such a 'going over' were counted as having an unhealthy practice. The final query concerned the respondent's history of falling. Those who fell frequently or even occasionally were classified as 'having had a fall'.

Findings

Falls and life-style choices

Table 3.1 provides a breakdown showing the frequency distribution of unhealthy life-style habits by age and by gender. Smoking and alcohol consumption are found to occur much more among men in the AGES sample than among women, but declines with age. However, older Japanese women in the study are much more likely than men to have exercised insufficiently and to have failed to have a physical examination, and those deficiencies increased with age. Overall the proclivity to fall increased with age, and was greater among women; for those aged over 75 the percentage having had a bad fall was 33.5 percent for men and as high as 43.0 percent for women.

Life-style choices, falls and socio-economic status

Table 3.2 shows the distribution of unhealthy habits by level of equivalent household income. With the exception of alcohol consumption, the percentage with unhealthy habits was significantly higher among those in the lower income bracket. Those in the highest income bracket drank the most, but not significantly more. As Table 3.3 shows, those with lower levels of education are generally more likely to make unhealthy lifestyle choices and to have falls. However,

Table 3.1: Prevalence of unhealthy habits and falls by gender and age group

	Men by age group					**Women by age group**				
	65–69	**70–74**	**75–79**	**80–84**	**85+**	**65–69**	**70–74**	**75–79**	**80–84**	**85+**
Number in sample (N)	4,452	4,164	2,295	1,370	644	4,884	4,701	3,567	2,071	983
Percentage who smoke every day	25.6	23.6	20.7	18.3	14.4	2.8	2.7	1.6	1.6	1.7
Percentage who drink 270 ml or more everyday	12.6	9.2	6.2	4.2	3.5	0.5	0.1	0.1	0.2	0.2
Percentage who walk thirty minutes or less per day	31.4	35.6	38.9	39.6	42.4	33.9	39.8	40.8	42.0	45.9
Percentage who have not had a physical examination	17.1	19.5	21.8	25.3	37.8	17.6	21.3	24.4	32.3	44.2
Percentage who have experienced a fall	18.0	23.8	30.3	35.0	44.7	27.8	36.2	42.1	42.6	47.7

Table 3.2: Age-adjusted prevalence rates of unhealthy habits and falls by level of income

	Men by income group (million yen)				**Women by income group (million yen)**			
	<2	**2–4**	**4+**	**p-value**	**<2**	**2–4**	**4+**	**p-value**
Number in sample (N)	5,501	5,364	1,239		5,896	4,411	1,201	
Percentage who smoke every day	23.9	21.9	23.0	*	2.7	1.9	2.3	*
Percentage who drink 270 ml or more everyday	8.9	9.1	10.2	n.s.	0.3	0.1	0.4	n.s.
Percentage who walk thirty minutes or less per day	38.1	33.0	31.5	***	40.3	36.0	36.5	***
Percentage who have not had a physical examination	24.1	15.8	16.1	***	24.9	19.1	20.1	***
Percentage who have experienced a fall	26.8	23.4	22.0	***	37.5	33.1	32.0	***

Notes:

1. All figures were adjusted for age using general linear models (GLMs)

2. F-tests were used to compare prevalence rates of unhealthy habits between income groups.

*: p = 0.05; ***: p = 0.001; n.s. = not significant.

Table 3.3: Prevalence of unhealthy habits and falls by years of education

	Men by years of education					Women by years of education				
	<6	**6–9**	**10–12**	**13+**	**p-value**	**<6**	**6–9**	**10–12**	**13+**	**p-value**
Number in sample (N)	414	7,515	4,041	1,815		1,073	9,087	5,185	813	
Percentage who smoke every day	23.6	22.8	24.1	18.9	***	4.7	2.3	1.8	1.9	***
Percentage who drink 270 ml or more everyday	11.5	9.1	8.8	8.0	n.s.	0.3	0.3	0.1	0.1	n.s.
Percentage who walk thirty minutes or less per day	47.3	35.8	34.8	33.9	***	41.8	39.2	37.1	39.3	*
Percentage who have not had a physical examination	34.6	23.0	17.4	14.5	***	32.2	24.5	19.9	18.9	***
Percentage who have experienced a fall	39.1	34.5	34.7	30.2	n.s.	40.5	30.8	28.4	33.6	***

Notes:

1. All figures were adjusted for age using general linear models (GLMs)
2. F-tests were used to compare prevalence rates of unhealthy habits between level of education.

*: $p = 0.05$; ***: $p = 0.001$; n.s. = not significant.

although the average for alcohol consumption varied in that way, the difference turned out to be statistically insignificant.

Subjective perceptions of well-being and life-style choices

Figure 3.1 shows how life-style generated habits heighten the likelihood of being depressed. For both men and women, a low level of self-assessed physical well-being, depression and low levels of happiness with life correlate positively (at $p < 0.01$) with lack of exercise, failure to have a physical examination and falling. At the same time, the level of physical well-being claimed in self-assessments correlates positively with the consumption of alcohol. Strong relationships with most of the unhealthy habits were found with depression, an outcome shown in Figure 3.1. One's history of psychological problems seemed to account for the biggest differences in whether the respondents to the AGES survey experienced a fall.

Residential settings

Table 3.4 shows a significant difference between urban and rural regions, with a larger proportion of the urban population having smoking habits. Also significant was the lower percentage of persons living in rural regions who had physical examinations. Differences in terms of exercise and falls by type of region were not significant. However, differences in SES were important. In regions characterized by lower SES scores, the older respondents did less exercise and were more likely to experience falls. They were also less likely to have had a physical check-up. Figure 3.2 shows the relationship between equivalent income and the percentage of those who have had such a check-up in men.

With regard to smoking, the socio-economic differences again come into play. In urban and semi-urban regions the rate of smoking is very high among the lower income groups (here defined as those with equivalent household incomes below 2 million yen), whereas the percentage who smoke declines as income increases. However, as shown in Figure 3.3, in rural-agricultural regions the lowest rate of smoking is found among those with incomes between 2 million and 3 million yen.

Respondents who did less exercise, however, were more likely to experience falls in every type of region. They were also less likely to have had a health check-up regardless of the type of region in which they were living. Figure 3.2 shows that for men there was a consistent

Figure 3.1: Percentage who have unhealthy habits or who have experienced a fall by level of depression

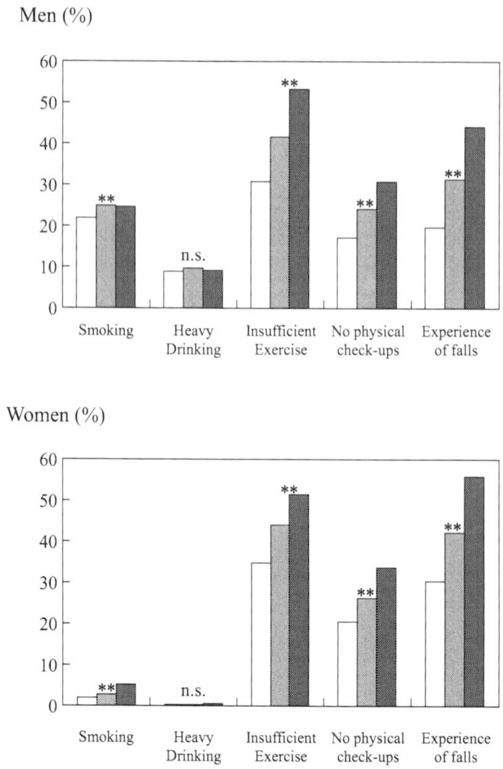

Notes.

1. The respondents were classified as 'not depressed', 'mild depression' and 'moderate to severe depression' using the GDS scale as introduced in Chapter 2. The following colors distinguish each type in the graph:

□ = no depression (N = 8,006 men or 8,438 women)

■ = mild depression (N = 2,878 men or 3,234 women)

■ = moderate to severe depression (N = 940 men or 1,038 women)

2. The figures were adjusted for age using general linear models (GLMs). F-tests were used to compare prevalence rates of the three groups by the extent of depression. Calculated p-values were shown with the following symbols:

** = $p < 0.01$

n.s. = no significance

3. Descriptions of the different habits and the experience of falling are provided in the text of the chapter.

Table 3.4: Prevalence of unhealthy habits by type of region

	Urban	Semi-urban	Rural-agricultural	p-value
Number in sample (N)	7,936	4,787	20,168	
Percentage who are smokers	14.4	13	12.2	**
Percentage who have had a physical examination	19.7	19.7	21.6	***

Notes.

1. All figures were adjusted for age, income levels and years of education, using general linear models (GLMs)

2. F-tests were used to compare prevalence rates of unhealthy habits between the groups by level of education.

**: p = 0.01; ***: p = 0.001

Figure 3.2: Relation between income and not having a physical examination among men by type of region[a, b]

Percentage of respondents who had not received a physical examination[c]

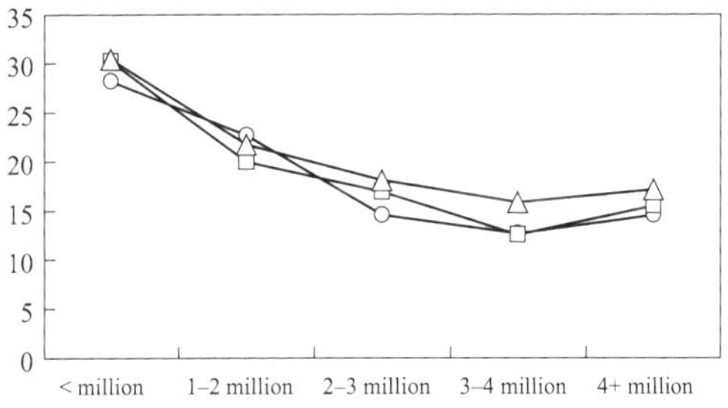

Equivalent household income (yen/year)

Notes.

a: Types of regions

—○— = urban

—□— = semi-urban

—△— = rural-agricultural

b: F-test with significant level 0.05 was used to compare prevalence rates of smoking of the income groups for each type of region. For all regions, a null hypothesis that all income groups had the same prevalence rates was rejected.

c: All figures were adjusted for age using general linear models (GLMs).

Figure 3.3: Relation between income and smoking among men by type of region[a, b]

Percentage of respondents who smoke[c]

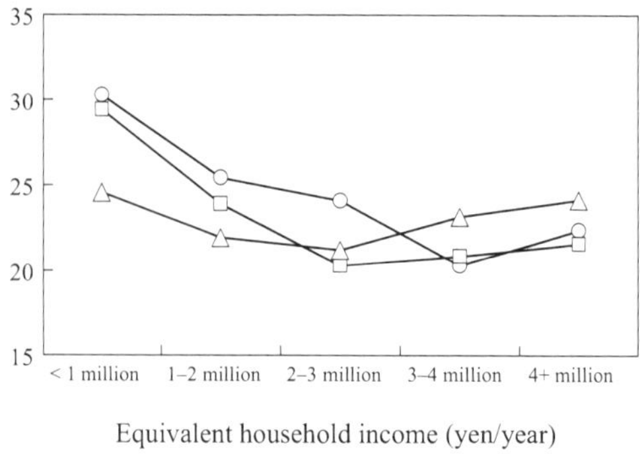

Notes.

a: Types of regions

–○– = urban

–□– = semi-urban

–△– = rural-agricultural

b: F-test with significant level 0.05 was used to compare prevalence rates of smoking of the income groups for each type of region. For urban regions, a null hypothesis that all income groups had the same prevalence rates was rejected; for semi-urban regions and rural-agricultural regions, however, the null hypothesis was not rejected.

c: All figures were adjusted for age using general linear models (GLMs).

relationship across regions between equivalent income and the percentage of those who have had a health check-up.

The data was also examined to see if there was a link between socio-economic status, life-style practices and the incidence of falls across regions. The data revealed significant differences in the average income, the prevalence of unhealthy life-style choices and falls for each of the regions.

Discussion

The findings presented above indicate that Japan's older citizens have experiences similar to those of their counterpart populations in Western Europe. Among citizens characterized by lower SES 'bad' habits seem to be more common: more smoking, less exercise, and fewer appointments for physical check-ups.

Smoking

The relationship of the level of education to smoking is more pronounced than that found for income. This has also been the findings of research on adults in Western Europe (Huisman, Kunst and Mackenbach 20005; Mackenbach 2006). Our findings are similar to those of Anzai et al. (2000) who found that more highly educated older men in the city were less likely to smoke. They found a similar relationship for older women, although the differences did not appear to be statistically significant. The larger AGES sample yielded a significant relationship between income and smoking in older women.

The relationship between smoking and the level of income was not simple. Respondents whose income was between 2 million and 4 million yen were least likely to smoke. This finding is different from that of a previous study of the Japanese population aged 25 to 54 (Fukuda, Nakamura and Takano 2005a). Our research indicated that for both men and women, those with the highest incomes were least likely to be smokers. The difference between the two sets of findings might be in the age group studied or in the fact that Fukuda et al. used five income groupings for their study whereas we used three.

Drinking

The connection between SES and drinking is not as clear as that for smoking. Marmot (1997) argues there is no simple causative relationship. In England, for example, research among those aged over 75 found that those who had a stable source of income were accustomed to imbibing moderate amounts of alcohol (Hajat, Haines, Bulpitt et al. 2004). In contrast, in the United States another survey of adults found that the heaviest drinkers were those with lower levels of education (National Center for Health Statistics 1998). In northern Italy De Vogli, Gnesotto, Goldstein et al. (2005) found no relationship between the excessive intake of alcohol and SES. Still other research from Israel (Neumark, Rahav and Jaffe 2003) revealed international cultural differences with the wealthy imbibing the most among the Arab community whereas within the Jewish community heavy drinking was most frequently found to occur among those with the least income. Chaix and Chauvin (2003) have suggested that the level of alcohol consumption is affected by the overall performance of the national economy. Considering the findings of these and other studies, it is not at all surprising that the AGES data also revealed no clear connection between moderate levels of drinking (e.g., imbibing the equivalent of 90 ml of alcohol per day) and SES. There is, however, as Mackenbach (2006) suggests, a need to rethink the way we define 'excessive drinking' or 'heavy drinking'. In Healthy Japan 21 'heavy drinking' was defined as the daily consumption of over 60 grams of alcohol per day, and sets 20 grams as a moderate standard (Ministry of Health and Welfare 2000).

Health check ups

The relationship between SES and having had a health check-up was strong. Those with lower SES were less likely to have had a health check-up, a finding that is consistent with those of Fukuda, Nakamura and Takano (2005b) for the population aged under 60. The reasons for that behavior have not been investigated, but we might speculate that the more educated are better able to deduce the benefits that flow from a health check-up. Check-ups also involve several costs and the better educated might be in a better position to afford the examination. If higher SES is reflected in lower rates of depression, it might also be the case that there is a psycho-social outlook whereby greater optimism about life course outcomes results in individuals being more willing to have a check-up.

Exercise

Similar to the situation surrounding health check-ups, across gender and age groups those with higher SES are more likely to engage in exercise. That was not the case in the earlier research by Anzai (2000), although the relationship between SES and exercise was found by Anzai to exist among men aged under 70. Reflecting the fact that lower SES is associated with higher levels of depression, it is interesting to note that the more psychologically sound individuals are more likely to partake in exercise and have physical check-ups. One can speculate further that those with lower SES profiles might live in places which are not suited to walking owing to traffic conditions or the built-up nature of the environment. Taking time to exercise properly is likely to bolster one's willingness to venture beyond the confines of one's residence. And, conversely, having the ability to be mobile can in itself serve to enhance one's psychological well-being. All these hypotheses require further examination.

Falls

The AGES data yield a slightly higher incidence of falls than previous research (Suzuki 2001). Compared to those with no falls, those who have had a fall are at a greater risk of falling again in the future, and should be candidates for a deliberate exercise program designed to strengthen lower back and thigh muscles. Again, we need to be cognizant of the fact that those with lower incomes and less education are more prone to fall. This view is in line with that surfacing from previous research in South Australia and in Kent, England (Gill, Taylor and Pengelly 2005; West, Hippislay-Cox, Coupland et al. 2004). We could not duplicate research in the United States and Sweden (Bacon and Hadden 2000; Farahmand, Persson et al. 2000) that showed a link between SES and broken thigh bones. There is a need in Japan to investigate the linkages between SES and bone fractures more generally.

SES is indirectly related to the factors that often occasion a fall. On the one hand is one's own medical situation characterized by other ailments, medication and a loss of physical abilities as age advances. On the other hand is the immediate environment in which one lives: slippery floors, high door sills and other unevenness under foot, loose floor coverings and electric cords that make it easy to stumble (Suzuki 2001). The AGES data reveal a correlation between falls and depression, but the chain of causation was not clear. Was it that falling led to a loss of mobility that was then found to be depressing, or was it that the depression was treated with medications that left patients less steady on their feet? This is another area for future research.

If low SES results in a higher risk of illness or falling, it makes sense that policy makers give some thought to the likely impact of SES. For example, if low SES is reflected in fewer visits for a check-up, the opportunity to introduce a preventative strategy is minimized. Accordingly, there is a danger that warning signs are missed (Hiramatsu, Kondō and Hirai 2009). If this is the case, policy makers can then focus on devising prevention programs that are easily accessed by persons with less education and lower levels of income. At the same time, policies are needed which direct resources to improve the immediate home and neighborhood environment in which less privileged citizens are living, and to programs that will assist with the maintenance of their health. In these regards as well, further research is needed.

Conclusion

Although there is some variation according to gender and age, overall the risk factors – smoking, lack of exercise, falls and the failure to have a physical check-up – were most prevalent among respondents with low levels of SES. Compared to those who do not suffer from depression, those who do are much more likely to have engaged in unhealthy practices. For men the relationship between smoking, SES, falls and other unhealthy habits varied from one region to another. It is, therefore, desirable to keep all of these facets in mind when devising programs to reduce the need for aged care among our senior citizens.

The relationship between years of education and a healthy lifestyle continues throughout adult life and deserves careful attention. That connection seems to follow each cohort after they graduate, enter the labor force, marry, have children and experience other big life-changing events as they age. When we think of policies to reduce the need for aged care among our older citizens, we need to consider the importance of promoting healthy practices in our schools and as people go through the processes of becoming young adults (Kuh and Ben-Shlomo 2004). As Davey-Smith (2003) argues, policy makers must give thought to the factors which work to generate different healthy practices among different socio-economic strata in our society.

Note

1. In Japan the adult population is advised to have a health check-up every year. Such a check-up includes a physical examination (including blood, urinary and faecal tests to screen for cancer and other illnesses) and an electrocardiogram to screen for cardiovascular problems (Tatara and Okamoto 2009).

Chapter 4

Dental, Oral and Nutritional Statuses

Miyo Nakade

Introduction

Maintaining oral health and preventing poor nutrition are key elements for living independently in one's senior years (Shinkai et al. 2001; Baba and Une 2005). "Enhancing oral health" and "improving nutrition" are both regarded as areas requiring great effort to minimise the need for long-term care of older people in the context of revising the long-term care insurance system in Japan (Ministry of Health 2005). Oral health and nutrition are closely related. Decreased oral health, such as impaired masticatory ability due to loss of teeth, can cause decline in food intake, resulting in poor nutrition in older people (Sheiham et al. 2002; Marcenes et al. 2003).

In the field of Japanese dentistry, the 8020 Movement was launched in 2000 as a national campaign on the basis that "If a person has 20 or more remaining teeth at the age of 80, he/she is able to maintain sufficient masticatory function for an independent dietary life". The importance of dental health for general health issues was also noted in "Japanese National Health Promotion in the 21st Century (Healthy Japan 21)" (Japan Health Promotion 2000). Oral health is associated not only with physical health but also self-rated health (Seida et al. 2002; Yoshida et al. 1997; Nakanishi et al. 1998; Ide et al. 2000). Occupation and irregular working hours reportedly have an influence on oral health behaviors, such as taking care of oral health or having a regular dentist (Fukai 2003). However, our extensive literature search found no studies that have investigated the relationship of such behaviors with years of education or income. The WHO suggested in "The World Oral Health Report 2003", that poor oral health, particularly in older people, increases the risk of general health problems and has an influence on nutritional intake or quality of life, and that poor and disadvantaged populations suffer from serious oral health problems despite worldwide improvements in oral health.

The occurrence of falls or hospitalisation over the past year and nonparticipation in leisure activities have been found to be significant predictors of poor nutritional status in independent older people (Kumagai et al. 2005) but few Japanese studies have focused on poor nutritional status in older community-dwelling people. The number of years of education is reportedly associated with nutritional intake status (e.g. energy sufficiency) (Yukawa 2004) but few studies have found a relationship between SES and poor nutritional status. Overseas, using a nutritional screening tool, MNA (Mini-Nutritional Assessment), a 1-year follow-up study of community-dwelling older people at risk of malnutrition reported the frequent occurrence of hospitalisation, falls and weight loss among subjects (Visvanathan et al. 2003). Another study found a strong relationship between nutritional status, psychological stress and self-rated health using MNA (Soini et al. 2004). In the UK, a nutritional study of city-dwelling homebound older people found that lower BMI (Body Mass Index) was associated with oral symptoms, male gender, increased age and fewer years of education (Ritchie et al. 1997). However, our extensive search of the literature found no studies that have reported area differences in dental, oral and nutritional statuses.

The purpose of this chapter is to grasp the dental, oral and nutritional statuses of older Japanese people, discuss the relationships of these statuses with two health indicators (depression and self-rated health), and examine the infrequently-reported relationships of these statuses and SES with a focus on area differences in these relationships.

Method

The current study used the data from the AGES Project (Aichi Gerontological Evaluation Study; Box 2) of which the study population was Japanese aged 65 and older who were not eligible to receive long-term care and were living at home throughout 15 municipalities (12 long-term care insurers). The subjects included in analyses were 17,034 respondents (mean age 73.7 ± 6.2 years; response rate 58.0 percent) to one of the three questionnaires used in the AGES Project and mainly consisted of dental, oral and nutritional items (see Appendix 1). Note that the number of cases included in each analysis differs depending on missing values for study variables.

Dental and oral statuses were assessed using: number of remaining teeth; mastication; presence of subjective oral health problems (e.g. pain, difficulty chewing, dry mouth, bad breath, etc.) and two oral health behaviors (taking care of oral health and having a regular dentist). Nutritional status was measured using the following risk indicators of malnutrition: BMI; decline in food intake (staple and subsidiary foods); weight loss (more than 3 kg over the past six months); and lack of eating pleasure (i.e., feel that eating is not a pleasure but bothersome). As for the risk indicators of malnutrition, question items were developed based on "Assessment for preventing poor nutritional status-Use of self-check list" (Sugiyama et al. 2000).

GDS (Geriatric Depression Scale; Box 7) and self-rated health (4 categories of response were reduced into 2 categories; Box 6) were used as psychological health indicators, while years of education and income were used as SES indices. (Income is adjusted for family size, obtained by dividing the household income [10,000 yen/year] by the square root of household size; Box 3.) Comparisons were also made based on the three regional classifications (see Chapter 1).

The general linear model in the statistical software SPSS was used for statistical analyses in which health indicators and SES indices were treated as explanatory variables and dental, oral and nutritional indicators were treated as objective variables. The results show values adjusted for age. Analysis was also performed by gender. Good oral health behaviors and decreased food intake were more prevalent in women but no other differences were observed between genders for the remaining variables. Thus, the results will be given regardless of gender.

Results

Distribution of dental, oral and nutritional statuses

The distribution of dental, oral and nutritional statuses by age group is shown in Table 4.1. The proportion of subjects with a sufficient number of remaining teeth or with no masticatory problems decreased with age. More than 40 percent of subjects in every age group were aware of their oral health problems. As to nutritional status, the proportion of subjects with a thin figure (BMI of less than 18.5), decreased food intake or weight loss increased with age. Among those aged 80 and older, the prevalence of thinness (BMI of less than 18.5) and weight loss was 15.1 percent and 13.4 percent respectively. This suggests approximately one in seven in this age group is at risk of malnutrition. In respect to the relationship between the number of remaining teeth and nutritional status, low BMI, weight loss and decreased intake of staple and subsidiary foods were significantly more frequent in those with fewer remaining teeth (Table 4.2). Though not shown in the table,

Table 4.1: Distribution of dental, oral and nutritional statuses by age group (%)

Age group (years)	No. of remaining teeth				Mastication				Presence of oral health problems		Taking care of oral health		Presence of regular dentist		BMI				Intake of staple foods		Intake of subsidiary foods		Weight		Lack of eating pleasure	
	N	≥ 20	≤ 19	Few	N	Can chew	Cannot chew well	Cannot chew	N	Yes	N	Yes	N	Yes	N	< 18.5	18.5–24.9	≥ 25.0	N	Decr.	N	Decr.	N	Decr.	N	Yes
65–69	4,733	36.8	38.7	24.5	4,764	93.7	5.9	0.5	4,458	43.4	4,760	91.2	4,689	85.1	4,604	4.8	67.8	27.4	4,701	32.0	4,674	25.4	4,652	7.3	4,642	3.3
70–74	4,680	24.4	38.2	37.4	4,708	91.7	7.9	0.4	4,292	44.6	4,688	92.0	4,553	86.1	4,449	6.4	68.4	25.2	4,579	39.6	4,514	32.1	4,464	7.7	4,419	5.1
75–79	3,442	14.9	33.1	52.0	3,461	90.1	9.3	0.6	3,127	45.3	3,454	91.6	3,325	83.2	3,247	9.7	69.0	21.3	3,329	47.0	3,265	37.9	3,186	9.2	3,176	7.1
80–84	1,903	10.8	24.1	65.1	1,917	86.9	11.7	1.5	1,737	44.9	1,923	91.7	1,829	78.1	1,686	15.1	68.0	16.9	1,839	48.9	1,784	42.7	1,734	13.4	1,705	8.2
85+	912	5.8	17.8	76.4	913	83.2	15.3	1.4	815	45.6	923	85.5	884	68.6	722	18.3	70.4	11.4	889	52.8	862	45.1	836	14.4	843	10.0

Notes. N = No. of subjects. Can chew = Can chew most foods; Cannot chew well = Cannot chew very well. Decr. = Decreased.

Table 4.2: Relationship between number of remaining teeth and nutritional status (%)

No. of remaining teeth	N	BMI < 18.5	p	Weight loss	p	Decreased intake of staple foods	p	Decreased intake of subsidiary foods	p
≥ 20	3,376	6.7	***	7.0	***	34.3	***	27.0	***
≤ 19	4,770	7.5		7.9		38.8		31.7	
Few	5,391	9.3		9.8		41.8		34.9	

Notes.
Results adjusted for age using the general linear model.
N = No. of subjects.
p = p-value. ***: $p < 0.001$.

the following differences were also observed between genders: 87.6 percent of men and 93.1 percent of women were reportedly taking care of oral health; 81.4 percent of men and 84.8 percent of women had a regular dentist; and 43.5 percent of men and 38.2 percent of women reported a decline in the intake of staple foods.

Relationships with depression and self-rated health

Table 4.3 shows the relationships of dental, oral and nutritional statuses with depression and self-rated health. Poor self-rated health, mild depression and moderate to severe depression were more prevalent among subjects with fewer remaining teeth or impaired masticatory ability, with 54.0 percent of those with masticatory problems rating their health status as "fair" or "poor". Though not shown in the table, depression was less frequent in those taking care of oral health or having a regular dentist. As to the risk indicators of malnutrition, subjects with a thin figure (BMI of less than 18.5) or weight loss more frequently reported mild depression, moderate to severe depression and poor self-rated health. Similar results were observed among those with a decreased food intake or a lack of eating pleasure.

Relationships with income and years of education

The relationships of dental, oral and nutritional statuses with income and years of education are shown in Table 4.4. The table gives the proportions of subjects with 20 or more remaining teeth and those with less than 20 remaining teeth, and the proportions of subjects with some masticatory and related problems.

Table 4.3: Relationships of depression and self-rated health with dental, oral and nutritional statuses (%)

		Depression (GDS)						Self-rated health	
	N	Not depressed	p	Mild depression	p	Moderate to severe depression	p	Fair or poor	p
No. of remaining teeth									
≥ 20	3,049	74.3	***	20.1	***	5.6	***	21.2	***
≤ 19	4,370	65.9		26.0		8.1		27.9	
Few	4,922	60.8		29.4		9.8		32.1	
Mastication									
Can chew most foods	11,345	68.1	***	24.7	***	7.2	***	25.6	***
Cannot chew very well or cannot chew	1,054	41.3		39.2		19.5		54.0	
BMI									
≥ 18.5	10,788	67.1	***	25.3	**	7.7	***	26.8	***
< 18.5	900	58.2		30.6		11.2		39.0	
Weight loss									
No	10,995	68.1	***	24.8	***	7.1	***	25.3	***
Yes	1,050	47.2		35.0		17.8		51.7	

Notes.

Results adjusted for age using the general linear model.

N = No. of subjects.

p = p-value. **: $p<0.01$, ***: $p<0.001$.

Geriatric Depression Scale (GDS 15-item version): "Not depressed (≤ 4 points)"; "Mild depression (5–9 points)"; "Moderate to severe depression (≥ 10 points)".

Self-rated health: Subjects who rated their current health status as "Fair" or "Poor".

The proportion of subjects with 20 or more remaining teeth was significantly higher in the higher income group, whereas the proportion of those with few remaining teeth or masticatory problems was significantly higher in the lower income group. The number of remaining teeth was associated with age and income (Figure 4.1). Weight loss was more prevalent in the lower income group but there was no significant relationship between income and thinness (BMI of less than 18.5).

Similar to income, the proportion of subjects with few remaining teeth or masticatory problems was higher in the less educated groups than in the more educated groups (i.e., those with less or more years of formal education). Though statistically non-significant, thinness (BMI of less than 18.5) was more prevalent in the group with the most years of education. Weight loss was significantly more frequent in the

Table 4.4: Relationships of income and years of education with dental, oral and nutritional statuses (%)

	Per capita equivalent income adjusted for family size (10,000 yen/year)[a]				Years of education				
	< 200	200–400	≥ 400	p	< 6	6–9	10–12	≥ 13	p
No. of subjects	5,355	4,353	1,019		552	7,358	4,315	1,208	
No. of remaining teeth									
≥ 20	23.0	29.7	33.3	***	23.4	22.1	27.7	33.0	***
Few	41.5	33.6	32.3	***	50.0	42.6	35.8	30.6	***
Mastication									
Cannot chew very well or cannot chew	10.1	6.8	5.9	***	14.4	9.7	6.3	5.7	***
BMI									
< 18.5	8.0	7.6	8.6	n.s.	7.5	8.2	7.8	9.0	n.s.
Weight									
Lost 3kg+ over the past 6 months	9.3	7.7	8.3	*	9.2	9.4	7.4	7.3	**

Notes.
Results adjusted for age using the general linear model.
p = p-value. *: $p < 0.05$, **: $p < 0.01$, ***: $p < 0.001$, n.s.: not significant.
a: Household income (10,000 yen/year) divided by the square root of household size.

less educated groups. Although not shown in the table, the higher the income or the more years of education, the higher the tendency towards good oral health behaviors ($p < 0.001$). In contrast, the lower the income or the less education, the greater the decline in food intake or the higher the tendency towards a lack of eating pleasure ($p < 0.001$).

Comparison of relationships with income and years of education by area type

Comparisons were then made to examine whether the relationships of dental, oral and nutritional statuses with income and years of education differ according to area type (Table 4.5). As to the number of remaining teeth, the proportions of subjects with 20 or more remaining teeth was significantly higher in the higher income group in all areas. Of particular importance is the finding that the number of remaining teeth varied greatly according to income as well as area type. For example, the proportions of subjects with few remaining

Box 8: International Comparison of Dental Conditions among Older People

Miyo Nakade

In Japan, the national survey of dental health is conducted every six years and reports on the prevalence of dental diseases. According to the report, the ratio of people who still have at least 20 original teeth at the age of 80 is rising gradually from 15.3 percent in the 1999 survey to 24.1 percent in the 2005 survey (Ministry of Health, Labour and Welfare 1999, 2005). An earlier survey of 2,000 people aged 80 found that 46.1 percent were edentulous and 10.2 percent had at least 20 remaining teeth. It reported that the average number of remaining teeth per person was 6.0 when edentulous subjects were included and 11.2 when edentulous subjects were not included (Andō 2000).

International comparative analysis is needed to determine whether these figures are better or worse than the international standard but the existing data was collected using surveys that targeted different age groups, survey years, geriatric dental health indicators and criteria and tabulation methods, making international comparison very difficult. For this reason, the International Collaboration Study II (ICS II) (Barnes and Leclercq 1994), an international comparative study conducted by WHO, is used for the present discussion of the dental health status of the Japanese in an international context. While it was a cross-sectional study, it did include generational surveys. The number of untreated decayed teeth in children (aged 12–13) was relatively high in Japan (Yamanashi region) (1.5), ranked sixth among seven regions. Japan also had a relatively high ratio of adults (aged 35–44) with periodontal disease (periodontal pocket 6 mm or more) (8 percent), ranked fifth among seven regions. However, Japan fared better and came second in terms of the number of lost teeth in older persons (aged 65–74) (2.4). It is possible to surmise based on the findings that tooth decay and periodontal disease are prevalent but older people have relatively high numbers of remaining teeth in Japan. The study included data compiled by socioeconomic status as well and found that the numbers of lost teeth in older people in different income levels were similar in Japan at 2.4 for low income, 2.4 for middle income and 2.2 for high income. In contrast, tooth loss varied considerably in the USA (Baltimore region) at 4.2 for low income, 2.1 for middle income and 1.1 for high income. Consequently, the average number of lost teeth was lower in Japan than in the USA although it was lower in the latter among high-income earners who enjoyed high levels of preventive care for tooth decay and periodontal disease. The difference is likely to have resulted from a difference in health insurance systems between Japan and the USA where access to dental treatment is easier under universal health insurance coverage regardless of income in the former and it is more difficult for many low-income earners with little or no health cover in the latter.

While dental disease is rarely life-threatening, its high prevalence places a heavy burden on Japanese society in terms of medical care costs (Aida and Kondō 2007). The dental health status of the older population depends on not only preventive efforts in their youth but also the level of dental care they receive. Since each country has its own co-payment rates for patients who use services covered by the public health care scheme (OECD 2005), the ramifications of the level of co-payment for socioeconomic strata are also relevant to the tooth retention status of older people in each country.

Figure 4.1: Relation between number of remaining teeth and income by age group

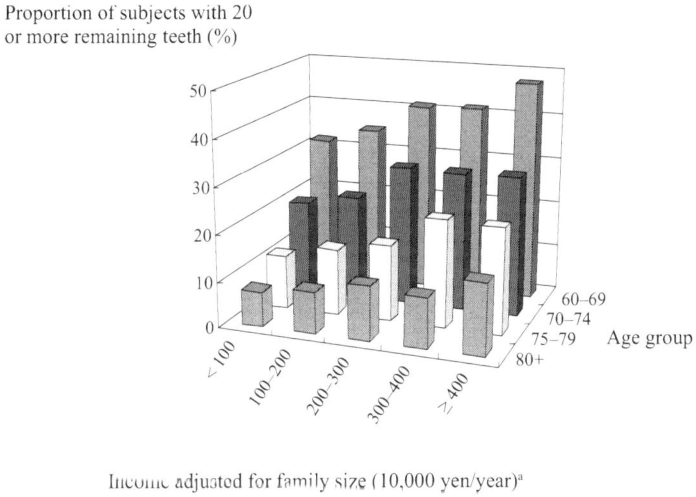

Note.
a: Household income (10,000 yen/year) divided by the square root of household size.

teeth differed between the income groups by 6.3–9.2 percent and differed between the urban and rural areas by 12.8–15.7 percent. Moreover, the proportion of subjects with few remaining teeth in the higher income groups in the rural areas was 35.9 percent, which is 6.5 percent higher than that of the lower income group in the urban areas

Table 4.5: Comparison of relationships of income and years of education with dental and oral status by regional type (%)

	Equivalent income adjusted for family size (10,000 yen/year)[a]	Type of area					
		Urban	p	Semi-urban	p	Rural	p
No. of subjects		1,880		1,114		7,733	
No. of remaining teeth							
≥ 20	< 200	29.9	***	29.0	*	21.0	***
	200–400	37.6		35.9		26.2	
	≥ 400	44.5		36.5		29.0	
Few	< 200	29.4	n.s.	29.7	n.s.	45.1	***
	200–400	25.2		25.4		37.5	
	≥ 400	23.1		28.4		35.9	
Mastication: Cannot chew very well or cannot chew							
	< 200	9.9	**	9.7	n.s.	10.3	***
	200–400	6.7		7.5		6.6	
	≥ 400	4.2		7.8		6.0	

	Years of education	Type of area					
		Urban	p	Semi-urban	p	Rural	p
No. of subjects		2,186		1,337		9,910	
No. of remaining teeth							
≥ 20	<6	33.9	**	29.6	n.s.	19.9	***
	6–9	31.6		29.3		19.2	
	10–12	36.2		34.6		25.0	
	≥ 13	42.0		37.9		29.5	
Few	< 6	34.2	*	51.5	***	53.8	***
	6–9	30.1		31.2		46.8	
	10–12	25.6		27.3		39.0	
	≥ 13	21.9		20.7		34.6	
Mastication: Cannot chew very well or cannot chew							
	< 6	9.2	*	17.6	**	15.2	***
	6–9	9.2		10.6		9.7	
	10–12	5.5		5.6		6.6	
	≥ 13	5.6		4.9		6.0	

Notes.

Results adjusted for age using the general linear model.

p = p-value. *: $p<0.05$, **: $p<0.01$, ***: $p<0.001$, n.s.: not significant.

a: Household income (10,000 yen/year) divided by the square root of household size.

Figure 4.2: Relationship between number of dental clinics and number of remaining teeth

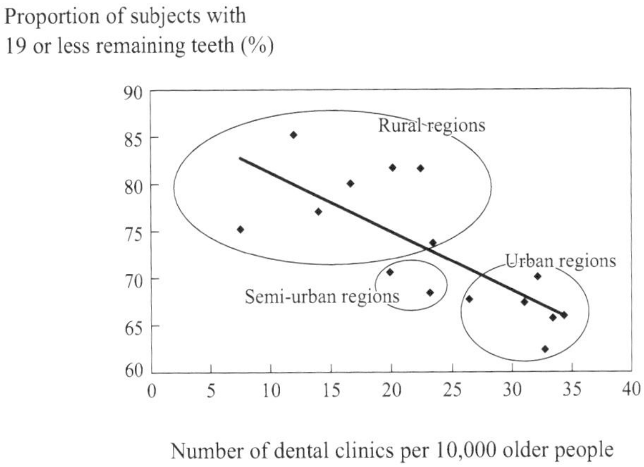

(29.4 percent). The proportions of subjects with impaired masticatory ability were significantly higher in the lower income group in both the urban and rural areas. With a few exceptions, there was also a significant relationship between mastication and years of education in all areas.

The rural regions appeared to have significantly lower rates of retaining teeth compared to the urban and semi-urban areas but the areas did not differ significantly in mastication. Figure 4.2 illustrates the relationship between the number of dental clinics per 10,000 older people (Ministry of Internal Affairs 2005) and the proportion of subjects with 19 or fewer remaining teeth in the areas investigated in this study (6 urban areas; 2 semi-urban regions and 7 rural regions).

As shown in the figure, there were fewer dental clinics and more subjects with 19 or fewer remaining teeth in the rural regions compared to the other regions.

Although not shown in the table, the relationships of thinness (BMI of less than 18.5) and weight loss to years of education and income did not significantly differ according to area type, with the exception that weight loss was significantly more prevalent in the less educated groups than in the more educated groups in the rural regions. The proportion of subjects taking care of oral health was not associated with years of education in the urban regions, whereas in the rural regions it was significantly higher in the more educated groups (by 9.2 percent) than in the less educated groups. Decreased food intake and lack of eating pleasure were significantly more frequent in the

Box 9: What is the 8020 Movement?
Miyo Nakade

In 1982, the World Dental Federation (FDI) and the WHO recommended a goal of having at least 20 functional teeth at the age of 65 and older (FDI 1982). In Japan, the then Ministry of Health and Welfare and the Japan Dental Association began to promote the 8020 Movement in 1987, and it has subsequently spread through every layer of the Japanese nation as a health promotion movement. The 8020 Movement promotes the retention of 20 or more original teeth at the age of 80. The number 8020 is based on the view that at least 20 original teeth are needed to maintain masticatory function and ensure independent dietary life (8020 Suishin Zaidan).

In 2000, the then Ministry of Health and Welfare formulated the Program for National Health Promotion in the 21st Century (Healthy Japan 21) with the extension of healthy life expectancy as the ultimate goal and incorporated 'dental health' into this program. This meant that the previously stand-alone dental health care system became part of the overall health care administration. The first item on the agenda was the prevention of tooth loss with 'at least 20 percent of the population aged 80 retaining at least 20 of their own teeth' as the target. Since 90 percent of tooth loss is caused by cavities and periodontal disease, 8020 can be regarded as a benchmark goal for life-long dental and oral health care. And thus, the minimum teeth retention of 20 is used as the indicator of dental and oral health status in this study.

lower income group as well as in the less educated groups in the rural regions but not so in the other regions.

Discussion

The purpose of this chapter is to grasp the dental, oral and nutritional statuses of older Japanese people, discuss the relationships of these statuses with the two psychological health indicators (depression and self-rated health), and examine the relationships of these statuses and SES with a focus on area differences in these relationships.

Of the subjects of this study, the proportions of those with 20 or more remaining teeth were lower in every age group compared to that of the National Survey of Dental Diseases conducted in 1999 (Ministry of Health and Welfare 1999). The target of "Healthy Japan 21" in 2010 is more than 20 percent of older people having 20 or more remaining teeth at the age of 80. Given the current finding that 14.9 percent of subjects aged 75–79 in 2003 had 20 or more remaining teeth, the target seems to be difficult to achieve in the short-term. As to nutritional status, the risk of malnutrition increased with age and was higher among those with fewer remaining teeth. An earlier study has reported that older people with fewer remaining teeth were at risk of long-term care dependence (Baba and Une 2005). The results of this study also suggest that the maintenance of remaining teeth can reduce the need for long-term care for older people.

Decreased number of remaining teeth and impaired masticatory ability were more frequent in subjects with mild depression, moderate to severe depression or poor self-rated health. Furthermore, subjects at risk of malnutrition more frequently reported mild depression, moderate to severe depression and poor self-rated health, whereas depression was less prevalent in those with good oral health behaviors. Previous studies have also reported positive relationships of the number of remaining teeth and health behaviors with subjective psychological and mental health (Fujimoto et al. 2004; Jingu et al. 2003; Akihusa et al. 2005).

The proportion of subjects with fewer remaining teeth or impaired masticatory ability was higher in the lower income group as well as in the less educated groups, whereas good oral health behaviors were more prevalent in the higher income group as well as in the more educated groups. Overseas studies have reported that the number of remaining teeth varied according to social class (Hanada et al. 2004; Vysniauskaite et al. 2005). The results of this study are consistent with those studies. Weight loss, decreased food intake and lack of eating pleasure were also more frequently reported in the lower income group as well as in the less educated groups. The finding that the proportion of subjects at risk of malnutrition or poor oral function was higher in the lower SES indicates the necessity for long-term care prevention measures in consideration of social class.

By regional type, the proportion of subjects with fewer remaining teeth or impaired masticatory ability was higher in the higher income group in the rural regions than in the lower income group in the urban regions. This suggests that dental and oral statuses vary greatly according to SES as well as regional type. Previous studies have reported regional differences in decreased basic activities of daily living (ADL) (Okumiya et al. 2005); participation in health check-ups (Mitsuhashi et al. 2003); and interests in daily life or quality of life (QOL) indices (Hayasaka et al. 2005) which are known to influence self-rated health. The results of this study also revealed regional differences in the dental, oral and nutritional statuses of older people, with the least desirable condition in rural regions. This may be due to uneven distribution of dental clinics and dentists with the highest concentration in urban regions, a possible scarcity of health care resources in rural regions, and the influence of inaccessible dental health services in rural regions. The regional difference in dental health resources may result from different levels of awareness of dental health behaviors from region to region. These issues await further investigation. Dental health behaviors are considered to be relatively easy to change as dental status is readily noticeable. In this regard, the promotion of dental check-ups or dental health classes in rural regions may be beneficial. Given the finding that regional social capital was associated with the number of remaining teeth (Aida et al. 2009), regional revitalisation which aims to increase social capital may produce favourable outcomes.

The results of this study confirmed the necessity of initiatives and support systems in consideration of social class and regional differences in order to effectively reduce the need for long-term care in older people as to their dental, oral and nutritional health.

Conclusions

The purpose of this chapter was to grasp the dental, oral and nutritional statuses of older Japanese people, discuss the relationships of these statuses with the two health indicators, and examine the relationships of these statuses and SES with a focus on regional differences in these relationships. The current analyses revealed negative relationships of dental, oral and nutritional statuses with psychological health and SES in older community-dwelling people. In comparison by regional type, dental, oral and nutritional statuses varied greatly according to SES as well as by regional type, with the least desirable state in rural regions. The differences in dental, oral and nutritional statuses were greater according to regional type than any health related factors examined in the other chapters. The results of this study suggest the necessity of long-term care prevention measures and intervention measures for environmental improvement based on the understanding of regional situations and should be taken into account when formulating such measures for older people to address their dental, oral and nutritional issues.

Chapter 5

Insomnia

Chiyoe Murata

Introduction

Approximately twenty to forty percent of the general adult population complains of sleep disturbance of some sort. Approximately seventeen percent of these adults are diagnosed with chronic insomnia (Vaz Fragoso and Gill 2007). Insomnia is a sleep disorder in which unsatisfactory quantities and quality of sleep continues for some period of time. Insomniac patients present with symptoms such as difficulty in falling asleep (difficulty initiating sleep: DIS), repeated sleep interruptions during nighttime (difficulty maintaining sleep: DMS), lack of satisfaction with the quality of sleep at awakening (poor perceived quality of sleep: PQS), and waking too early in the morning (early morning awaking: EMA) (Vaz Fragoso and Gill 2007; National Center on Sleep Disorders Research 1998).

Sleep is essential to maintaining sound brain and body functions, and thus to the quality of daily life. Studies have confirmed that sleep disorders, including insomnia, are strongly associated with various physical and mental disorders, with some disorders being preceded by insomnia (Riemann and Voderholzer 2003). Others studies have reported that chronic insomnia is a risk factor for stroke, myocardial infarction and other cardiovascular diseases, as well as being associated with depression and cognitive disorders (National Center on Sleep Disorders Research 1998; Rieman and Voderholzer 2003; Richards et al. 2005). In some studies, twenty percent of those who seek medical attention for insomniac complaints have reported depression, while ninety percent of depressed patients have sleep disorders (Stepnowski and Ancoli-Israel 2008). According to a report from the USA, residents who had insomnia at the time of the survey and continued to complain of insomnia one year later were 39.8 times more likely to develop depression than those without insomnia (Ford and Kamerow 1989). The Japanese Ministry of Health, Labour and Welfare (2004) has recognized the importance of screening for and countermeasures against depression. Since depression is a significant risk factor for the development of conditions requiring long-term care (Stuck et al. 1999), identifying the factors involved in sleep disorders, particularly insomnia, in the older population may prevent various health problems and thus avoid or delay the conditions requiring long-term care.

According to a national epidemiological survey conducted by Doi et al. (2000), the age-adjusted prevalence of insomnia in the general adult population aged twenty or above was 17.3 percent in men and 21.5 percent in women. In particular, the population aged eighty or above showed extremely high age-adjusted prevalence, with 30.5 percent and 40.3 percent of men and women, respectively, suffering from insomnia. In this older population aged eighty or above, 10.2 percent of men and 21.8 percent of women were regularly using sleeping pills. Insomnia among older people has become a real and substantive health issue in Japan, where the population aged sixty-five or above accounted for 22.3 percent of the entire population in 2008 (Ministry of Health, Labour and Welfare 2008).

In this study, we investigated the prevalence of insomnia in the local older population and analyzed the potential associations of insomnia with age, health status and lifestyles. While an association between socioeconomic status (SES) and depression has been reported (see Chapter 2), there has been no research from Japan indicating an association between SES and insomnia. We therefore investigated whether an association can be observed between SES and insomnia after controlling for depression.

Method

The survey was conducted on older persons aged sixty-five or above who lived at home, had not been certified as requiring long-term care, and who resided within the fifteen target municipalities (corresponding to twelve nursing care insurers which were local governments governing these municipalities). The study population consisted of 14,925 subjects (6,751 men and 8,174 women with mean ages [± S.E.] of 73.2 ± 5.98 years and 73.8 ± 6.27 years, respectively) who responded to the surveys asking questions about insomnia (see the Appendix at the end of this book: the dementia version; and the family and abuse version) out of the three types of surveys (see Chapter 1) used in the Aichi Gerontological Evaluation Study (AGES) project (see Box 2).

A subject was defined as having insomnia if he/she responded yes to the question, "Do you have any of the following problems with your sleep?: difficulty falling asleep at night (DIS); waking repeatedly at night (DMS); or lack of satisfaction with the quality of sleep when you wake up in the morning (PQS)." Using an age-adjusted general linear model, associations were evaluated between insomnia and the following factors: age; lifestyles (smoking, alcohol consumption, a habit of midday napping, and the number of hours spent walking each day); health status (conditions under treatment and self-rated health status [see Box 6]); depression as assessed by GDS-5 (5-item Geriatric Depression Scale, see Box 7) (a score of five points or higher was defined as having a mild depression); SES (years of education and equivalent income [see Box 3]; and regional classification (urban, semi-urban or rural [see Chapter 1]). For variables representing SES, we used years of education and equivalent income, which is income per capita obtained by dividing annual household income by the square root of the number of household members. In addition, since depressive patients have shown high rates of insomnia (Vaz Fragoso and Gill 2007; Sukigawa et al. 2003), an analysis was conducted to determine if an association can be observed between income or years of education and insomnia after adjusting for GDS-5 scores.

Finally, in order to determine whether the association between insomnia and depression still remains after controlling for the influence of various factors, an analysis was conducted by dividing the study population into the "depression-free" group, the "mild depression" group and the "severe depression" group, whose GDS-5 score ranges were: 4 or lower; between 5 and 9; and 10 or higher, respectively. Since gender differences in sleep have been established (Vaz Fragoso and Gill 2007; National Center on Sleep Disorders Research 1998; Doi et al. 2000), all analyses were conducted separately for men and women.

Results

Prevalence of insomnia in different age and gender groups

Table 5.1 shows that the percentages of older persons who complained of difficulty initiating sleep (DIS), difficulty maintaining sleep (DMS) and poor perceived quality of sleep (PQS) were 22.3 percent, 46.5 percent and 23.0 percent, respectively, in men and 33.8 percent, 47.4 percent and 25.0 percent, respectively, in women, with significantly more subjects having complained of insomnia in older age groups

Table 5.1: Prevalence of insomnia in different gender and age groups (%)

Age group (years)	No. of subjects (persons)	DIS		DMS		PQS		Any one symptom	
		Men	Women	Men	Women	Men	Women	Men	Women
p-value		< 0.001	< 0.001	< 0.001	< 0.001	< 0.001	< 0.01	< 0.001	< 0.001
65–69	4,629	15.6	30.5	38.0	41.9	20.7	23.5	44.1	50.6
70–74	4,475	22.4	32.9	46.1	45.3	21.5	26.0	52.6	53.3
75–79	3,224	26.7	35.5	51.7	50.9	25.4	24.8	57.5	57.6
80–84	1,759	29.1	39.0	57.3	53.3	27.2	25.5	63.2	59.6
85 +	838	32.0	38.5	60.2	60.1	28.9	28.0	66.6	65.4
Total	14,925	22.3	33.8	46.5	47.4	23.0	25.0	52.4	54.8

The p-value represents the result of the chi-square test to detect significant differences between different age groups.

($p < 0.001$, see Box 10). As many as 52.4 percent and 54.8 percent of the older men and women, respectively, had one or more of the above three symptoms. More women complained of insomnia than men, even after controlling for age.

Factors associated with insomnia

Table 5.2 shows the associations between health status and insomnia. Significantly more older people with conditions under treatment complained of insomnia ($p < 0.001$). Older people who evaluated their own health status as "fair" or "poor" or who had a mild depression were more likely to have insomnia.

Table 5.3 shows the associations between insomnia and lifestyles. A higher proportion of men who smoked had DIS. Daily consumption of approximately 270 mL or more of alcoholic beverages (which corresponds to approximately 30 grams of pure alcohol) was associated with a higher prevalence of DMS in both older men and women and that of PQS in women only. A significantly higher proportion of older subjects who walked less than 30 min daily on average had insomnia than those who walked at least 30 min daily ($p < 0.001$). Subjects who regularly took a midday nap were more likely to complain of insomnia.

Table 5.4 shows the associations of insomnia with years of education, income and regional type. Lower incomes and less education were both associated with more complaints of insomnia in the older population, with a similar association being observed for both men

Table 5.2: Age-adjusted associations between health status and insomnia (%)

	No. of subjects (persons)	DIS		DMS		PQS	
		Men	Women	Men	Women	Men	Women
Conditions under treatment							
p-value		< 0.001	< 0.001	< 0.001	< 0.001	< 0.001	< 0.001
No	2,317	12.8	20.4	31.1	32.0	13.5	14.8
Yes	11,104	24.5	36.5	50.1	50.5	25.1	27.2
Self-rated health status							
p-value		< 0.001	< 0.001	< 0.001	< 0.001	< 0.001	< 0.001
Good	10,101	15.9	27.1	39.3	40.8	16.7	18.6
Poor	3,946	37.6	51.3	63.4	64.2	38.4	42.0
Mild depression (GDS ≥ 5)							
p-value		< 0.001	< 0.001	< 0.001	< 0.001	< 0.001	< 0.001
No	7,772	15.6	25.8	38.7	38.9	16.0	18.1
Yes	3,735	32.3	46.0	58.4	60.6	35.6	38.5

All figures and p-values in the table were calculated based on a general linear model. The number of subjects varies due to missing data.

and women. As for regional type, in women only, the prevalence of DIS were higher in the following order: urban > semi-urban > rural. However, no clear regional differences were observed in DMS or PQS.

Table 5.5 shows an analysis of whether the association between SES and insomnia is still observed after controlling for depression scores in addition to age. In both men and women, the significant associations observed in the model with age adjustment only were either eliminated or considerably weakened after controlling for depression scores. This tendency was more marked in men.

Figure 5.1 shows an analysis of whether insomnia is observed at higher percentages in groups with higher depression scores after controlling for the factors which showed a significant association with insomnia in Table 5.2. In both men and women, higher depression scores were significantly associated with higher proportions of subjects complaining of insomnia ($p < 0.001$).

Discussion

While a higher proportion of women than men complained of insomnia in this study, the same tendency has been reported in clinical settings

Table 5.3: Age-adjusted associations between lifestyles and insomnia (%)

	No. of subjects (persons)	DIS		DMS		PQS	
		Men	Women	Men	Women	Men	Women
Smoking							
P-value		< 0.01	< 0.05	< 0.001	n.s.	n.s.	n.s.
Never smoked	8,807	20.6	33.0	47.0	46.9	23.4	24.8
Smoked in the past but stopped	3,183	21.6	40.1	48.7	49.3	23.1	26.3
Currently smoking	1,496	25.3	37.4	42.1	39.6	21.9	24.7
Drinking							
P-value		n.s.	n.s.	< 0.001	n.s.	n.s.	< 0.05
Nil or < 270 mL	13,358	22.2	33.4	45.4	47.0	22.8	24.8
≥ 270 mL daily	560	23.0	30.6	57.6	49.8	22.4	47.3
Walking hours							
P-value		< 0.001	< 0.001	< 0.001	< 0.001	< 0.001	< 0.001
≥ 30 min daily	8,154	19.4	30.6	43.4	44.3	19.8	22.4
< 30 min	4,450	27.2	38.1	51.6	50.1	28.1	28.8
Napping habits							
P-value		< 0.05	< 0.05	< 0.001	< 0.001	< 0.001	< 0.001
No	8,504	21.1	32.8	42.9	45.2	20.9	23.2
Yes	5,589	23.8	35.1	51.5	50.3	25.4	28.0

n.s.: Not significant.
All figures and p-values in the table were calculated based on a general linear model.
The number of subjects varies due to missing data.

that treat sleep disorders (Vaz Fragoso and Gill 2007; National Center on Sleep Disorders Research 1998). In a Dutch study conducted with subjects aged fifty or above, more women than men had DIS, DMS and PQS, with the cause of DMS being nocturia in men and anxiety in women (Middelkoop et al. 1996). Aging causes deterioration of the quality of sleep by reducing the duration of slow wave sleep (SWS) (i.e. non-REM [non-rapid eye movement] sleep, which means deep sleep that corresponds to stages 3 and 4 of the four stages of deep sleep) (Vaz Fragoso and Gill 2007). This tendency appears to be more marked in men; in women, the quality of sleep has been reported to be relatively maintained despite aging, with the duration of SWS not always being reduced (Doi et al. 2000; Japanese Ministry of Health, Labour and Welfare, 1994). The influence of hormones has been suggested as one

Table 5.4: Age-adjusted associations of insomnia with income, years of education and regional type (%)

	No. of subjects (persons)	DIS		DMS		PQS	
		Men	Women	Men	Women	Men	Women
Equivalent income (yen/yr)							
P-value		< 0.001	< 0.001	< 0.001	< 0.001	< 0.001	< 0.001
Low (≤ 2 mil.)	5,371	25.5	36.9	50.9	50.2	25.8	27.4
Middle (2–4 mil.)	4,533	19.0	29.3	43.1	43.1	20.1	22.5
High (≥ 4 mil.)	1,085	19.2	23.0	42.3	38.9	23.4	19.9
Years of education							
P-value		< 0.001	< 0.001	< 0.001	< 0.001	< 0.001	< 0.001
< 6 yrs	598	24.8	37.5	56.9	52.2	29.8	29.7
6–9 yrs	7,785	24.0	36.4	49.0	50.2	24.6	26.9
10–12 yrs	4,457	20.9	30.0	42.1	42.8	20.7	21.6
≥ 13 yrs	1,162	16.3	24.1	42.3	35.5	18.3	21.2
Regional type							
P-value		n.s.	< 0.05	n.s.	n.s.	n.s.	n.s.
Urban	2,182	21.6	30.8	46.7	44.5	24.4	24.7
Semi-urban	1,252	21.0	33.0	43.2	47.4	20.5	26.0
Rural	9,588	22.6	34.5	46.9	47.9	22.9	24.9

n.s.: Not significant.
All figures and p-values in the table were calculated based on a general linear model.
The number of subjects varies due to missing data.
Equivalent income: Household income divided by the square root of the number of household members.

possible reason why more women complain of subjective insomnia despite the above findings, since sleep disorders are particularly common in postmenopausal women (Stepnowski and Ancoli-Israel 2008). According to a study of a representative sample of the Taiwanese population aged fifteen or above (Chen et al. 2005), the gender differences in insomnia could not be explained solely by women's social roles, such as household chores. Analyses of gender differences in sleep may be necessary in order to devise effective countermeasures against sleep disorders.

Strong associations with insomnia were observed in health-related indices and lifestyles, such as the presence/absence of conditions under treatment, self-rated health status, depression, smoking and alcohol consumption. It has been confirmed that nicotine contained

Table 5.5: Age- and depression score-adjusted associations of insomnia with income and years of education (%)

	No. of subjects (persons)	DIS		DMS		PQS	
		Men	Women	Men	Women	Men	Women
Equivalent income(yen/yr)							
P-value		n.s.	< 0.001	n.s.	n.s.	< 0.01	n.s.
Low (≤ 2 mil.)	5,371	21.6	33.4	46.6	46.6	22.2	25.1
Middle (2–4 mil.)	4,533	20.1	30.2	43.9	44.5	22.1	24.0
High (≥ 4 mil.)	1,085	22.6	26.1	46.4	43.0	28.1	24.0
Years of education							
P-value		n.s.	< 0.05	n.s.	< 0.001	n.s.	n.s.
< 6 yrs	598	18.0	30.2	47.3	46.5	21.6	26.6
6–9 yrs	7,785	20.9	34.0	45.7	47.8	22.1	25.4
10–12 yrs	4,457	21.9	30.7	43.7	43.9	22.7	22.9
≥ 13 yrs	1,162	18.0	27.5	43.1	37.2	20.6	25.6

n.s.: Not significant.

All p-values and figures in the table have been adjusted for age and GDS scores using a general linear model.

The number of subjects varies due to missing data.

Equivalent income: Household income divided by the square root of the number of household members.

in cigarettes, a large amount of alcohol, and some medical drugs have the property of exciting nerves, leading to insomnia (Vaz Fragoso and Gill 2007; National Center on Sleep Disorders Research 1998). It is also possible that the pain and psychological anxiety of having certain health problems might affect sleep.

Consistent with a report that low daytime physical and mental activity levels is associated with insomnia (Vaz Fragoso and Gill 2007), the present study has found more complaints of insomnia among older subjects who walk less than 30 minutes per day. Low levels of physical activity and social relationships are risk factors for conditions requiring long-term care (Stuck et al. 1999). One study has reported that DMS is associated with a deterioration of cognitive and physical functions (Richards et al. 2005). This process is likely to involve sleep disorders which reflect a certain aspect of brain functions. In this respect, an intervention study conducted in the USA has reported that the quality of sleep among older people with cognitive disorders was significantly improved by providing opportunities for social activities (Richards et al. 2005). Further research is required

Figure 5.1: Associations between depression and insomnia after adjustment for age, conditions under treatment, self-rated health status, lifestyles, income and years of education

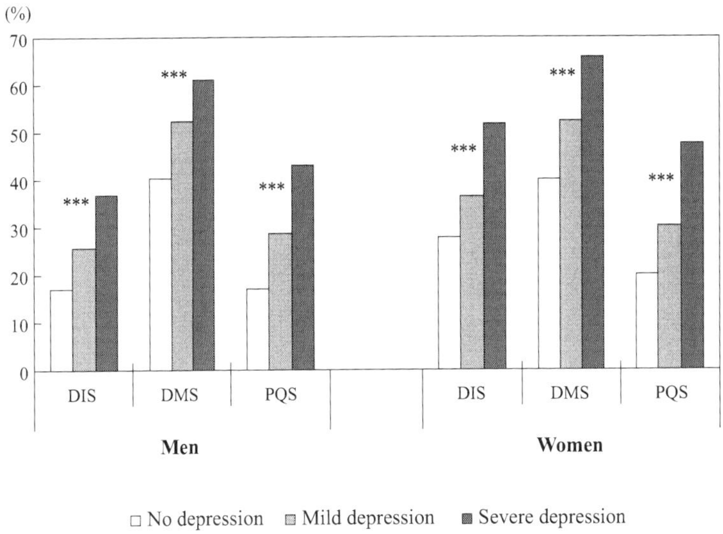

Notes.

The three depression score groups: Subjects whose GDS-15 scores (which range from 0 to 15) were 0–4, 5–9 and 10 or higher were divided into the "no depression", "mild depression" and "severe depression" groups, respectively.

Adjusted variables: age, presence/absence of conditions under treatment, self-rated health status, alcohol consumption, smoking, presence/absence of napping habits, walking hours, equivalent income and years of education.

***: $p < 0.001$ (p-value for the difference in prevalence of insomnia between the three depression score groups).

to determine whether, in the general population, approaches intended to prevent conditions requiring long-term care, such as increasing opportunities for social exchanges, will increase physical and mental activity levels, leading to improved QOL by reducing insomnia.

While a higher proportion of subjects who habitually took a midday nap complained of insomnia, one study reported that such a habit reduces the development of dementia (Chen et al. 2005). Another study, however, has suggested that daytime sleepiness is a risk factor for the development of dementia (Richards et al. 2005). Evidence from psychiatric clinical settings also suggests that older people with daytime sleepiness tend to have sleep-wake cycle disorders (Vaz Fragoso and Gill 2007). In order to determine whether or not daytime

Box 10: A Global Perspective on Insomnia in Japan's Older Population

Chiyoe Murata

Symptoms of insomnia include: difficulty initiating sleep (DIS), difficulty maintaining sleep (DMS), early morning awakening (EMA) and poor perceived quality of sleep (PQS) (American Psychiatric Association 1994). Causes of the high prevalence of sleep disorders in older people include the increase of health problems due to aging, in addition to physiological changes caused by aging (Vaz Fragoso and Gill 2007). Insomnia and other sleep complaints or disturbances are associated with poor prognosis in the general older population, in such terms as death, depression, dementia, heart disease and other conditions requiring long-term care (Vaz Fragoso and Gill 2007).

Of all sleep complaints, the prevalence of insomnia is particularly high among older people. In the USA, of the population aged sixty-five or above, 43–50 percent had DIS or DMS (Vaz Fragoso and Gill 2007). In a Dutch study using a representative sample, the prevalence rates of DIS and DMS in the general resident population aged sixty or above were 4.8–13.3 percent and 19.0–36.7 percent, respectively, in men and 19.3–28.8 percent and 28.8–30.1 percent, respectively, in women (Middelkoop et al. 1996). In comparison, in Japan, a study conducted by Doi et al. (2000) revealed that the proportions of persons aged sixty or above with any one of DIS, DMS and PQS were 20.5–30.5 percent in men and 20.3–40.3 percent in women. Another Japanese study has found that the prevalence of insomnia (which was represented by the percentage of those who scored six points or higher in the 17-item Japanese version of Pittsburgh Sleep Quality Index [PSQI-J]) in a population aged sixty-five or above was 37.3 percent (Sukegawa et al. 2003).

napping is a desirable lifestyle practice, further detailed analyses by longitudinal cohort studies are warranted, including analyses of bedtime and wake time.

Higher proportions of older subjects with lower SES complained of insomnia. Reports from studies conducted in Japanese and foreign occupational groups indicate that sleep disorders are more common in groups with lower SES (Akerstedt et al. 2002; Moore et al. 2002; Sekine et al. 2006; Kagamimori et al. 2009). However, only a small number of studies have analyzed the potential associations between sleep disorders and SES among the older population. Of these, an Italian study conducted by Geroldi et al. (1996) has reported that in subjects aged seventy-five or above, the prevalence of insomnia was lower in those whose longest-held occupation was white collar work compared to those whose longest-held occupation was blue collar work. In the present study, differences in the prevalence of insomnia were observed in the general older population depending on SES, such as household income and years of education. However, adjusting for depression scores considerably weakened the association between insomnia and SES. This suggests a possibility that the higher prevalence of insomnia in the groups of older subjects with low SES is due to the higher prevalence of depression in these groups (see Chapter 2; Murata et al. 2008; Lorant et al. 2003). It is not entirely clear whether insomnia precedes depression or can be a cause of depression. However, the possibility that insomnia may be improved with appropriate treatment suggests that many cases of depression may be improved by treating insomnia.

Summary

In the older population, differences were observed in the prevalence of insomnia depending on age, gender, self-rated health, lifestyles and SES. Being older, female, and in poorer health were all associated with more insomniac complaints. Even after controlling for age, the associations were observed between insomnia and unhealthy lifestyles, such as smoking, daily consumption of 270 ml or more of alcoholic beverages, and short walking hours. Older subjects with a habit of taking a midday nap also showed high rates of insomnia. While higher proportions of older subjects with lower SES complained of insomnia, adjusting for depression scores in addition to age weakened or eliminated the significant association between insomnia and SES. This suggests that the higher rates of insomnia among older people with lower SES can be considerably explained by the higher prevalence of depression in these persons. No clear differences were observed in the prevalence of insomnia depending on regional classification.

As an approach to help older people suffering from insomnia, longitudinal studies are necessary to determine whether smoking cessation, reduction of alcohol consumption, promotion of physical and social activities, and improvement of depression will lead to good quality sleep.

Chapter 6

Sense of Coherence (SOC) as Stress-Coping Ability

Kiyoko Yoshii

Introduction

People use various health resources in order to maintain good health (Yamazaki 2003; Sugisawa and Shibata 2000). In this context, 'health resources' means materials, information, human relationships and so on that people can make use of in order to maintain their health. For instance, if one becomes critically ill, the more money and personal connections he/she has, the more likely he/she is able to escape death or becoming disabled by consulting an appropriate medical institution. These health resources consist of external and internal resources (Yamazaki 2003; Taylor and Seeman 1999). Well-known internal resources include locus of control and self-efficacy (see Box 9). Another internal resource that has recently been receiving attention in Japan is a stress-coping ability known as 'SOC' (Yamazaki 2003; Antonovsky 1987; Kondō 2004).

What is SOC?

SOC stands for 'sense of coherence' (Antonovsky 1987). This concept was developed by medical sociologist Aaron Antonovsky, who investigated the characteristics of people who did not fall ill despite much stress, but stayed well by taking advantage of their negative experiences. Antonovsky referred to the characteristics of these people as SOC. SOC consists of three components: 'comprehensibility', a sense that you can understand events in your life; 'manageability', a belief that you can take care of things by yourself or with help from others; and 'meaningfulness', a belief that overcoming difficulties is meaningful and worthwhile. Since persons with a strong SOC are likely to be able to deal well with and overcome many stressful events, in Japan SOC is also referred to as a 'stress-coping ability' or 'health maintaining ability' (Yamazaki 2003). In this chapter, SOC will also be referred to as 'stress-coping ability', as this gives us a clear image of the role played by SOC. Previous studies have found that people with a strong SOC are less susceptible to health damage caused by stressful events (Takayama et al. 1999), and they have lower mortality and disability rates (Poppius et al. 2003; Surtees et al. 2003; Avlund et al. 2003; Suominen et al. 2005).

Antonovsky conceptualized SOC and developed it into scales so that SOC would be applicable not only to America and other western countries but also to countries with different histories and cultures. For instance, 'manageability', a belief that you will eventually manage things successfully, includes not only the western, individualistic concept that you can deal with everything by yourself, but also the eastern way of successfully overcoming problems by getting help from others. As an example of a culture with this approach to problem management, Antonovsky cites Japan. Antonovsky also describes the characteristics of life experiences of Japanese and Jewish people in their adolescence as producing firm family bonds, strong bonds of love and interdependence between mother and children, and, at the core of these, education and achievements as a value and goals. Antonovsky argues that this kind of life experience nurtures a strong SOC. Antonovsky's conceptualization of SOC, then, rests on an empirical claim, which needs to be tested through concrete studies of SOC in Japan.

SOC is not supposed to be a special personal characteristic; but is, instead, considered to be learnt from the environment in which one grows up, especially through life experiences during adolescence and early adulthood. According Antonovsky, a strong SOC is formed in a person if: there has been a proper degree of consistency in the life course since birth (consistency); the load imposed has been appropriate – neither too light nor too heavy (load balance); and he/she has had many life experiences in which he/she felt able to participate in important decision-making (participation in shaping outcome). For instance, compared to blue-collar workers such as manual laborers, white-collar workers such as clerical or managerial workers are more likely to find themselves in a position to conduct work that influences the organization's decision-making, and thus have more opportunities for 'participation in shaping outcome'. As for 'load balance', while blue-collar workers tend to conduct work that does not require high skills and can be done by anyone (underload), white-collar workers tend to be given opportunities to work on important tasks and enhance their skills, a situation that helps to enhance their SOC as a stress-coping ability. Furthermore, while SOC is enhanced through repeated experiences in which the person coped well with the stressors encountered, having knowledge and sufficient money to deal with them are, according to Antonovsky (1987) important resources leading to successful stress coping. Overseas studies, mainly on adolescents and adults, have demonstrated that socioeconomic status, which is a focus of this book, is one of the factors influencing SOC (Lundberg 1997; Geyer 1997; Smith et al. 2003).

SOC and socioeconomic status (SES)

In studies on socioeconomic disparities in health, internal resources, including stress-coping ability (SOC), is considered a pathway in the mechanism by which SES and health are related to one another (Taylor and Seeman 1999; Kondō 2004). This view has been reduced to a hypothesis that a person with a higher SES has a stronger SOC, which makes him/her healthier. Several studies supporting this hypothesis have been reported (Ing and Rutter 2003; Kosteniuk and Dickinson 2003).

What significance, then, does SOC have for older people? An older person must adjust to many changes in life, including: reduction of his/her role, such as retirement from work; acceptance of aging; and loss of people close to him/her. SOC is expected to play a major role in living well during the final stages of life, by coping with changes in a flexible manner and maintaining physical and mental health. To this end, an older person's well-being should be understood to be pluralistic, including aspects such as physical and cognitive functions, mental health and social relationships (Lawton 1982). From this perspective, having a strong SOC, such as an ability to find meaning in life (meaningfulness) or confidence that you can deal with the things that are happening in your life (manageability), has been used to provide indices of good QOL in older persons (Smits et al. 1995; Steiner et al. 1996; Takkinen and Ruoppila 2001).

Since Yamazaki (1999; Antonovsky 1987) introduced Antonovsky's *salutogenesis* (lit. 'health-origin') and SOC to Japan, many Japanese studies have adopted SOC scales or the concept of SOC. However, most of these studies targeted a general adult population, workers or students. No socio-epidemiological studies on SOC have as yet targeted an older population.

This chapter analyzes the potential associations between SES, SOC and certain health indices based on survey data on an older population aged sixty-five or above who do not have conditions requiring long-term care. Specifically, analyses will be conducted on the following points: (i) Is a higher SES associated with a stronger SOC?; (ii) Is a stronger SOC associated with better health index scores, and can a strong SOC alleviate negative effects of stressful life events on the health indices?; (iii) Can the association between SES and the health indices be explained by the association between a higher SES and a stronger SOC?; and (iv) Is SOC associated with other health-related factors, such as lifestyles and social relationships? In addition, differences in SOC by regional type will also be analyzed. Since the formation of SOC is considered to be influenced not only by personal life experiences but by the group characteristics of the community the person has lived in, such as its stability or norms (Antonovsky 1987), it is expected that each regional type used in this book has some group characteristics that result in differences in SOC.

Method

Subjects

This analysis used data from the Aichi Gerontological Evaluation Study (AGES; see Box 2) project conducted in 2003 on the older population (either random or complete samples of persons aged sixty-five or above who had not been certified as requiring long-term care) residing in fifteen municipalities in three Japanese prefectures (number of persons who returned responses: 32,891; response rate: 55.2 percent).

Variables used in analyses

Stress-coping ability (SOC)

Antonovsky (1987) created questionnaires intended to measure personal SOC levels. His SOC scales have been used in many countries, including Japan, and their reliability and validity have been confirmed (Antonovsky 1993; Erikson and Lindstrom 2005; Togari and Yamazaki 2005). The present study used a short, 13-item SOC scale (corresponding to Question 5 of the Appendix). A higher score indicates a stronger SOC (range, 13–91; α coefficient, 0.91). The mean SOC (± S.D. [standard deviation]) score was 63.2 (±12.5) points. In the following analyses, whenever SOC scores are categorized, they are converted to variables based on the following tertile groups: the low score group (56 points or lower); middle score group (57 to 69 points); and high score group (70 points or higher).

Health indices

Self-rated health status (a four point scale from 'excellent' to 'poor') and depression (15-item GDS, see Boxes 6 and 7, respectively).

SES indices

Years of education and equivalent income (i.e., income per capita obtained by dividing annual household income [in 10,000 yen/year] by the square root of the number of household members) (see Box 3).

Analytical methods

Since both SES and the health indices are strongly associated with age, the influence of age must be eliminated in order to assess the associations correctly. Thus, in each association analysis of any two variables, a general linear model method of the SPSS statistical software was used to obtain age-adjusted figures and significance levels.

Results

Association between SES and SOC

Table 6.1 shows the association between the SES indices and SOC scores. In both men and women, a significant association was observed between higher SES indices (years of education and income) and higher SOC scores ($p < 0.001$). In men, for instance, while the group with thirteen or more years of education had a mean SOC score of 66.6 points, those groups with ten to twelve years, six to nine years and less than six years of education had progressively lower mean SOC scores, namely, 65.2, 62.6 and 58.7 points, respectively. The association between years of education and SOC scores and that between income and SOC scores were found to be independent of each other (data not shown). For example, persons with the same years of education had significantly different SOC scores depending on their income levels.

Verification of the functions of SOC as stress-coping ability – Does a stronger SOC provide better health?

While SOC is also referred to as a stress-coping ability or health maintaining ability, are persons with higher SOC scores really in better health? In addition, are they more likely to maintain their health under stress? In this section, these two points are analyzed using self-rated health status and depression as the health indices.

Direct effect of SOC as a stress-coping ability on the health indices – Does a person with a stronger SOC have better health index scores?

An analysis was conducted to find any differences in the proportion of persons with good self-rated health status (i.e., those who rated their health status as 'excellent' or 'good') and that of persons who

Table 6.1: Association between SOC scores and years of education/ income

	Men			Women		
	n (persons)	SOC scores	p-value	n (persons)	SOC scores	p-value
Years of education						
< 6 yrs	262	58.7	***	684	58.2	***
6–9 yrs	5,875	62.6		6,311	61.6	
10–12 yrs	3,556	65.2		4,158	64.6	
≥ 13 yrs	1,663	66.6		702	65.3	
Equivalent income (yen/yr)[a]						
< 1.5 million yen	2,314	61.0	***	2,848	60.3	***
1.5–3.0 million yen	5,021	63.9		3,877	63.0	
> 3.0 million yen	2,974	66.7		2,541	65.5	

All figures have been age-adjusted using a general linear model. n: Number of subjects analyzed.

a: Household income (in 10,000 yen/year) divided by the square root of the number of household members.

***: $p < 0.001$

are not severely or mildly depressed (i.e., those whose 15-item GDS score was four points or lower) between the three SOC score groups (Table 6.2). In both men and women, the groups with higher SOC scores (i.e., higher stress-coping ability levels) had a significantly higher proportion of persons with good self-rated health status and higher proportion of persons who are not severely or mildly depressed. In men, for example, the proportion of persons with good self-rated health status was progressively higher in higher SOC score groups, namely, about 60 percent, 70 percent and 80 percent in the low, middle and high SOC score groups, respectively ($p < 0.001$).

The results described thus far have shown that a person with higher SES (number of years and income) has a higher SOC score, and that a person with a higher SOC score is in better health status. Chapter 2 has indicated that a person with higher SES has a better health status (Yoshii et al. 2005). Can the association between higher SES and better health index scores be explained by the association between higher SES and a stronger SOC as a stress-coping ability? Figures 6.1-a and 6.1-b show the association between SES and self-rated health status in each of the three SOC score groups. The significant association between SES and self-rated health status was maintained with some exceptions across all three SOC score groups. This indicates that the

Table 6.2: SOC scores and self-rated health status/depression

	SOC	n (persons)	Age-adjusted %	p-value
Men				
Self-rated health status = Excellent/Good				
	Low group	3,627	61.2	***
	Middle group	3,807	71.7	
	High group	3,818	81.2	
No depression	Low group	3,242	45.5	***
	Middle group	3,422	71.1	
	High group	3,503	89.3	
Women				
Self-rated health status = Excellent/Good				
	Low group	4,095	61.8	***
	Middle group	4,032	74.9	
	High group	3,631	82.7	
No depression	Low group	3,472	43.9	***
	Middle group	3,476	72.7	
	High group	3,208	89.0	

All figures have been age-adjusted using a general linear model.
n: Number of subjects analyzed.
***: $p < 0.001$
No depression: Persons whose 15-item GDS scores were 4 points or lower.

association between SES and self-rated health status can be explained in part, but not in whole, by the differences in SOC scores associated with SES. Similar results were obtained when depressive state was used as the objective variable.

Buffer effect of SOC as a stress-coping ability – Is a person with a stronger SOC more resistant to the negative effects of stressful life events on health?

If SOC has a stress buffering effect (i.e., a mitigating effect on the impact of stress) as is hypothesized, the results should demonstrate that persons with higher SOC scores are more likely to maintain their health despite the presence of strong stressors, while those with lower SOC scores are more likely to experience deterioration in their health status in the presence of only minor stressors. Figure 6.2 shows the results of an analysis of the association between the number of

Box 11: Locus of Control and Self-efficacy

Kiyoko Yoshii

Locus of control refers to an individual's perception about where control over outcomes resides (Rotter 1996). People are divided roughly into those with an 'internal control orientation', who believe that outcomes depend on their own behavior and efforts, and those with an 'external control orientation', who believe that outcomes depend on others and destiny. For instance, a person who believes that his/her health can be improved by his/her own behavior and efforts has an internal control orientation, while a person who believes that his/her health depends on his/her physician or destiny and cannot be improved by him-/herself in any way has an 'external control orientation'. In general, having an 'internal control orientation' has been considered more desirable for the maintenance of health.

According to Bandura's (1997) self-efficacy theory, a stronger belief that you will 'succeed' in an activity (i.e., self-efficacy) is associated with a higher possibility of successfully performing the activity. For example, even though one knows that smoking cessation will reduce health damage, it would be difficult to successfully quit smoking if one has no specific confidence or prospect that one can quit smoking. In this example, successful smoking cessation can be made easier by enhancing self-efficacy for smoking cessation, through such means as starting from an achievable level and repeating successful experiences (successful performances), gaining self-confidence by listening to successful quitters (vicarious experience), and receiving encouragement to continue from reliable persons (verbal persuasion).

stressful life events (i.e., seven types of events, including retirement from work, loss of a spouse, etc., see question 4 in the Appendix) experienced in one year and the proportion of persons in a depressive state in each of the three SOC score groups. In the groups with lower SOC scores, the proportion of persons with depression increased to a greater degree with an increasing number of stressful life events, while in the high SOC score group no such increase in the proportion of persons with depression was observed. This supports the hypothesis that persons with a stronger SOC as a stress-coping ability are more likely to maintain their health in the presence of many stressors. Note that when self-rated health status was used as the objective variable, no such stress buffering effect was observed.

Figure 6.1a: Association between years of education and self-rated health status in each of the three SOC groups

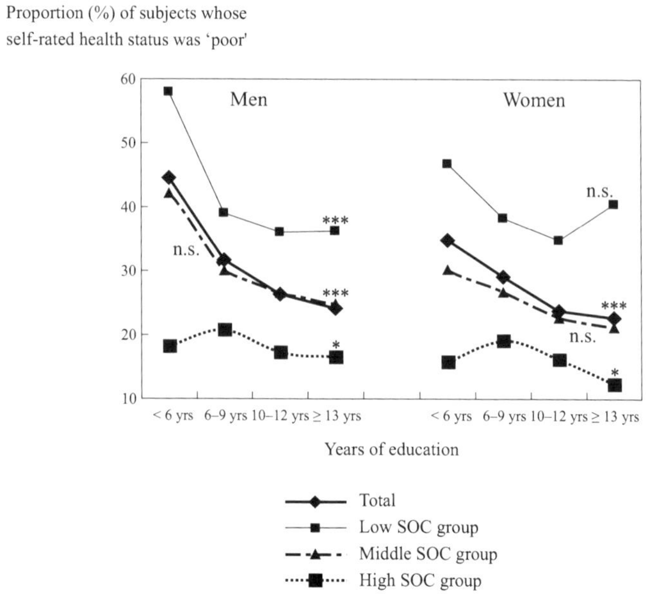

Notes.

Figures indicate results adjusted for age using a general linear model.

P-values indicate age-adjusted results of a test conducted in each group to check for differences in the proportion (%) of subjects whose self-rated health status was 'poor' between different categories of years of education and equivalent income.

Proportion (%) of subjects whose self-rated health status was 'poor' includes: Persons whose self-rated health status was either 'fair' or 'poor'.

Equivalent income (household income [in 10,000 yen/year] divided by the square root of the number of household members) low: < 1.5 million yen; middle: 1.5–3.0 million yen; high: > 3.0 million yen.

*: $p < 0.05$; ***: $p < 0.001$; n. s.: not significant.

Associations between SOC and indices of lifestyles/social relationships

Antonovsky (1987) suggested the possibility that a person with a stronger SOC may engage in healthier behavior and have richer human relationships. This possibility has been demonstrated by various researchers (Nakamura et al. 2003; Kimura et al. 2001; Krantz and Ostergren 2004). Table 6.3 shows the association between SOC scores and the indices of lifestyles/social relationships that have been reported thus far in this book. While no significant associations were

Figure 6.1b: Association between income and self-rated health status in each of the three SOC groups

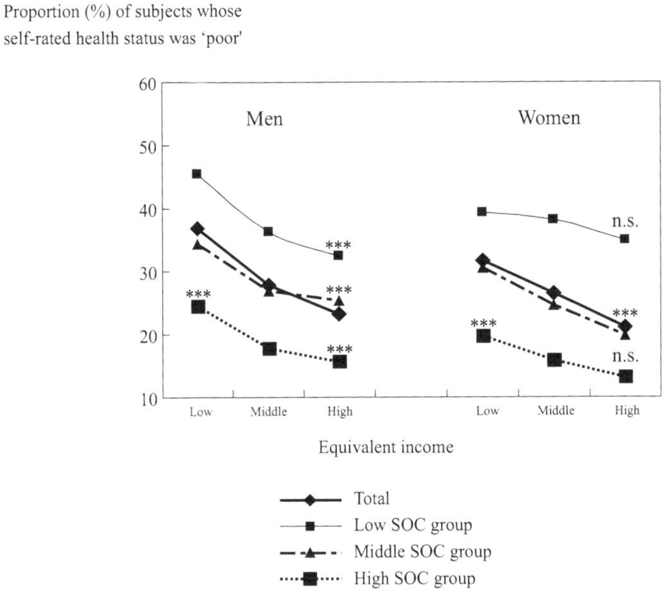

Notes.

Figures indicate results adjusted for age using a general linear model.

P-values indicate age-adjusted results of a test conducted in each group to check for differences in the proportion (%) of subjects whose self-rated health status was 'poor' between different categories of years of education and equivalent income.

Proportion (%) of subjects whose self-rated health status was 'poor' includes: Persons whose self-rated health status was either 'fair' or 'poor'.

Equivalent income (household income [in 10,000 yen/year] divided by the square root of the number of household members) low: < 1.5 million yen; middle: 1.5–3.0 million yen; high: > 3.0 million yen.

***: $p < 0.001$; n. s.: not significant.

observed between SOC scores and smoking or alcohol consumption, the groups with lower SOC scores had significantly higher proportions of persons who had not had a health checkup, or who had nineteen or less remaining teeth, or who walked less than thirty minutes per day. In addition, these groups had significantly higher proportions of persons who had few exchanges with friends or family members living apart, or who went out less frequently, or who had no hobbies, or who provided or received no support.

As in other chapters in this book, an analysis was conducted on the potential association between SOC scores and regional types. In men,

Figure 6.2: Association between the number of stressful life events and depression

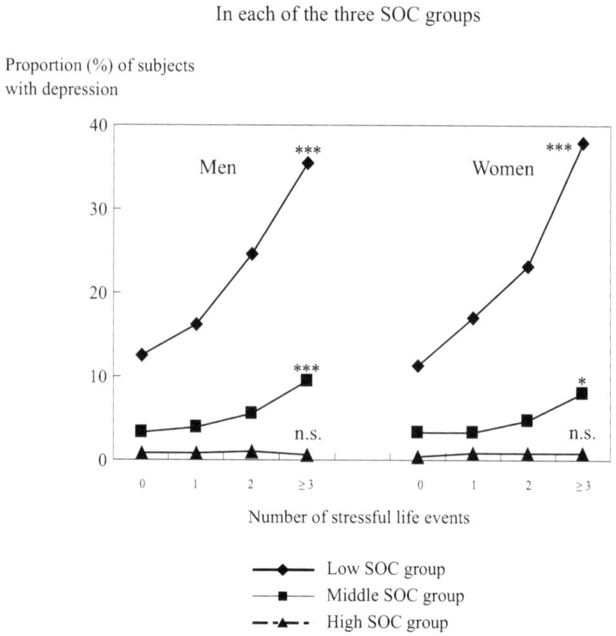

Notes.

Figures indicate results adjusted for age using a general linear model.

P-values indicate results of a test conducted in each group to check for differences in the proportion (%) of subjects with depression between different categories of the number of stressful life events.

Persons with depression: Persons whose 15-item GDS scores were 10 points or higher.

Seven stressful life events: retirement from work; loss of a spouse; loss of a close relative, family member or friend; contracting a major disease; house-moving or other changes in the living environment; increased financial difficulty; and starting caring for a family member.

*: $p < 0.05$; ***: $p < 0.001$; n. s.: not significant.

the urban regions had significantly higher SOC scores than the rural and semi-urban regions (data not shown). However, these significant regional differences disappeared when income differences were added to the analysis. This means that the higher mean SOC score of men in the urban regions was due to a larger number of persons with higher incomes than in the other regions (Kondō et al. 2005). When persons with the same level of income were compared, no differences in SOC scores were observed between different regional types.

Discussion

There have been few studies in Japan on SOC in the older population, and no analysis has been conducted on the association between SOC and SES. The results of the present analyses have demonstrated the following. First, different levels of SOC as a stress-coping ability were observed in the Japanese older population, as has been the case with other populations, depending on SES (years of education and equivalent income) (i.e., persons with higher SES had a stronger stress-coping ability). As described above, it is considered that the level of a person's SOC as a stress-coping ability depends on the quality of his/her life experiences and his/her successful stress-coping experiences (Antonovsky 1987). Assuming that years of education has an impact on one's occupation and living environment which, in turn, are reflected in his/her income later in life, this significant association between SES and SOC is understandable.

Second, SOC was strongly associated with health index scores independently of SES (i.e., the groups with higher SOC scores were in better health status). These results do not support the hypothesis that the association between higher SES and a stronger SOC explains the socioeconomic disparities in health status. As seen in Figure 6.1, even persons with the same level of SES showed considerable differences in health index scores depending on their SOC level. This suggests that there are tertiary factors determining the SOC levels of persons with the same level of SES (for instance, the quality of family relationships or social relationships). If such factors are revealed, there is a possibility that even persons with lower SES may be able to improve their SOC, which may lead to better health outcomes.

Third, higher SOC scores were significantly associated with better scores of lifestyle/social relationship indices which have been considered to be associated with health. These results suggest the possibility that good lifestyles and social relationships of persons with a strong stress-coping ability might be beneficial to health.

We have thus far interpreted the results assuming that 'a stronger SOC brings better health'. Conversely, however, we could interpret that 'better health brings a stronger SOC.' In Antonovsky's model, the relationship between SOC and health is reciprocal in the first place, with a stronger SOC leading to better health and good health being regarded as one resource for successful stress coping. In the case of older people,

Table 6.3: Association between SOC scores and indices of health-related habits/social relationships

	Smoking: Yes			Alcohol consumption: ≥ 30g/day			Physical Examination: No		
	n	%	p-value	n	%	p-value	n	%	p-value
Men									
Low SOC group	1,871	24.4	n.s.	1,902	10.3	n.s.	1,878	20.4	**
Middle SOC group	2,081	22.9		2,116	8.6		2,085	16.6	
High SOC group	2,176	23.4		2,213	8.6		2,190	17.0	
Women									
Low SOC group	1,983	3.4	n.s.	2,023	0.3	n.s.	1,995	23.9	***
Middle SOC group	1,968	2.6		2,002	0.2		1,982	18.0	
High SOC group	1,838	2.6		1,858	0.2		1,821	19.9	

	Outing: < Once/week			Hobby: None			Emotional support: No receipt		
	n	%	p-value	n	%	p-value	n	%	p-value
Men									
Low SOC group	1,879	5.9	***	1,838	27.4	***	1,893	18.7	***
Middle SOC group	2,096	3.7		2,054	18.4		2,107	12.7	
High SOC group	2,168	2.5		2,139	15.1		2,205	10.6	
Women									
Low SOC group	2,015	5.0	***	1,925	34.2	***	2,038	8.5	***
Middle SOC group	2,001	2.2		1,933	24.0		2,012	4.8	
High SOC group	1,845	2.7		1,776	17.5		1,862	3.6	

	Walking: < 30 min/day			Social contact with family members living apart: < Once/week			Social contact with friends: < Once/week		
	n	%	p-value	n	%	p-value	n	%	p-value
Men									
Low SOC group	1,810	39.3	***	1,883	57.0	***	1,895	55.2	***
Middle SOC group	2,017	33.0		2,086	53.8		2,106	48.6	
High SOC group	2,105	31.8		2,167	49.2		2,192	43.0	
Women									
Low SOC group	1,809	40.7	***	1,983	48.5	**	2,021	37.7	***
Middle SOC group	1,819	37.3		1,971	44.7		2,007	33.0	
High SOC group	1,672	32.9		1,792	42.6		1,850	28.9	

Table 6.3: continued

	Emotional support: No provision			Emotional support: No receipt			Instrumental support: No provision		
	n	%	p-value	n	%	p-value	n	%	p-value
Men									
Low SOC group	1,887	21.4	***	1,905	6.6	***	1,890	9.9	***
Middle SOC group	2,097	15.6		2,123	3.6		2,110	6.1	
High SOC group	2,202	16.5		2,215	2.0		2,203	5.6	
Women									
Low SOC group	2,023	15.0	n.s.	2,028	11.7	***	2,009	10.4	***
Middle SOC group	1,996	12.5		2,012	5.9		1,996	7.4	
High SOC group	1,849	13.3		1,863	3.5		1,848	5.9	

Figures indicate results adjusted for age and presence of disease (0 and 1 indicate the absence and presence, respectively, of disease).
**: $p < 0.01$; ***: $p < 0.001$; n.s.: not significant.

it is quite possible that a sudden disease or disability may result in a deteriorated SOC. Further longitudinal studies to demonstrate the level of causal association of SOC with health are needed.

As described in the Introduction, longitudinal studies have shown that a higher SOC is associated with a lower probability of death or disability. This indicates that focusing on older people's SOC is meaningful from the perspective of preventing conditions requiring nursing care and the extension of healthy life expectancy. While Antonovsky's theory suggests that SOC does not change significantly after adulthood is reached (Antonovsky 1987), subsequent experimental studies have demonstrated that SOC scores do change after adulthood (Takayama et al. 1999; Smith et al. 2003; Nilson et al. 2003). There have also been reports of intervention studies demonstrating improvements in SOC scores after interventions such as a stress management program (i.e., eight weekly sessions of mental training, including relaxation, and massage) (Haraldsson et al. 2005) and exercise (i.e., ten months of three times weekly sessions of aerobics) (Kohut et al. 2005). Few studies have been conducted with respect to changes in or effects of interventions on SOC scores in older age. It seems worthwhile to further investigate the possibility of improving SOC scores and health status in older people by using approaches that would help them find meaning in their lives or achieve more successful stress coping.

Summary

This study focused on SOC as a stress-coping ability in older people and analyzed the associations between SOC and indices of SES and health. Higher SES (years of education and equivalent income) was significantly associated with a stronger SOC. A stronger SOC was significantly associated with better self-rated health status and lower occurrence of depression. However, while the hypothesis that 'the association between higher SES and a stronger SOC explains socioeconomic disparities in health status' was supported in part, this was not able to explain everything. A strong SOC alleviated negative effects of stressful life events on health (depression). A stronger SOC showed a positive association with better results of the indices of lifestyles and social relationships.

Chapter 7

Hobby Activities

Tokunori Takeda

Introduction

Older people have more free time as a result of retirement from activities they used to be responsible for, such as work, household duties and social activities. Older people reportedly spend their time in increased hours of sleep, watching TV, listening to the radio, and resting (NHK Broadcasting Culture Research Institute 2005). How they spend their increased free time is considered to be important not only for QOL but also in terms of preventing the conditions that require long-term care. Various studies have shown that hobbies and recreational activities (hereinafter referred to as "hobby activities"), which engage people in various intellectual activities and social networks, are factors involved in preventing the onset of housebound behavior and dementia (Wilson et al. 2002; Verghese et al. 2003; Scarmeas et al. 2001; Colette et al. 1995; Wang et al. 2002). In Western countries, several reports have indicated that hobby activities are positively associated with life satisfaction and a sense of well-being and may alleviate anxiety and a sense of helplessness in the older people (Kelly and Steinkamp 1987; Wynne and Groves 1995; Herzog et al. 1998; Ragheb 1993). In Japan, cross-sectional studies have reported an association between hobby activities and the maintenance and improvement of physical functions and QOL, increased outings and social participation, and better psychological status (Anme et al. 2006; Fujita et al. 2004; Takeda et al. 2005). For instance, the results of a survey of a general older population consisting of approximately 3,000 persons living in one municipality demonstrated that, compared to those who had no hobbies, those who did have hobbies showed higher psychological QOL, such as significantly higher life satisfaction, significantly better self-rated health status, a significantly better self-rated sense of well-being, and a lower rate of depression (Takeda et al. 2005).

However, since these earlier studies analyzed older people living in specific regions, different results might be obtained in different countries or regions. For instance, the proportion of older people who use hobby activities as a means of socializing with neighbors was 25.4 percent, 24.4 percent, 18.5 percent, 18.1 percent and 15.3 percent in Japan, Korea, Germany, the USA and Sweden, respectively (Naikakufu [Japanese Cabinet Office] 2002). Furthermore, the proportion of older people who report feeling fulfilled when absorbed in hobbies is different in different countries (38.1 percent, 15.8 percent, 46.5 percent, 42.9 percent and 33.2 percent in Japan, Korea, Germany, the USA and France, respectively) (Japanese Cabinet Office 2005).

In Japan, few studies have reported the actual conditions of hobby activities or trends in the type of hobby activities, or the associations between hobby activities and psychosocial aspects, in older people residing in multiple regions. There have also been surprisingly few surveys on the types of hobby activities and other recreational interests of older community-dwelling people who are targeted by long-term care prevention projects. Furthermore, only a limited number of studies have reported an association between socioeconomic status (SES) and hobby activities.

Hence, this chapter has three objectives: (i) to examine the conditions of hobby activities in older community-dwelling people in multiple regions; (ii) to analyze the associations between hobby activities and psychological aspects, such as depression and self-rated health status; and (iii) to clarify the association between hobby activities and SES.

Method

Data from the Aichi Gerontological Evaluation Study (AGES) project were used. This project targeted older people aged sixty-five or above who had not been certified as requiring long-term care and who resided within fifteen municipalities (corresponding to twelve long-term care insurers which were local governments in these municipalities) in three Japanese prefectures. Of these older people, the present study targeted 26,628 persons (mean age, 73.3 ± 6.1 years) who responded to the survey questions about hobbies.

This chapter reports the following: (i) whether or not subjects conduct hobby activities and the purposes and nature of their hobby activities; (ii) the associations between hobby activities and psychosocial factors; (iii) the association between hobby activities and SES; and (iv) regional differences in hobby activities.

i. Subjects were asked to choose any number of hobby activities from the following multiple-choice items: sporting activities;

cultural activities; musical activities; creative activities; horticultural activities; audiovisual activities; sightseeing activities; and investment/gambling activities. Only 9,250 subjects responded to the question about the purposes of hobby activities since this question was included only in the dementia version of the survey (See Appendix 1). Choices included: to improve skills; to enjoy; to socialize with others; to stay fit; and to stave off dementia. Each item was assessed using a two-point scale (i.e. whether or not the purpose is important to the subject) (See Appendix 1).

ii. Of the psychological factors, depression was assessed using the 15-item Geriatric Depression Scale (GDS) (Burke et al. 1991; see Box 7). Subjects were classified into two groups as follows: those whose GDS scores were lower than five points were classified as the 'no depression' group; and those whose GDS scores were five points or more were classified as the 'mild depression/moderate to severe depression' group. In terms of self-rated health status (see Box 6), subjects were classified into two groups as follows: those who chose the item 'excellent' or 'good' were classified as the 'good health' group; and those who chose the item 'fair' or 'poor' were classified as the 'poor health' group. The self-rated sense of well-being was assessed using the 11-item version of the Philadelphia Geriatric Center (PGC) Morale Scale (Lawton 1975). Subjects whose scores were nine points or higher and those whose scores were lower than nine points were classified as the 'high well-being' group and the 'middle/low well-being' group, respectively. In terms of life satisfaction, subjects were classified into the 'satisfied' group and the 'unsatisfied' group. As for the frequency of meeting friends, subjects were classified into the 'at least once weekly' group and the 'less than once weekly' group.

iii. With respect to SES, income was represented by equivalent income. In addition, subjects were classified into four strata according to their years of education.

iv. In terms of regional classification (see Chapter 1), target regions were classified into urban, semi-urban and rural regions, based on their population density on inhabitable land and proportion of persons employed in primary industries. Statistical analyses were conducted using the SPSS software. The associations of hobby activities with the psychosocial factors described above, income, and years of education were analyzed by using the chi-square test and other tests. A general linear model was used to adjust data for age.

Results

Conditions of hobby activities

Table 7.1 shows the proportions of subjects who had hobbies. Overall, about 70.1 percent of subjects had hobbies. The proportion varied by age groups, though: 76.5 percent of the 65–69-year-old group had hobbies, with the proportion decreasing with increasing age, down to as low as 52.1 percent in the 85 years or older group. A comparison between the three regional types found that the proportion of subjects who had hobbies was 77.5 percent, 76.6 percent and 65.1 percent in the urban, semi-urban and rural regions, respectively, with the more urban regions having a significantly higher proportion of subjects who had hobbies ($p < 0.001$).

Table 7.2 shows the nature of hobby activities. In the entire subject population, audiovisual activities, including TV watching and radio listening, were pursued by the highest proportion of respondents, with the proportion exceeding 90 percent in both men and women. This was followed by cultural activities such as reading and calligraphy, sightseeing activities such as travelling and tours of old Buddhist temples, and horticultural activities such as gardening and crop cultivation, each showing a proportion of approximately 40 percent to 50 percent. Compared to women, men showed significantly higher proportions of subjects who conducted cultural and horticultural activities, or investment/gambling activities, such as stock investment and pachinko ($p < 0.001$). On the other hand, women showed significantly higher proportions of subjects who conducted musical activities such as karaoke, choral singing and playing an instrument, or creative activities such as handicraft and painting ($p < 0.001$).

The comparison between the three regional types (Table 7.2) revealed no major differences in the proportions of subjects conducting audiovisual, sightseeing, horticultural or musical activities. However, more urban regions showed higher proportions of subjects conducting cultural, sporting, creative and investment/gambling activities.

Table 7.3 shows the purposes of different hobby activities. In all activities, 'to enjoy' and 'to socialize with others' were both considered to be important by as high as 30 percent to 44 percent of both men and women subjects, indicating the importance of psychological purposes. In contrast, 'to stay fit' and 'to stave off dementia', which are related to long-term care prevention, were considered to be important by as few as 20 percent of subjects. Significantly higher proportions of men than women considered these two purposes important ($p < 0.001$). Of

Table 7.1: Proportions of subjects with hobbies by age and region type (%)

Age group	All subjects (n = 26,628)			Urban (n = 6,966)			Semi-urban (n = 4,124)			Rural (n = 15,538)			p-value
	Total	Men	Women	Total	Men	Women	Total	Men	Women	Total	Men	Women	
65–69 yrs	76.5	78.4	74.4	83.0	84.6	81.2	83.1	85.3	80.9	70.6	71.1	69.8	***
70–74 yrs	71.1	73.8	68.3	78.4	81.2	75.6	75.8	78.6	73.2	66.5	68.7	64.1	***
75–79 yrs	67.2	70.1	64.4	76.5	80.0	73.0	72.7	74.9	70.6	62.1	64.5	59.7	***
80–84 yrs	60.9	66.5	57.1	70.2	73.5	68.7	69.7	73.4	65.9	57.2	62.4	52.0	***
≥ 85 yrs	52.1	55.7	49.5	57.8	63.6	52.3	62.7	67.9	57.8	48.6	51.1	46.3	***
Total	70.1	72.9	67.5	77.5	80.3	75.0	76.6	79.4	73.9	65.1	67.0	63.0	***

All figures indicate results adjusted for age using a general linear model. N: number of subjects.

P-values indicate the significance of difference between the total results of the three regional types. ***: $p < 0.001$.

Table 7.2: Nature of hobby activities by regional type (%)

	Total			Urban			Semi-urban			Rural		
Hobby activity	**Men**	**Women**	**p-value**	**Men**	**Women**	**p-value**	**Men**	**Women**	**p-value**	**Men**	**Women**	**p-value**
Number of subjects analyzed (n = persons)	9,085	9,455		2,899	2,551		1,571	1,576		4,615	5,328	
Audiovisual activities	92.3	93.4	n.s.	93.3	93.7	n.s.	92.8	94.2	n.s.	91.6	93.1	n.s.
Cultural activities	50.9	44.9	***	52.3	41.4	***	52.0	39.8	***	47.9	41.8	***
Sightseeing activities	44.5	44.1	n.s.	44.9	44.9	n.s.	45.4	41.7	*	42.0	43.8	n.s.
Horticultural activities	45.0	38.0	***	45.1	39.2	***	43.1	35.1	***	43.1	36.8	***
Sporting activities	37.1	38.2	n.s.	39.4	41.9	n.s.	38.2	41.4	n.s.	33.8	35.4	n.s.
Musical activities	30.1	39.0	***	30.4	40.6	***	28.8	43.3	***	30.2	36.8	***
Creative activities	32.3	37.5	***	34.8	40.4	***	32.7	37.8	**	28.9	34.7	***
Investment/gambling activities	25.7	7.8	***	29.8	11.3	***	31.7	9.3	***	21.4	7.5	***

Figures indicate results adjusted for age using a general linear model.

*: $p < 0.05$; **: $p < 0.01$; ***: $p < 0.001$; n.s.: not significant.

Audiovisual activities: TV watching, radio listening, video watching, etc. Cultural activities: reading, calligraphy, activities using personal computers, etc. Sightseeing activities: traveling, tours of old Buddhist temples, etc. Horticultural activities: gardening, crop cultivation, etc. Sporting activities: ground golf, Japanese croquet, walking, etc. Musical activities: karaoke or choral singing, instrument playing, etc. Creative activities: handicraft, painting, etc. Investment/gambling activities: stock investment, pachinko, speedboat racing, etc.

those who considered the purpose of improving skills to be important, women characteristically showed higher (but not significantly) proportions than men. In both men and women, higher proportions of subjects who worked on horticultural and sightseeing activities did so for some important purpose. Conversely, lower proportions of subjects who conducted cultural activities did so for some important purpose.

Associations between hobby activities and psychosocial factors

Table 7.4 shows the associations between whether or not subjects conducted hobby activities and psychological aspects, such as depression and self-rated health status. Significantly higher proportions of subjects who had hobbies were in a more desirable psychological status, which were represented by 'no' depression as assessed by the GDS, 'good' self-rated health status, a 'satisfied' status in terms of life satisfaction, and a 'high' sense of well-being as assessed by the PGC Morale Scale which assesses the self-rated sense of well-being ($p < 0.001$). In addition, significantly higher proportions of those with hobbies than those without met their friends at a frequency of once or more per week ($p < 0.001$), which represents an indicator of rich social networks.

The comparison between the three regional types revealed that lower proportions of subjects living in rural regions than in urban regions were 'satisfied' in terms of life satisfaction and had a 'high' self-rated sense of well-being. In contrast, the rural regions showed higher proportions of subjects who met their friends once or more per week, indicating more active personal interaction in the rural regions.

Associations between hobby activities and income/years of education

Figure 7.1 shows the associations between having hobbies and income/years of education. The proportions of subjects who had hobbies were higher in groups with higher income and more years of education. For instance, while subjects who had hobbies accounted for 45.2 percent of the group whose income level was below two million yen and with less than six years of education, the proportion of subjects with hobbies doubled to 91.4 percent in the group with thirteen years or more of education and whose income level was four million yen or above. A comparison between the income groups and the years of education groups revealed that, in each of the three income level groups, more

Table 7.3: Purposes of hobby activities by activity types (%)

Purpose of hobby activities	Cultural			Sightseeing			Horticultural			Sporting			Musical			Creative		
	Men	Women	p-value	Men	Women	p-value	Men	Women	p-value	Men	Women	p-value	Men	Women	p-value	Men	Women	p-value
Number of subjects analyzed (n = persons)	1,926	1,647		2,124	2,312		2,085	2,000		1,398	1,373		1,119	1,442		1,202	1,466	
To improve skills	23.4	25.8	n.s.	33.9	35.5	n.s.	35.6	38.0	n.s.	32.9	32.0	n.s.	29.0	28.9	n.s.	21.4	25.1	n.s.
To enjoy	31.2	27.0	**	42.3	38.7	***	44.1	41.7	***	39.6	35.1	***	32.5	27.0	***	32.1	25.6	***
To socialize with others	30.6	24.5	***	40.0	33.8	***	41.0	36.4	***	35.2	28.0	***	27.1	22.3	***	28.7	21.9	***
To stay fit	23.6	18.9	***	30.0	26.7	***	29.3	26.1	n.s	24.0	19.9	**	24.1	20.5	***	23.3	20.0	***
To stave off dementia	22.6	15.2	***	30.2	23.6	***	31.2	23.3	***	26.4	18.1	***	21.2	16.6	***	29.1	22.5	***

Figures indicate results adjusted for age using a general linear model.

*: $p < 0.05$; **: $p < 0.01$; ***: $p < 0.001$; n.s.: not significant.

Table 7.4: Associations between having hobbies and psychosocial factors by regional types (%)

	Total			Urban			Semi-urban			Rural		
Psychosocial factor	**Hobbies: yes**	**Hobbies: no**	**p-value**	**Hobbies: yes**	**Hobbies: no**	**p-value**	**Hobbies: yes**	**Hobbies: no**	**p-value**	**Hobbies: yes**	**Hobbies: no**	**p-value**
Number of subjects analyzed (n = persons)	18,540	8,088		5,450	1,516		3,147	977		9,943	5,595	
Depression: no	49.4	27.3	***	50.3	26.4	***	49.8	27.8	***	48.1	27.9	***
Self-rated health status: good	72.4	57.3	***	72.3	57.7	***	72.9	59.0	***	72.1	55.3	***
Life satisfaction: satisfied	77.7	66.3	***	79.0	69.2	***	80.0	69.2	***	73.9	60.7	***
Self-rated sense of well-being: high	50.1	34.0	***	52.0	34.6	***	51.1	35.8	***	47.3	31.6	***
Meet friends: ≥ once/week	46.6	32.1	***	44.9	25.2	***	47.1	34.0	***	48.3	37.1	***

Figures indicate results adjusted for age using a general linear model.

***: $p < 0.001$

Figure 7.1: Associations between having hobbies, equivalent income and years of education

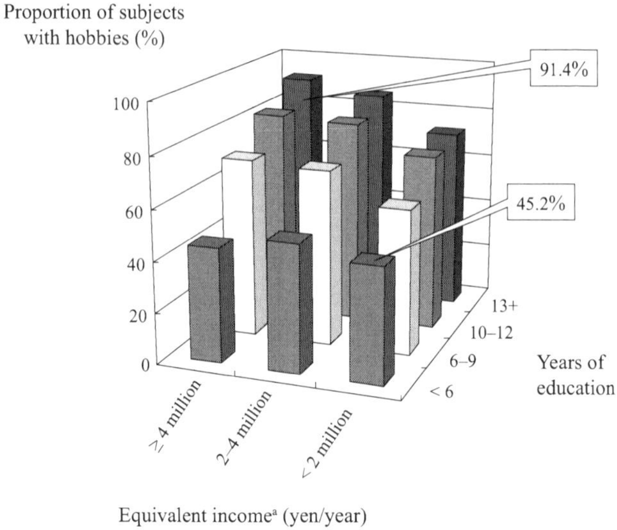

Notes.
All columns indicate results adjusted for age using a general linear model.
a: Obtained by dividing household income (in 10,000 yen/year) by the square root of the number of household members.

education was associated with a higher proportion of subjects who had hobbies. However, in the group who had less than six years of education, higher income was associated with a lower proportion of subjects who had hobbies, indicating that years of education might have a stronger influence.

Discussion

Conditions of hobby activities

While approximately 70 percent of all subjects had hobbies, the proportion of subjects with hobbies decreased with increasing age. Consistent with earlier studies (Takeda et al. 2005), the present study confirmed a tendency that the proportion of persons who had hobbies decreases considerably with increasing age. Further studies are warranted to investigate whether this simply represents effects of biological factors caused by aging or a birth cohort effect.

Nature of hobby activities

With respect to the nature of hobby activities, audiovisual activities were conducted by over 90 percent of all subjects who conducted hobby activities. While audiovisual activities may look passive, they seem to be conducted not only for recreational purposes but also to obtain information such as news.

A higher proportion of men than women conducted cultural activities such as reading and calligraphy, and horticultural activities such as gardening. However, a higher proportion of women than men conducted musical activities such as karaoke singing and playing an instrument, and creative activities such as handicraft and painting. In terms of the purposes of hobby activities, psychological aspects that are normally expected of hobby activities, such as enjoyment and socializing with others, were regarded as more important than the prevention of conditions requiring long-term care. There was a tendency for more women than men to consider the purpose of improving skills important. These results suggest that long-term care prevention projects should not provide uniform programs but conduct assessments of individual participants and provide different programs to different participants depending on their age and gender (Anme et al. 2006; Fujita et al. 2004; Takeda et al. 2005) and that these programs should be intended to keep participants sociable (Glass et al. 1999; Steinbach 1992).

Associations between hobby activities and psychosocial factors

Consistent with our previous report (Takeda et al. 2005), the large-scale data of the present study, in which the number of subjects and of target municipalities were increased from the previous study, confirmed the reproducibility of the associations between hobby activities and psychological aspects, with higher proportions of subjects with hobbies than those without showing better psychological status, such as an absence of depression and good self-rated health status. Since the present study analyzed cross-sectional survey results, there is a possibility that the above findings were caused by the fact that more subjects in a good psychological condition worked on hobby activities. Even assuming this is true, however, the above findings do indicate that persons without hobbies are more likely to be in a poor psychological status. This means that hobby activities may serve as a screening tool to identify persons who should be targeted by long-term care prevention projects. There have also been reports indicating a possibility that inactivity in terms of hobby or recreational activities is a risk factor for the development of dementia and poor life prognosis (Wilson et al. 2002; Verghese et al. 2003; Scarmeas et al. 2001; Colette et al. 1995; Wang et al. 2002; Steinbach 1992; Kondō et al. 1994). In a five-year cohort study using the same AGES data as used in the present study, compared to subjects without hobbies, those with hobbies showed a high odds ratio of 2.2 for living a healthy lifespan without conditions which are accompanied by dementia and requiring long-term care (Takeda et al. 2007). This seems to indicate the high significance of utilizing hobby activities in long-term care prevention projects.

Association between hobby activities and income/years of education

The analysis of the association between hobby activities and income/years of education revealed that groups with lower income and fewer years of education had higher proportions of subjects without hobbies. The analysis of the association between income and years of education demonstrated that, in each of the three income level groups, more years of education were associated with a higher proportion of subjects with hobbies compared to those with six or fewer years of education. In addition, in each of the years of education groups, higher income was associated with a higher proportion of subjects who had hobbies. These results indicate that years of education and income are both associated with having hobbies independently of each other. It is likely that the number of years of education results in differences in subsequent life experiences and income which, in turn, influence whether or not hobbies are pursued later in life. The promotion of long-term care prevention projects utilizing hobby activities seems to require planning and the introduction of programs which take fully into account not only gender and age but also income and years of education, all part of the background of participants' lives.

Hobby activities and regional differences

In each of the age groups, the proportion of subjects who had hobbies tended to be higher in urban regions and lower in rural regions. Regional differences were also observed in the nature of hobby activities. Since many older people regard their occupation as a hobby or purpose of life (Takeda et al 2005), there is a possibility that people in different regions may have different understandings of hobby activities. Another possibility is that environmental differences may influence people's cultural, sporting and investment/gambling activities, since rural regions provide fewer places or opportunities for these activities (Kishi et al. 1994).

In older people living in urban regions, more subjects with hobbies were in a good condition in terms of life satisfaction and self-rated sense of well-being. In contrast, for those living in rural regions, lower proportions of subjects with hobbies were in good condition in these terms, suggesting a possibility that some factor other than hobby activities is related to their psychological aspects. The present analysis found that older people living in more rural regions met their friends more frequently, which indicates a possibility that rich social networks may be associated with a good psychological condition more strongly than hobby activities are. Further studies are warranted to analyze these possibilities.

Summary

Approximately 70 percent of older community-dwelling people have hobbies, and this proportion decreases with increasing age. A comparison of the three regional types revealed that a higher proportion of older people living in urban regions than rural regions had hobbies.

An analysis of trends in the nature of hobby activities found that higher proportions of men than women conducted cultural, horticultural and investment/gambling activities, while higher proportions of women than men conducted musical and creative activities, confirming gender differences in the nature of hobbies pursued. An analysis of the purposes of hobbies revealed a tendency for older people to emphasize enjoyment and socializing with others. As for the associations between psychological indices and hobbies, more subjects with hobbies than those without were in good condition in all indices, including depression, self-rated health status, life satisfaction and self-rated sense of well-being. An analysis of the associations between hobby activities and income/years of education confirmed that higher income levels and more years of education are associated with a higher proportion of subjects with hobbies.

Hobby activities in older people were found to be associated with their psychological QOL, income and years of education, indicating a possibility that an early assessment of whether older people have hobbies may help the identification of persons with high risk of conditions requiring long-term care and may help provide interventions to reduce such risk.

Chapter 8

Housebound Behavior (*tojikomori*)

Hiroshi Hirai

Introduction

The term 'housebound' refers to a state in which an individual rarely has outings, social interaction is impoverished, and physical, psychological and social functioning are low. However, the term housebound is used differently overseas than in the context of home help service provision in Japan.

According to Hatono (2000), the term housebound is often used overseas in a sense which is roughly synonymous with individuals receiving nursing care at home rather than in a hospital or residential facility (Pasternak et al. 1999; Newman and Smith 1989). It refers to a state whereby a person cannot go out due to health reasons. As noted by Shinkai (2000), it is standard for this definition to include individuals whose health has already deteriorated to such an extent that they require long-term care.

In contrast, in Japanese Frailty Prevention Services for the Elderly circles, housebound behavior (*tojikomori*) is conceptualised as a risk factor for a decline in health that will eventually necessitate long-term care. Takeuchi was the first to propose this concept of housebound in Japan (Takeuchi 1984) in reference to an older person who does not go out of the house although they retain the capacity to do so. Such behavior leads to reduced mental and physical activity which in turn progresses to the development of a 'disuse syndrome' and deterioration in health that necessitates long-term care.

While ill-health may lead to housebound behavior, a number of studies of healthy cohorts have reported that an infrequency of outings poses a risk for deteriorating health that may necessitate long-term care (Yoshii 2004; Shinkai et al. 2005; Hirai et al. 2009).

The term housebound is currently defined using four main indices: (1) range of daily activities (Imuta et al. 1998); (2) mobility (Kono 2000); (3) frequency of outings (Hatono et al. 2001; Shinkai et al. 2005; Yokoyama et al. 2005); and (4) the presence and frequency of social interaction (Watanabe et al. 2003; Sugihara 2004; Harada et al. 2005). It is defined using one or a combination of these indices. The current fashion is to define housebound behavior solely via the frequency of outings. In recent years, however, there have been efforts to define a number of varieties of housebound behavior such as 'spatially housebound' or 'social isolation' using multiple indices including the frequency of outings or social interaction (Sugihara 2004; Harada et al. 2005).

Much of the previous research on housebound behavior has sought to elucidate the characteristics of housebound older people and related factors. The majority of these have analyzed the physical, psychological and social environmental factors highlighted by Takeuchi as relating to housebound behavior. With the exception of research by Imuta et al. (1998), Sugihara (2004), and Harada et al. 2005), there has been little effort to investigate how levels of income or education might relate to housebound behavior. Further, Shinkai identifies 'regional' factors – the distance to public amenities or the frequency of public transport – as social-environmental factors which relate to housebound behavior (Shinkai 2000). However, investigations of the effects of regional factors have been stymied by the absence of large-scale studies targeting multiple regions and the difficulty in making comparisons between studies due to inconsistencies in how the term housebound has been defined.

In the present chapter, no single definition of housebound will be used. Rather, a number of relatively simple indices relating to housebound behavior will be employed to enable comparisons with previous research, highlight the prevalence of each definition, and elucidate the relevance of income and education. The aim of this chapter is to compare the relationship between the prevalence of housebound behavior, income, and level of education as a function of regional type by using data from the Aichi Gerontological Evaluation Study (AGES) project which targeted fifteen local governments differing in regional characteristics.

Method

A total of 59,622 older people were posted a survey to complete and return via post. The participants resided in twelve nursing care insurance districts (fifteen local governments), were sixty-five years of age or older, and had not been subject to a care-needs assessment. Since participants completed and returned the survey themselves, it is conceivable that any housebound individuals unable to leave their abode to return the survey would be among those who failed to respond. Hence, it is important to note that it was not possible to get a complete picture of housebound behavior by region. A total of 32,891 people returned the survey (response rate: 55.2 percent) and were analyzed, but the number of cases in each analysis differs due to missing values.

In the present chapter, frequency of outings and frequency of social interaction were used as indices of housebound behavior. Frequency of outings was divided into four categories: 'almost every day'; 'two to three times a week'; 'about once a week'; and 'hardly ever'. The frequency of social interaction was defined as either the frequency of social interaction with family members living separately or with relatives or, alternatively, as the frequency of social interaction with friends. The frequency of social interaction was then divided into seven categories: 'almost every day', 'two to three times a week'; 'usually every week'; 'one to two times a month'; 'a few times a year'; 'hardly ever'; and 'I don't have family who live separately or friends'.

Labels have been abbreviated as follows. For frequency of outings, with higher frequency being 'about once a week', responses of 'hardly ever' were labelled 'less than once a week'. For frequency of social interaction, the responses 'one to two times a month', 'a few times a year', 'hardly ever', and 'I don't have family who live separately or friends' were all labelled 'less than weekly'.

As shown in Figure 8.1, five definitions of housebound behavior are used in the present chapter. These are: (A) 'housebound where outings are infrequent'; (B-1) 'housebound where social interaction with friends is infrequent'; (B-2) 'housebound where social interaction with family who live separately or with relatives is infrequent'; (C) 'broad definition of housebound behavior'; and (D) 'narrow definition of housebound behavior'.

(A) refers to people whose frequency of outings is less than weekly. (B-1) refers to people whose frequency of social interaction with friends is less than weekly while (B-2) refers to people whose frequency of social interaction with family who live separately or with relatives is less than weekly. (C) refers to individuals with either infrequent outings (less than weekly) or with infrequent social interaction (i.e. both social interaction with friends, and social interaction with family who live separately or with relatives is less than weekly). (D) refers to individuals with both infrequent outings (less than weekly) and infrequent social interaction (i.e. both social interaction with friends, and social interaction with family who live separately or with relatives is less than weekly).

Figure 8.1: Prevalence of housebound behavior according to five definitions

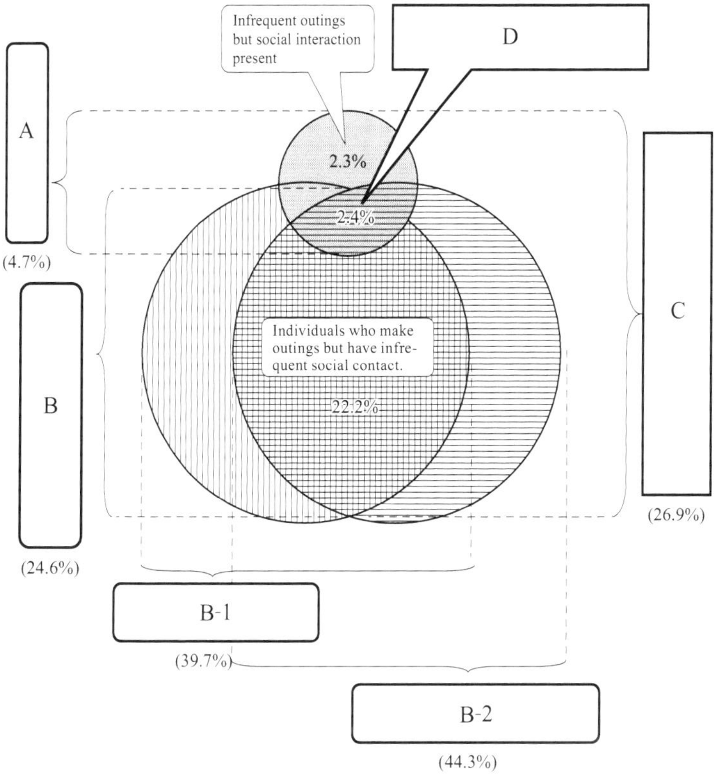

Legend.

A. Housebound where outings are infrequent

B. Individuals with infrequent social contact with both family who live separately & friends.

C. Broad definition of housebound behavior. Either outings or social contact is infrequent.

D. Narrow definition of housebound behavior. Infrequent outings & social interaction.

B-1. Housebound where social interaction with friends is infrequent

B-2. Housebound where social interaction with family who live separately or with relatives is infrequent

First, the prevalence of each type of housebound behavior was calculated by age-bracket, sex, and household type. Next, the relationships between the prevalence of each type of housebound behavior and health indices (subjective assessment of health – see Box 6); depression (Geriatric Depression Scale (GDS) – see Box

7), income, years of education and regional type were investigated. Equivalent income was used for the income variable and calculated by dividing household income by the square root of the number of household members (see Box 3). Finally, the relationship between housebound behavior, income and years of education was analyzed by community type (Chapter 1).

Analyses were conducted using the General Linear Model in the Statistical Package for the Social Sciences (SPSS) software with 'age', 'health' 'income' and 'years of education' as predictor variables and housebound behavior as the dependent variable.

Results

Prevalence of housebound behavior by definition

The prevalence of housebound behavior differed considerably according to the four definitions from 26.9 percent by the broad definition (C) to 2.4 percent by the narrow definition (D). As shown in Table 8.1, there was a greater proportion of individuals with infrequent outings (A) in the younger age group (65–69 age bracket) for men at 3.5 percent compared to women at 2.2 percent. However, this trend was reversed in the 80–84 age bracket with women more likely to have less frequent outings than men at 8.5 percent and 6.2 percent respectively. Overall, there were fewer women who had infrequent social interaction with friends (B-1) with 48.0 percent of men falling into this category compared to 33.6 percent of women. As age increased, there was a decrease in the prevalence of individuals who had infrequent social interaction with family who lived separately (B-2), pointing to the support such family members provide to older people. Housebound prevalence by the broader definition indicates that men have about a 10 percent higher overall frequency of social interaction (men at 32.8 percent compared to women at 21.7 percent).

Type of household & housebound behavior

In addition to older people who are voluntarily housebound, the housebound population may also include people whose outings and social interactions are restricted by family members out of health concerns, fear of accidents, and similar reasons (Yasumura 2006). Table 8.2 shows the prevalence of each type of housebound definition by household type after correcting for age. By almost all definitions, there were significantly fewer instances of housebound behavior in

Table 8.1: Basic distribution of housebound behavior according to each definition (%)

	Males						Females					
			Infrequent social interaction						Infrequent social interaction			
Age	**n**	**Infrequent outings**	**Friends**	**Separated family**	**Broad definition[a]**	**Narrow defintion[b]**	**n**	**Infrequent outings**	**Friends**	**Separated family**	**Broad definition[a]**	**Narrow defintion[b]**
65–69	4,405	3.4	46.9	49.8	30.1	1.3	4,745	2.2	33.0	43.3	18.4	0.9
70–74	3,997	4.2	45.6	49.0	29.5	1.7	4,508	3.1	32.1	42.5	18.4	1.0
75–79	2,802	5.5	48.3	47.8	30.1	2.5	3,390	4.0	32.8	39.6	18.9	1.6
80–84	1,291	6.1	50.3	45.2	31.0	2.8	1,920	8.2	33.2	41.1	22.7	2.7
85 +	592	15.7	59.0	39.8	35.6	6.9	908	18.4	46.6	39.5	32.0	8.3
Total	13,087	4.9	47.7	48.3	30.2	2.1	15,471	4.6	33.5	41.8	19.8	1.7

Notes.

a: Broad definition of housebound behavior: Either less than weekly outings or less than weekly social interaction with friends, relatives or family who live separately.

b: Narrow definition of housebound behavior: Both (1) less than weekly outings and (2) less than weekly social interaction with friends, relatives or family who live separately.

individuals who lived alone compared to an increase in prevalence in individuals who lived with their children.

Housebound behavior & health indices

Figure 8.2 shows the relationship between housebound behavior and depression scores (GDS). Across all definitions, there is an increase in the prevalence of housebound behavior as depression increases in severity. In a similar pattern to depression scores, an analysis of self-rated health scores revealed a significantly higher prevalence of housebound behavior in older people who were experiencing undesirable psychological circumstances.

Income, education & housebound behavior (Table 8.3)

In men, no matter which definition was used, housebound behavior was correlated with income and years of education. There was a lower prevalence of individuals who were 'housebound where outings are infrequent' in the cohort with high levels of income and education. While the phenomenon of being 'housebound where social interaction with friends is infrequent' was the least prevalent in high-income individuals, it was the most prevalent in the highly educated group. Education and equivalent income thus demonstrated different relationships by this definition of housebound behavior. Housebound behavior as defined by infrequent social interaction with family living separately or with friends was the most prevalent in highly educated individuals, demonstrating an inverse relationship compared to when it was indexed by frequency of outings. The relationships between housebound behavior and income and years of education were weaker in women compared to men.

Housebound behavior & regional differences

The three regional types used in the AGES project (see Chapter 1) were compared with each other. All values were corrected for the effects of age since rural regions are disproportionately affected by the effects of an aging population (Table 8.4). For both men and women, there was a greater prevalence of individuals who had infrequent outings in rural regions and a greater prevalence of individuals who had infrequent social interaction with friends in urban regions. These regional differences were, however, small. There was no significant difference between regions with respect to social interaction with

Table 8.2: Type of household & distribution of housebound behavior according to each definition (adjusted for age) (%)

	Males						Females					
			Infrequent social interaction						Infrequent social interaction			
	n	Infrequent outings	Friends	Separated family	Broad definition[a]	Narrow defintion[b]	n	Infrequent outings	Friends	Separated family	Broad definition[a]	Narrow defintion[b]
Live alone	601	2.5	40.8	51.8	25.4	1.0	2,523	3.3	26.8	39.6	14.6	0.9
Only older people	6,519	4.3	48.3	50.5	31.7	2.1	4,932	3.7	34.4	43.8	20.6	2.0
With children	3,087	5.8	51.6	57.2	37.8	3.7	3,782	5.4	36.6	49.3	25.6	2.8
Three-generations	3,180	4.8	43.3	51.5	31.1	2.7	4,310	5.3	34.2	46.2	24.2	2.4
Other	279	8.8	48.2	52.0	33.8	6.8	460	5.4	31.9	42.4	22.6	3.1
p-value[c]		***	***	***	***	***		***	***	***	***	***

Notes.

a: Broad definition of housebound behavior: Either less than weekly outings or less than weekly social interaction with friends, relatives or family who live separately.

b: Narrow definition of housebound behavior: Both (1) less than weekly outings and (2) less than weekly social interaction with friends, relatives or family who live separately.

c: *** = $p < 0.001$.

Figure 8.2a: Prevalence of depression & housebound behavior by definition (males)

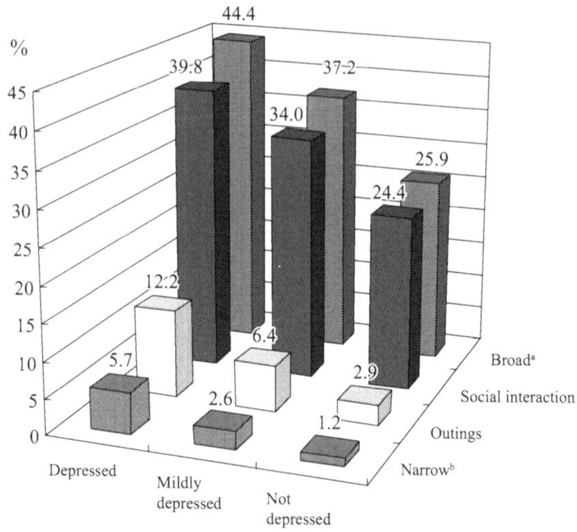

Notes.

a: Broad definition of housebound behavior: Either less than weekly outings or less than weekly social interaction with friends, relatives or family who live separately.

b: Narrow definition of housebound behavior: Both (1) less than weekly outings and (2) less than weekly social interaction with friends, relatives or family who live separately.

family members for either sex. There was a higher prevalence of housebound men, using the broad definition, in urban regions while there was a higher prevalence of housebound women, using the narrow definition, in rural regions. However, the sample from which the AGES data was obtained was not representative of Japan as it did not include data from the so-called 'major cities' in which population density exceeds 3,000 people per square kilometre. It is therefore important to note that any relationship between the prevalence of housebound behavior and urban versus rural regions cannot be generalised to Japan as a whole.

Regional type, education & housebound behavior

Figures 8.3 and 8.4 show the prevalence of different definitions of housebound behavior as a function of regional type and years of education, respectively. Individuals with infrequent outings were significantly more prevalent in the cohort with the lowest education

Figure 8.2b: Prevalence of depression & housebound behavior by definition (females)

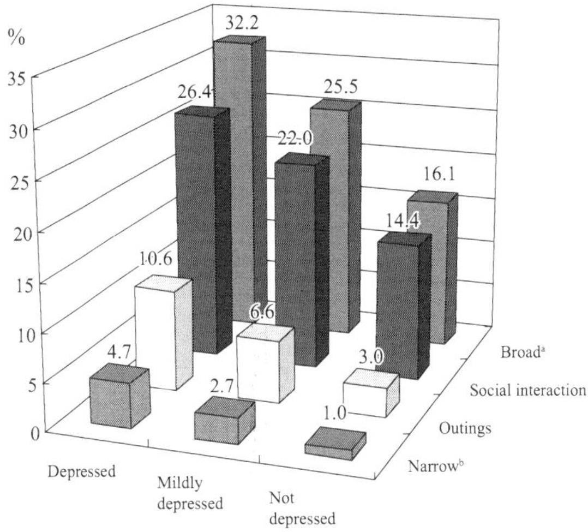

Notes.

a: Broad definition of housebound behavior: Either less than weekly outings or less than weekly social interaction with friends, relatives or family who live separately.

b: Narrow definition of housebound behavior: Both (1) less than weekly outings and (2) less than weekly social interaction with friends, relatives or family who live separately.

levels across all regional types. Further, in the cohort with 6 to 9 years of education, the proportion of housebound behavior was significantly higher in rural compared to urban regions, although only by a few percent (Figure 8.3). In contrast, the reverse relationship was seen in rural regions where individuals were more likely to have infrequent social interaction with friends the higher their level of education. Further, in the cohorts with 6 to 9 years and 10 to 12 years of education respectively the relationship to the frequency of outings index observed was the complete opposite (Figure 8.4) with a 5 percent to 6 percent lower prevalence of housebound individuals in rural compared to urban regions.

Discussion

The present chapter analyzed the prevalence of housebound behavior in the older population according to five different definitions. Depending on the definition used, frequency of housebound behavior

Table 8.3: Income, education & prevalence (%) of housebound behavior according to each definition (adjusted for age)

	Males						Females					
			Infrequent social interaction						Infrequent social interaction			
	n	Infrequent outings	Friends	Separated family	Broad definition[a]	Narrow defintion[b]	n	Infrequent outings	Friends	Separated family	Broad definition[a]	Narrow defintion[b]
Equivalent income[c]												
< 2 million yen	4,880	5.2	48.6	51.2	33.0	2.7	5,232	4.4	33.9	44.1	21.4	2.0
2–4 million yen	4,950	3.6	47.6	53.8	32.0	2.3	4,059	4.0	33.1	46.3	21.7	1.6
≥ 4 million yen	1,147	2.9	43.8	51.6	28.9	1.3	1,083	4.1	36.2	47.3	23.2	2.4
p-value[d]		***	*	*	*	*		n.s.	n.s.	*	n.s.	n.s.
Yearsof education												
< 6	271	11.5	50.1	51.2	35.2	4.9	578	10.4	36.7	42.4	25.8	4.8
6–9	5,646	4.8	45.9	49.5	30.3	2.7	5,525	4.5	33.2	43.7	21.2	1.9
10–12	3,452	3.6	48.7	54.1	33.4	1.9	3,640	2.9	34.6	48.0	21.9	1.4
≥ 13	1,608	2.7	51.2	59.4	35.6	1.9	631	3.7	33.1	46.3	21.2	1.8
p-value[d]		***	**	***	**	**		***.	n.s	***	n.s	***

Notes.

a: Broad definition of housebound behavior: Either less than weekly outings or less than weekly social interaction with friends, relatives or family who live separately.

b: Narrow definition of housebound behavior: Both (1) less than weekly outings and (2) less than weekly social interaction with friends, relatives or family who live separately.

c: Equivalent income: calculated by dividing the annual household income by the square root of the number of people in the household

d: n.s.: Not significant; *: $p < 0.05$; **: $p < 0.01$; ***: $p < 0.001$

Table 8.4: Community type & prevalence (%) of housebound behavior according to each definition (adjusted for age)

Community type	Males						Females					
			Infrequent social interaction						Infrequent social interaction			
	n	Infrequent outings	Friends	Separated family	Broad definition[a]	Narrow defintion[b]	n	Infrequent outings	Friends	Separated family	Broad definition[a]	Narrow defintion[b]
Urban	3,517	3.9	52.8	54.7	35.3	2.3	3,318	3.3	36.2	45.9	23.0	1.6
Semi-urban	1,917	4.8	50.3	52.9	33.9	2.8	2,077	3.8	33.9	44.6	21.0	2.1
Rural	7,098	5.4	45.0	51.0	31.3	2.9	8,982	5.2	32.6	44.9	21.4	2.3
p-value[c]		**	***	**	**	n.s.		***	**	n.s.	n.s.	*

Notes.

a: Broad definition of housebound behavior: Either less than weekly outings or less than weekly social interaction with friends, relatives or family who live separately.

b: Narrow definition of housebound behavior: Both (1) less than weekly outings and (2) less than weekly social interaction with friends, relatives or family who live separately.

c: n.s. = Not significant; * = $p < 0.05$; ** = $p < 0.01$; *** = $p < 0.001$.

Figure 8.3: Prevalence of individuals with infrequent outings by years of education & regional type (adjusted for age)

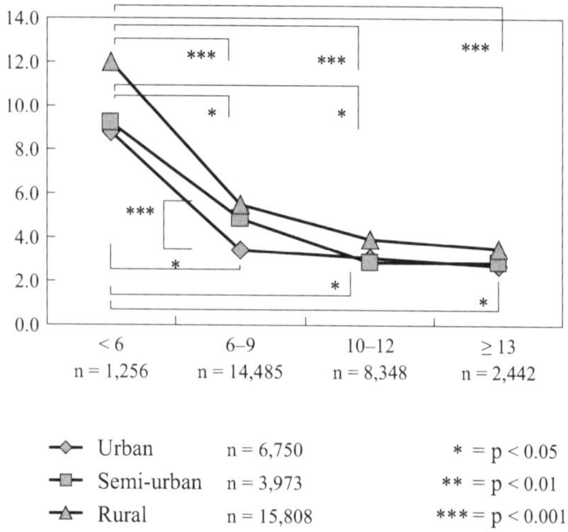

differed by between 2.4 percent and 26.9 percent. While Sugihara (2004) and Harada et al. (2005) also used multiple definitions of housebound behavior, the prevalence observed in the present study was two to three times greater than that observed by Sugihara (2004) (7.4 percent–14.2 percent) or Harada et al. (2005) (4.3 percent–14.2 percent). Moreover, since it is conceivable that some individuals who failed to respond were themselves housebound and therefore did not return the survey by post, it is likely that the actual proportion of housebound older people is greater than the figures cited here.

In terms of household type, across almost all definitions, housebound behavior was less prevalent when individuals lived alone than in other household types. While this relationship is similar to that seen in the findings of Sugihara (2004) and Harada et al. (2005), other researchers such as Yokoyama et al. (2005) and Watanabe et al. (2003) report no difference in the prevalence of housebound behavior as a function of household type. Even if an individual were living alone, it is conceivable that the circumstances would differ depending upon whether or not the person's family lived nearby and provided support. Future studies that take account of these issues are required.

Earlier research (Nakata et al. 2002; Kurihara and Katsura 2003) analyzed the relationship between housebound behavior and the subjective assessment of health, depression and other health indices and reported results similar to those found in the present study. That

Figure 8.4: Prevalence of individuals with infrequent social interaction with friends by years of education & regional type (adjusted for age)

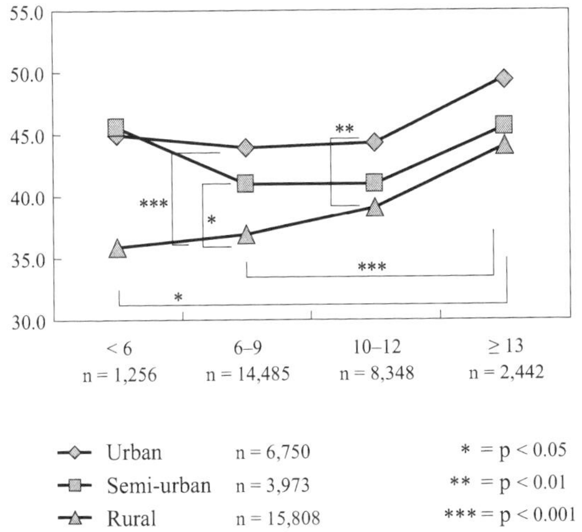

is, in almost all studies, most older housebound people are found to have poor health or, alternatively, many people with poor health are found to be housebound.

Gilbert et al. (1992), Imuta et al. (1998), Hatono (2001), Sugihara (2004) and Harada et al. (2005) have all analyzed the relationship between income, education and housebound behavior. Gilbert et al. (1992) demonstrated that housebound behavior as defined by frequency of outings is more prevalent in cohorts with lower levels of education and fewer savings. Harada et al. (2005) defined housebound behavior using frequency of outings and range of behavior and reported a relationship with income consistent with the current findings.

Sugihara (2004) and Harada et al. (2005) defined 'interpersonal housebound behavior' according to the frequency of social interaction and the frequency of participation in group activities (community organisations, interest groups and similar associations) and found it was more prevalent in individuals with lower incomes. The present study only used frequency of social interaction in its definition of housebound behavior and did not include frequency of participation in group activities. Nevertheless, consistent with past research, the current study did find a relationship between housebound behavior and income and education in men. No significant relationship was observed, however, in women. Sugihara (2004) and Harada et al. (2005) did not

Box 12: International Comparison of Housebound Behavior (Social Isolation)

Hiroshi Hirai

The present chapter has operationalised 'housebound behavior' (*tojikomori* in Japanese) using frequency of outings and frequency of social interaction.

The frequency of outings is the most often used definition of housebound behavior in Japan. While some overseas research also uses this index in the definition of housebound behavior (Gilbert et al. 1992; Ganguli et al. 1996), it was not possible to locate data which would allow for an international comparison. It may simply be the case that infrequent outings alone is not recognised as an issue.

Overseas, infrequent social interaction is generally thought of as 'social isolation' rather than housebound behavior. Social isolation has been recognised as a problem by the Social Exclusion Unit's (SEU) (Office of the Deputy Prime Minister, UK) publication of 2006, which treats it as a contributor to 'social exclusion' for older people alongside poverty, poor health and the need for nursing care. The World Values Survey has established research criteria for social isolation which allows for a comparison between OECD countries. Figure 8.5 shows the proportion of people who responded to a question concerning the amount of contact and social interaction they had with people other than friends, colleagues or family with the responses 'none at all' or 'extremely rarely'. The data is not limited to older people (65 years plus) but includes all age groups. Japan has the highest proportion at 15.3 percent.

analyze their data according to sex. The current study found, however, that housebound behavior as defined by infrequent social interaction was less prevalent in women than in men by about 10 percent. This speaks to the necessity of conducting sex-specific analyses. Further, Harada et al. (2005) demonstrated that 'psychologically housebound' individuals as defined by their subjective feelings of isolation were more prevalent in low income cohorts but less prevalent in cohorts with lower levels of education. While the heterogeneity of the indices used makes comparisons problematic, these findings do suggest that, depending upon the definition of housebound used, low levels of income and education do not always demonstrate a relationship with housebound behavior.

Figure 8.5: The proportion (%) of people with a minimal amount of contact with people other than their friends, colleagues or family

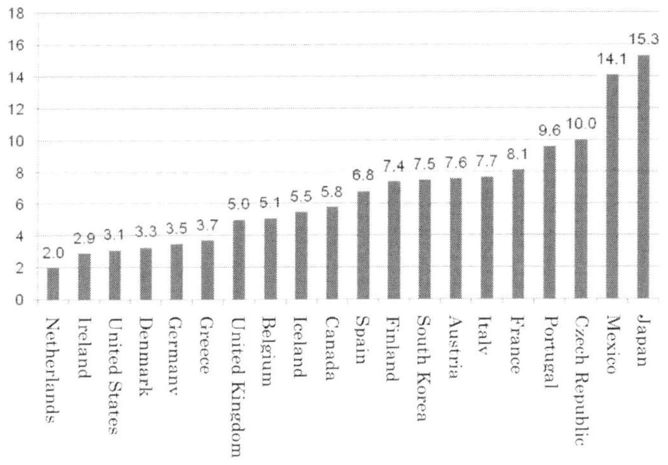

Source: World Values Survey 2000 data: Society at a glance: OECD social indicators (2001).

While Shinkai (2000) has pointed out the necessity of taking regional factors into account, there has been very little research which has considered such factors. Hatono et al. (2001) analyzed intra-regional differences according to whether a locale was either 'sea-facing' or 'mountain-facing' since they found that, in the end, these factors exerted the greatest effect. Research by the Japanese Cabinet Office (2002) and by Torii et al. (2005) demonstrates that regional differences exist when considering the prevalence of older people who go out only infrequently. The Cabinet Office research used the location of respondents to compare regional attributes between 'major cities', 'medium-sized cities', 'small cities' and 'towns & villages'. Torii et al. (2005), in contrast, classified all of Ehime prefecture as either 'urban' or 'town/village areas'. They demonstrated results consistent with the findings of the present study, namely, that the prevalence of individuals who go out infrequently increases as the environment becomes less urban. Shinkai et al. (2005) compared Yoita-machi in Niigata prefecture with Hatoyama New Town in Hatoyama-cho, Saitama prefecture, and found the reverse relationship, namely, that there were more housebound individuals in the relatively more urbanized Hatoyama-cho. It is conceivable, however, that rather than reflecting the distinction between urban and rural areas, this reflected the distinct community make-up of planned, suburban "new town" developments which lack historical community ties.

The present study found differences in the prevalence of housebound behavior as a function of income, years of education and regional type and distinctive relationships between these factors. Sex also had a unique influence on the relationships between these factors. Such findings attest to the existence of different types of housebound behavior which readily emerge as a function of income, education, regional type and sex. This in turn indicates the necessity of considering income, education level, regional factors and sex in any future interventions by home help service providers and, moreover, flags the importance of developing distinctive intervention protocols.

Conclusions

This study illustrates the prevalence of housebound behavior according to multiple definitions and found in excess of a tenfold difference – from 2.4 percent to 26.9 percent – depending upon the definition used.

In terms of the relationship between housebound prevalence and income, years of education and regional factors, other chapters have highlighted the prevalence of individuals in 'undesirable states' in cohorts with low levels of income and education and in older people residing in rural areas (Chapter 5). In contrast, the reverse phenomenon is seen with housebound behavior. Housebound behavior in men, as defined by infrequent social interaction with friends or family members living separately, is more prevalent in the cohort with the highest level of education and in more urbanised regions. The sex-based differences are also noteworthy in comparison to the other chapters. Not only are there close to 10 percent fewer women than men who are 'housebound where social interaction is infrequent', women are mostly unaffected by the impact of income or years of education. Further, the frequency of social interaction with friends remains, in women, resistant to decline even with increasing age. This finding supports the stereotype that women may have higher levels of communication skills.

Such a finding would be consistent with research by Okubo et al. (2005) who found that older men were less likely to participate in services which emphasised social interaction, such as community centres. According to Okubo et al. (2005), men prefer a selection of goal-oriented activities and tend to participate in services planned by men in which men play a central role. In order to increase the number of opportunities for men to interact socially, it may be possible to create an impetus for social interaction within other services in which the objectives are clear. Alternatively, men could be encouraged to become involved in the planning and administration of services by tapping into neighbourhood community associations, senior citizens associations or other such organisations in which men already participate and using these as a base. A number of places already have male participation at 30 percent to 40 percent. These include Inami-cho in Hyogo prefecture in which neighbourhood community associations and senior citizen associations are run autonomously and can be used as base organizations (Takeo 2004). Kyonrodan leisure and welfare facilities for the older population in South Korea, some of which have sex-specific activity centres, are another example (Saito et al. 2007).

The current findings highlight the importance of being mindful of differences in income, education, regional factors and sex in order to develop more effective Frailty Prevention Services for the Elderly initiatives in the future.

Chapter 9

Abuse

Etsuko Katō

Introduction

Since the 1980s, developed countries have led the way in recognising elder abuse as a social problem (Steinmetz 1988). The problem of "elder abuse" was highlighted in Japan in 1987 when medical doctor and public health centre head Yoshihiko Kaneko published findings from a fact-finding study (Yoshihiko 1987). Following this, a number of research organisations across Japan conducted fact-finding research on elder abuse, mainly with a focus on domestic abuse (Elderly Treatment Workgroup 1994, 1997, 1998, 2000; Takasaki et al. 1999; Osaka Elder Abuse Prevention Workgroup 1997; Tatara 1999, 2000). From the late 1990s there was an increase in the number of case reports from people involved in the care of older people. There was also increased interest in elder abuse, particularly in the most effective form for interventions to take (Takasaki et al. 1998). Then, in Autumn 2003, the Institute for Health Economics and Policy conducted a nation-wide survey on elder abuse (hereafter, the 'National Survey', published 2004) under the auspices of the Ministry of Health, Labour and Welfare. The National Survey conducted a detailed analysis of the 1991 cases brought to attention mainly by home care providers. It mapped out the characteristics of abusers and their victims, potential background factors to the abuse, and what could be done to help, among other factors.

However, the National Survey and research conducted by various research organisations targeted older people who required assistance with everyday activities. The nature of abuse in older people who did not require everyday assistance or who require everyday assistance but who were not utilising long-term care insurance services was unclear. The National Survey did not highlight the prevalence of elder abuse in communities or highlight the characteristics of victims based on a comparison with individuals not being abused, leaving such issues open for future research.

Large-scale community surveys on elder abuse have been conducted in the United States (Pillemer and Finkelhor 1988), the United Kingdom (Ogg and Bennett 1992), Canada (Podnicks 1992) and the Netherlands (Comijs et al. 1998), all of which are gradually adopting anti-abuse systems informed by the prevalence of abuse and similar factors. In order for municipalities to develop effective measures to counter elder abuse, it is imperative for Japan to ascertain the prevalence of victims at a local government level – including information on older people not requiring assistance – and the nature of such abuse, background factors and other relevant information (Watanabe 2005).

Accordingly, the present chapter focuses on older people who have not been subject to a care insurance long-term assessment. It investigates the nature of physical, psychological and financial abuse and analyses community differences in the psychological or financial status of victims, their level of education and victim prevalence. In addition, another aim is to discuss measures for the early identification of cases of abuse.

Method

Subjects

The subjects comprised regular people who resided in twelve long-term care insurance districts (fifteen local governments) in three prefectures, were sixty-five years of age or older, and had not been subject to a care-needs assessment.

Individuals subject to analyses were people who had responded to the 'family relationships & abuse' survey (See Appendix) which was one of the three surveys used in the AGES (Aichi Gerontological Evaluation Study; see Box 2) project. This survey contained detailed questions on family relationships and abuse in addition to the basic questions common to all participants. The survey was sent to 29,373 people with responses received from 17,257 people (response rate of 58.8 percent).

Respondents were asked to rate whether or not they required assistance with walking, bathing or toileting using one of three responses; 'no assistance', 'require some assistance', and 'require comprehensive assistance'. Of the 17,257 people who responded, a total of 15,655 people (90.7 percent) responded with 'no assistance' to all three questions and were deemed 'independent'. A total of 624 participants (3.6 percent) responded to the questions with either 'require some assistance' or 'require comprehensive assistance' and were classified as the 'assistance-required' group.

Ethical considerations

The proposal for the present research was approved by the Nihon Fukushi University Research Ethics Committee. Specifically, information provided by the relevant local government bodies was coded prior to delivery so that the researchers were not privy to any personal information.

Questions on abuse

In the present study, participants were asked whether they had experienced physical abuse, psychological abuse or financial abuse. The questions are detailed below.

Physical abuse & psychological abuse

Respondents were asked, 'Have you ever been subject to any of the following by someone in your family?': (1) 'Physical violence such as being punched, being kicked, having an object thrown at you or being locked up?'; (2) 'Any action which has upset your self-respect such as being yelled at, being subject to offensive remarks, or being ignored for a long time?'. In response to these two questions, participants responded with one of the following: 'never', 'once or twice', 'sometimes', and 'often' (see Appendix).

Participants who responded with 'once or twice', 'sometimes', and 'often' were then asked, 'Did you talk to somebody about it?' and given five options to choose from: friend or acquaintance; family or relative; doctor; police; and other (multiple responses permitted). In addition, people who responded with, 'I did not talk to anybody,' were then asked, 'Would you like to talk to somebody who can be trusted?'

Financial abuse

Participants were asked to respond with, 'yes' or 'no' to the question: 'Has someone (including family members) used or taken your savings or pension without your permission?' Participants who responded 'yes' were also asked to indicate their relationship with the other party from the following three relationships: 'a family member who lives with me'; 'relative or family member who lives separately'; or 'acquaintance, friend or neighbour' (multiple responses permitted). In the present study, participants who responded ‘never’ with respect to physical abuse and psychological abuse were categorised as ‘no abuse’ while participants who responded ‘once or twice’ were categorised as ‘suspected abuse’. Participants who responded ‘sometimes’ or ‘often’ were categorised as ‘abused’. For financial abuse, participants who responded ‘no’ were categorised as ‘no abuse’ while participants who responded ‘yes’ were categorised as ‘abused’.

Questions on the psychological health of abuse victims

In order to investigate the relationship between abuse and the psychological health of older people, comparisons were made with respect to self-rated health, subjective happiness and depression.

For self-rated health, participants were asked to choose to respond to the question, ‘How is your health at the moment?’ with one of four responses: ‘poor’, ‘fair’, ‘good’ or ‘excellent’ (see Box 6). For subjective happiness, the following were used: the Philadelphia Geriatric Centre Morale Scale (hereafter the ‘PGC’) (Lawton 1972) which is comprised of the three subscales of (1) ‘attitude toward aging’, (2) ‘agitation’ and (3) ‘lonely dissatisfaction’; and the 15-item Geriatric Depression Scale (hereafter the ‘GDS’; see Box 7) (Sheikh and Yesavage 1986).

The Statistical Package for the Social Sciences (SPSS) was used for statistical analyses with chi-squared analyses used to examine categorical differences. The sample size varied with each analysis due to the removal of individuals who failed to respond.

Results

Sample demographics

A total of 45.6 percent of the participants were men while 54.4 percent were women (see Table 9.1). The mean age was 73.2 years for men and 73.8 for women. In terms of household, 11.0 percent lived by themselves, 40.0 percent lived in a household of two people while 48.5 percent lived in a household with three or more members. A total of 60.9 percent had nine or less years of schooling while 58.5 percent had an equivalent income – which takes into account the number of household members – of two million yen or less (see Box 3). A total of 23.7 percent of participants rated their own health as ‘fair’ while 5.2 percent responded with ‘poor’.

Table 9.1: Sample demographics

	Number of respondents	%	Average
Total	17,257		
Gender and age			
Male	6,908	45.6	
Age			73.2
Female	8,242	54.4	
Age			73.8
Household type			
Living alone	1,663	11.0	
Two people	6,112	40.0	
Three or more	7,327	48.5	
Schooling years			
9 or less	9,337	60.9	
10 or more	5,991	39.1	
Equivalent income (million yen)[a]			
2 or less	6,197	58.5	
More than 2	5,906	41.5	
Self-rated health			
Excellent	1,159	7.2	
Good	10,252	63.9	
Fair	3,809	23.7	
Poor	830	5.2	
Self-rated happiness	13,336		6.83
Depression (GDS)	12,295		3.83

Note. a: Per annum household income divided by the square root of the number of people in the household.

Prevalence of abuse victims

Of the 17,257 people who responded (see Table 9.2), 2,805 people were classified as having been 'abused' physically, psychologically or financially (16.3 percent, 95 percent confidence interval, 15.7 percent–16.8 percent) while 1,555 people were classified with 'suspected abuse' (9.0 percent; 95 percent confidence interval, 8.5 percent–9.4 percent) and 10,784 people were classified with 'no abuse' (62.5 percent; 95 percent confidence interval, 61.8 percent–63.2 percent).

Prevalence of abuse victims as a function of their physical condition

After removing people who had failed to respond as to whether they required assistance with walking, bathing or toileting, 16,279 people

Table 9.2: The proportion of abuse victims

	N	%	Confidence interval
Abused	2,805	16.3	15.7–16.8
Suspected abuse	1,555	9.0	8.5–9.4
No abuse	10,784	62.5	61.8–63.2
No response	2,113	12.2	11.6–13.7
Total	17,257	100	–

Table 9.3: The proportion of abuse victims: independent and assistance-required groups

	Independent		Assistance-required		
Abuse type	N	%	N	%	p-value
Physical, psychological or financial					**
No abuse	11,722	74.9	440	70.5	
Abuse or suspected abuse	3,933	25.1	184	29.5	
Physical					**
No abuse	13,823	95.8	498	94.0	
Abuse or suspected abuse	613	4.2	32	6.0	
Psychological					**
No abuse	11,156	78.1	401	76.5	
Abuse or suspected abuse	3,127	21.9	123	23.5	
Financial					**
No abuse	13,897	93.2	487	86.8	
Abuse or suspected abuse	1,020	6.8	74	13.2	

**: $p < 0.01$

remained (see Table 9.3). Abuse was suspected in 25.1 percent of the independent group and in 29.5 percent of the assistance-required group. A comparison was made between the independent group and the assistance-required group of the prevalence of combined 'abused/suspected abuse' cases by abuse type. For the independent group and the assistance-required group respectively the prevalence was 4.2 percent and 6.0 percent for physical abuse, 21.9 percent and 23.5 percent for psychological abuse, and 6.8 percent and 13.2 percent for financial abuse. While there was significantly more abuse in the assistance-required group, abuse was also seen in the independent group.

Prevalence of abuse victims by sex

There was a higher prevalence of both 'abuse' and 'suspected abuse' for physical and psychological abuse in women than in men (see Table 9.4). Conversely, financial 'abuse' was more prevalent in men than in women.

Household type, perpetrators of abuse, and abuse victims

Table 9.5 shows the relationship between the presence of abuse and household type by dividing physical and psychological abuse into the two groups of 'no abuse' and 'abuse/ suspected abuse' combined, and by dividing financial abuse into 'abuse' and 'no abuse'. Across all types, abuse was relatively more prevalent in households of two people.

Of the 1,094 people who had experienced financial abuse, a total of 512 people (response rate 46.8 percent) responded with respect to their relationship to the perpetrator of abuse, with 556 responses collected. Of these, a total of 459 of the 512 people (89.6 percent) reported that the perpetrator of the abuse was 'a family member who lives with me', 78 people (15.2 percent) reported that the perpetrator was a 'relative or family member who lived separately' and 19 people (3.7 percent) reported that the perpetrator was an 'acquaintance, friend or neighbour'.

Psychological health, income & education of abuse victims

For all abuse types, the 'abuse/suspected abuse' combined cohort was in significantly poorer psychological health compared to the 'no abuse' group (see Table 9.6). This group also had a higher number of people responding with 'poor' for self-rated health while subjective happiness was low and depression prevalent.

The only statistically significant difference with the years of education factor was for financial abuse, with 'abuse' more prevalent in individuals with an education of nine years or less. Abuse was significantly more prevalent in the cohort earning an equivalent income of two million yen or less across all types of abuse.

Abuse prevalence by regional type

There were no significant differences as a function of regional type for physical abuse (see Table 9.7). For psychological abuse, individuals who met the 'abuse/suspected abuse' combined criteria were more prevalent in semi-urban regions. Financial abuse was significantly more prevalent in urban compared to rural regions, with the rate of 'abuse' at 6.7 percent in rural regions, 7.5 percent in semi-urban regions, and 8.7 percent in urban regions.

Table 9.4: Prevalence of abuse victims by gender

	Male		Female		
Abuse type	N	%	N	%	p-value
Physical, psychological or financial					n.s.
No abuse	5,132	74.3	6,063	73.6	
Abuse or suspected abuse	1,776	25.7	2,179	26.4	
Physical					**
No abuse	6,542	97.4	7,347	94.2	
Abuse or suspected abuse	178	2.7	450	5.7	
Psychological					**
No abuse	5,411	81.0	5,769	74.9	
Abuse or suspected abuse	1,270	19.0	1,932	25.1	
Financial					**
No abuse	5,973	90.0	7,601	96.1	
Abuse	666	10.0	311	3.9	

Note: Non-response cases are excluded.
**: $p < 0.01$; n.s. = Not significant.

Table 9.5: Household type, perpetrators of abuse, and abuse victims

	Living alone		Two people		Three or more people		
Abuse type	N	%	N	%	N	%	p-value
Physical, psychological or financial							**
No abuse	1,237	84.3	4,364	71.6	5,630	73.6	
Abuse or suspected abuse	230	15.7	1,729	28.4	2,020	26.4	
Physical							**
No abuse	1,250	96.3	5,531	95	6,955	96.1	
Abuse or suspected abuse	48	3.7	292	5.0	285	3.9	
Psychological							**
No abuse	1,092	84.9	4,404	76.4	5,570	77.6	
Abuse or suspected abuse	194	15.1	1,359	23.6	1,607	22.4	
Financial							**
No abuse	1,353	97.1	5,408	92.1	6,800	92.7	
Abuse	41	2.9	464	7.9	532	7.3	

Note: Non-reponse cases are excluded.
**: $p < 0.01$.

Table 9.6: The psychological health, educational background and equivalent income of abuse victims

	All abuse[a]					Physical abuse					Psychological abuse					Financial abuse				
	None		Abuse[b]			None		Abuse[b]			None		Abuse[b]			None		Abuse[b]		
	N	%	N	%	p-value	N	%	N	%	p-value	N	%	N	%	p-value	N	%	N	%	p-value
Self-rated health					**					**					**					**
Excellent	941	81.2	218	18.8		1,059	97.6	26	2.4		918	85.6	155	14.4		1,034	92.7	82	7.3	
Good	7,802	76.1	2,450	23.9		9,139	96.2	360	3.8		7,479	79.4	1,938	20.6		9,165	93.6	626	6.4	
Fair	2,680	70.4	1,129	29.6		3,259	94.4	194	5.6		2,491	73.2	913	26.8		3,320	91.9	293	8.1	
Poor	562	67.7	268	32.3		684	92.6	55	7.4		521	71.7	206	28.3		693	90.1	76	9.9	
Self-rated health (PGC)					**					**					**					**
High (9+)	3,670	82.5	780	17.5		4,138	97.7	99	2.3		3,626	85.9	595	14.1		4,122	94.7	230	5.3	
Ordinary (4–8)	4,485	74.1	1,565	25.9		5,520	96.3	214	3.7		4,448	78.2	1,239	21.8		5,460	93.1	404	6.9	
Low (<4)	1,750	61.7	1,086	38.3		2,390	90.6	227	9.4		1,690	65	911	35.0		2,466	91.7	246	8.3	
Depression (GDS)					**					**					**					**
None	6,512	79.1	1,721	20.9		7,760	97.0	236	3.0		6,605	83.1	1,346	16.9		7,580	94.3	457	5.7	
Mild depression	2,067	67.1	1,012	32.9		2,767	94.1	173	5.9		2,104	72	820	28.0		2,716	91.2	261	8.8	
Moderate to severe depression	517	52.6	466	47.4		821	89.9	102	11.1		519	56.2	404	43.8		851	90.0	95	10.0	
Years of education					n.s.					n.s.					n.s.					**
9 or less	6,872	73.6	2,465	26.4		8,484	96.8	388	3.2		6,860	78	1,931	22.0		8,493	92.2	715	7.8	
10 or more	4,456	74.4	1,535	25.6		5,577	95.8	243	4.2		4,486	77.8	1,279	22.2		5,587	94.4	355	5.6	

Equivalent income (million yen)					*					**					**					**
Less than 2	4,456	71.9	1,741	28.1		5,548	95.1	285	4.9		4,417	76.4	1,364	23.6		5,618	91.6	514	8.4	
More than 2	4,432	75.0	1,474	25.0		5,476	96.0	227	4.0		4,460	78.6	1,217	21.4		5,577	94.0	357	6.0	

Notes.

a: All abuse = Physical, psychological or financial abuse.

b: Abuse = Abuse or suspected abuse.

*: $p < 0.05$, **: $p < 0.001$, n.s.: not siginificant.

Table 9.7: Abuse prevalence by regional type

Abuse type	Urban		Semi-urban		Rural-agricultural		p-value
	N	%	N	%	N	%	
Physical, psychological or financial							*
No abuse	1,863	73.0	1,097	72.1	9,202	75.4	
Abuse or suspected abuse	690	27.0	424	27.9	3,003	24.6	
Physical							n.s.
No abuse	2,255	95.5	1,319	94.6	10,747	95.9	
Abuse or suspected abuse	107	4.5	75.0	5.4	463	4.1	
Psychological							**
No abuse	1,828	77.4	1,043	75.5	8,686	78.5	
Abuse or suspected abuse	535	22.6	338	24.5	2,377	21.5	
Financial							**
No abuse	2,250	91.3	1,348	92.5	10,786	93.3	
Abuse	214	8.7	109	7.5	771	6.7	

*: $p < 0.05$; **: $p < 0.01$; n.s.: not significant.

Seeking advice on abuse & identifying advisors

Table 9.8 shows, for actual and suspected physical/psychological abuse, whether an individual sought advice on the abuse and, when advice was sought, the identity of the advisor/s.

A total of 30.7 percent of people who had experienced physical abuse sought advice while the proportion for psychological abuse was 24.2 percent. However, a total of 50.7 percent had not spoken to anyone about being physically abused. The proportion for psychological abuse was 65.7 percent.

When advice was sought for both physical and psychological abuse, it was most often sought from a 'friend or acquaintance'. Further, of the people who responded with, 'I did not talk to anybody', 22.9 percent of the victims of physical abuse and 16.1 percent of the victims of psychological abuse responded that they would like to talk to somebody who could be trusted.

Points for consideration

The following three points should be taken into consideration when interpreting the results from the present study.

Table 9.8: Identity of advisers by abuse type

	Physical abuse		Psychological abuse	
	N	%	N	%
Consulted with someone (multiple answers)	198	30.7	717	24.2
with friends or acquaintances	193	97.5	523	72.9
with family members or relatives	86	43.4	252	35.1
with doctors	12	6.0	11	1.5
with police	8	4.0	10	1.3
other	5	2.5	16	2.2
Not consulted	327	50.7	1947	65.7
No response	120	18.6	301	10.1

Abuse criteria

There is no consensus in either Japan or overseas on criteria for abuse (Brownwell et al. 2004; Decalmer and Glendenning 1998). Accordingly, it is difficult to clearly elucidate the criteria which would define the type of action – or neglect as the case may be – and its severity and frequency before the term 'abuse' can be applied. A multifaceted approach to such criteria is desirable, one that considers whether an older person's rights have been violated, whether it could be foreseen that their life might be put in danger, or whether their health or livelihood might be compromised (Editorial Committee on the Rights of the Elderly and the Disabled 2006).

In the present study, in order to ascertain whether abuse existed or not, a number of specific behaviors were listed – being kicked, being yelled at, or having one's savings or pension taken – and participants were asked to confirm whether they had experienced any of these. It should be noted, however, that this approach is wholly reliant on self-report and is not an objective measure.

Prevalence of abuse

The present study did not restrict responses in relation to abusive behavior to a certain period, such as 'the past year'. Consequently, it is possible that the cohort experiencing 'abuse' may have responded so because they had been abused in the past although they were not experiencing abuse at the current point in time.

Participant bias

Data was collected in the present study by posting surveys. However, it was not possible to ascertain whether an older person who did not respond (see Box 20) for any number of reasons had experienced abuse. Some of these reasons may have included: the fact that the person had dementia; that the survey had been left somewhere in the house and had not reached the participant; or that the person was depressed and lacked the motivation to complete the survey, among other possible reasons.

On the topic of dementia, however, the sample upon which the analyses were conducted had responded to a survey of 16 pages in length or more, had returned the completed survey in the envelope supplied, and were able to post it. This suggests that the sample subjected to analysis did not include older people with dementia severe enough to prohibit them from understanding the questions or responding appropriately.

Discussion

The present study has three main characteristics: (1) it targeted older people who had not been subject to a care-needs assessment; (2) it was a large-scale study with 17,257 people subjected to analysis and used a region-representative sample which included either all people within an insurance district or a random sample; and (3) it investigated the nature of abuse as perceived by older people themselves. A discussion of the results follows.

While prevalence studies on elder abuse conducted in the West from the 1980s through to the 1990s (Pillemer and Finkelhor 1988; Ogg and Bennett 1992) have targeted community representative samples, they have not compared prevalence rates between participants who are independent with their activities of daily living (ADL) compared to those requiring long-term care, as was done in the present study. Further, while telephone-based research on the prevalence of abuse has been conducted in Sweden and Denmark (Tornstam 1989), Canada (Podnicks 1992) and other locations, again, this has not compared prevalence rates between participants who are independent with their ADLs compared to those requiring long-term care.[1]

In the present study, a total of 16.3 percent (95 percent confidence interval, 15.7 percent–16.8 percent) of older people who had not been subjected to a care-needs assessment for long-term care insurance had experienced either physical, psychological or financial abuse.

When the independent and the assistance-required groups were examined separately, 16.0 percent (95 percent confidence interval, 15.4 percent–16.5 percent) of the independent group reported abuse while 22.1 percent (95 percent confidence interval, 18.9 percent–25.4 percent) of the assistance-required group reported abuse, with abuse significantly more prevalent in the assistance-required group. In 2000, the same year in which the present study was conducted, the AGES project conducted a survey on 5,918 older people requiring care who were using long-term care insurance services. The proportion of older people in which abuse (physical, psychological and financial abuse, and abandonment) was suspected was 20.8 percent (95 percent confidence interval, 19.0 percent–21.0 percent) which was significantly higher than for the participants in the present study who had not been subjected to a care-needs assessment (Kato 2004). These results suggest an increase in abuse when regular assistance or long-term care is required.

In terms of the relationship between abuse, sex and household type, financial abuse was more prevalent in men, while two-person households were more common in the 'abuse/suspected abuse' combined cohort compared to the 'no abuse' group. In comparison to physical abuse and neglect which are readily observable, financial abuse is difficult for bystanders to observe. Many middle-aged people do not consider the act of a spouse or child using or taking an older person's savings or pension for their own purposes without the older person's permission to be abuse (Takekuma and Shono 2006). However, the group who had experienced financial abuse had significantly poorer psychological health than the group reporting no abuse. Given the fact that a person who has had their savings or pension stolen is troubled by this act, it is important to raise awareness that the act of using or taking an older person's savings or pension without their permission is injurious to their self-respect. Further, the psychological health of the physical and psychological 'abuse/suspected abuse' combined cohort was poorer than the 'no abuse' group. Depression, in particular, is a risk factor for a deterioration in functioning that necessitates long-term care (Comijs et al. 1998). This highlights the necessity of immediately developing anti-abuse measures from the perspective of home care service provision as well.

With regards to the relationship between abuse, years of education and income, more research has been done on child abuse than on elder abuse. Research on child abuse has found a higher prevalence among lower social classes such as those experiencing poverty or the unemployed (Stuck et al. 1999). Pelton (1978) noted that the claim that abuse is not related to social class is a myth which ignores the evidence. The standpoint of abuse victims is different in child abuse compared to elder abuse. Further research is required on how differences such as those stemming from poverty or low academic achievement relate to abuse. The findings from the present study seem to suggest that regional characteristics, in some way, relate to abuse. Currently, each local government is putting together a response to elder abuse based on their individual circumstances. Another reason for drilling down into the relationship between abuse and regional characteristics is that it is important from the perspective of drafting policy and hence remains a subject for future research.

Further, the very fact that neglecting to respond to abuse has the potential to exacerbate it only highlights the necessity of early identification and carrying out an appropriate intervention (Kato et al. 2004). The present study found that advice was most frequently sought from friends and acquaintances. The problem here lies in whether the friends or acquaintances recognize the content of the discussion as abuse and is promptly able to link the person into an appropriate service (Tsunoda 2006). Local governments need to do a number of things in the future. They need to conduct an awareness campaign on elder abuse which targets a wide cross-section of the general community. They also need to establish services which victims of abuse feel safe to approach for advice and to ensure these services have a high profile amongst residents.

Summary

The present study found that a total of 16.3 percent of older people who have not been subject to a care-needs assessment for long-term care insurance had experienced physical, psychological or financial abuse. Physical and psychological abuse was more prevalent in women while financial abuse was more prevalent in men. Abuse was related to poor mental health and was more prevalent in cohorts with lower income levels, and in semi-urbanised communities.

An important challenge for future policy is the development of an anti-abuse framework which also takes into account the needs of older people who have not been subject to a care-needs assessment. Other challenges include the prompt establishment of an abuse counselling service and a corresponding public awareness campaign.

Note

1. The research on prevalence rates of elder abuse in different countries (Research Review Committee 2004; Plillemer and Finkelhor 1988; Ogg and Bennett 1992) reports rates of 3.2 percent, 5.6 percent and 4 percent respectively. Comijs et al. (1998) reports a prevalence rate over the past year of 5.6 percent. However, since these studies used different definitions of abuse and used different sampling and research methods, it was not possible to conduct an international comparison.

Chapter 10

Marital Status and Health

Kei Suemori

Introduction

Research conducted in Japan and elsewhere has demonstrated that multiple factors have a combined effect on older people's health. These include socioeconomic factors (e.g. educational background and income), lifestyle factors (e.g. time spent walking and alcohol consumption), and social network factors (e.g. the provision of social support) (Berkman and Kawachi 2000).

In studies of health promotion, the main focus tends to be on physical functioning, such as increasing muscle strength, addressing malnutrition, and improving speech, feeding and swallowing. Naturally these efforts are important, but a broader view of the social environments and lifestyles which help to maintain and improve older people's health is also important. In particular, determining how to create and sustain older people's social networks is key to forging social environments and lifestyles which support older people's health (Berkman and Syme 1979; House et al. 1982).

One social network factor that can impact upon older people's health is family. Previous research has demonstrated a relationship between marital status and older people's health. This has been shown, for instance, in overseas research which has found lower levels of depression in individuals with a spouse than those without (Verbrugge 1979; Ross and Mirowsky 2002).

The correlation between older people's marital status and health has been investigated, to some degree, in research conducted overseas. Little research has been done in Japan, however, to investigate the relationship between marital status and health in the older population. The aim of the present chapter is to investigate precisely this. Specifically, the present study aims to elucidate aspects of the relationship between the types of household, marital status, marital satisfaction and older people's health on the basis of AGES data.

Basic statistics on married people in Japan and the United States

Prior to reviewing previous research and conducting the set analyses, a brief overview will be made of the proportion of married people across Japan and the United States. The proportion of married people across Japan and the United States is shown in Figure 10.1 by sex although it should be noted that a close comparison is not possible since the research was conducted across different periods. First, the proportion of married people will be compared across Japan and the United States for individuals 15 years and older.

If we initially consider men, we note that the rate is 61.8 percent in Japan and 57.3 percent in the United States, with the proportion of married men slightly higher in Japan. For women, the values are 58.2 percent in Japan and 52.4 percent in the United States, with the proportion of married women again higher in Japan than in the United States. It is evident that the proportion of married people is higher in Japan than in the United States for both men and women.

Next, the proportion of married people will be considered solely for those individuals 65 years and older, the focus of the current research. For men, the values were 83.1 percent in Japan and 74.8 percent in the United States. For women, the values were 45.5 percent in Japan and 38.6 percent in the United States. In both Japan and the United States, the proportion of married men is higher in individuals of 65 years of age or older when compared to the total population (above 15 years of age). It should be noted, however, that the proportion of

Figure 10.1: Percentage of married people in the USA and Japan by sex

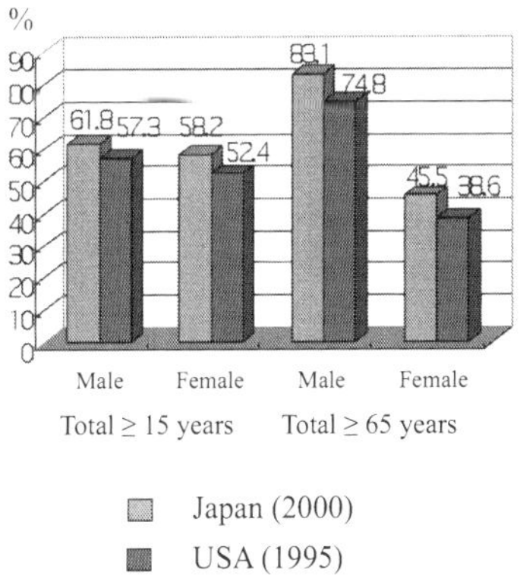

Source: National Institution of Population and Social Security Research (Japan)

married women is lower in individuals of 65 years of age or older when compared to the total population. While sex differences exist, the fact remains that there is a higher proportion of both men and women 65 years of age or older who are married in Japan than in the United States.

This comparison suggests that, while the same fundamental pattern in the proportions of married people is observable in both Japan and the United States, the proportion of married people is higher in both men and women in Japan than in the United States.

Theoretical background & prior research

Marital status and health: Three hypotheses

Much research has examined the relationship between families and health. The relationship between marital status and health has attracted considerable interest (Ross and Mirowsky 1990; Aseltine and Kessler 1993). Research has demonstrated that in comparison to unmarried people, in general, married people have lower mortality rates, lower morbidity rates, and better mental health (e.g. higher self-rated health, lower distress etc.) (Grundy and Holt 2000).

However, there has not been adequate research highlighting the process by which marital status leads to health inequalities (Joung et al. 1998). Consequently, research in recent years has focused on explaining the process by which health gaps emerge as a result of marital status. The pertinent issues raised above give rise to three major theoretical hypotheses explaining the link between marital status and health.

The first hypothesis is referred to as the 'protection hypothesis' (Ren 1997). This hypothesis suggests that marriage has a positive impact on a person's health by providing economic stability, encouraging spouses to adopt healthy behaviors, and by providing emotional support.

The second hypothesis is the 'loss hypothesis', which suggests that, rather than marriage having a protective effect, the loss of a spouse has a deleterious effect on health which, as a result, makes it appear that married people have better health outcomes. The differences between the 'loss hypothesis' and the 'protection hypothesis' can be found in their respective conceptualisations of marriage. According to the 'loss hypothesis', marriage in and of itself has fundamentally no impact on improving health but, rather, any health-related discrepancies resulting from marital status emerge primarily as a result of losing a spouse.

There is empirical research to support the 'loss hypothesis'. In recent years, there has been a move in research away from the dichotomy of people 'with' and 'without' a spouse. Instead, the 'without a spouse' category has been broken down into the finer grained distinctions of 'unmarried', 'divorced' and 'widowed'. After doing this, research has failed to find any health differences between unmarried individuals and married people, but has found that divorced/widowed individuals have lower health statuses (Williams et al. 1992).

The third hypothesis is the 'selection hypothesis'. This hypothesis proposes that married individuals are not healthier, but rather it is easier for someone who is healthy to find and keep a spouse. In a sense, the 'selection hypothesis' inverts the causal relationship of the 'protection hypothesis'. The logic of the 'selection hypothesis' is not that an individual is healthy as a result of being married but, rather, that a person is married because they are healthy.

In recent years, a longitudinal study has yielded support for this hypothesis. The longitudinal research has revealed that individuals with poor levels of health are 1.5 times more likely to divorce. While the authors of this paper concede that more research is required, they state that, in relation to divorce at the very least, the 'selection hypothesis' more or less fits (Joung et al. 1998). Other authors have commented that, from the outset, unhealthy people are more likely to marry unhealthy people thus increasing the risk of being widowed which, again, would lower their level of health (Joung et al. 1998).

In summary, differences in health based on marital status lend support to the 'loss hypothesis' and the 'selection hypothesis' but less so to the 'protection hypothesis'. Previous research conducted overseas has found that low levels of health in the divorced/widowed cohort give rise to differences in marital status (put the other way, there is no clear difference between being unmarried or being married). This research has also demonstrated that it is easier for healthy people to stay married.

The three hypotheses discussed above are the basic theories used to explain health differences based on marital status. The present study will investigate which of these three hypotheses is the most appropriate. Arguments on sex differences will be introduced next.

Sex differences

Some arguments on sex differences state that the emergence of disparities in health due to marital status is heterogeneous across the population. Previous research has found that married men enjoy greater health benefits from marriage than do women. This can be explained by the fact that, in many modern societies, there are sex differences in the performance of care. Often women are left to bear the burden of child-rearing and nursing-care while men are relieved of these familial responsibilities such that marriage tends to afford men more benefits.

The present research is the first large-scale study in Japan investigating marital status and older people's health. The present analyses will examine the relationship between a person's marital status and their health as well as whether sex differences exist.

Method

The present study drew on three data sets to examine associations between household type, marital status and health. The present analyses employed data from a survey centered on questions relating to family in particular. (A total of 15,125 surveys were distributed and 8,067 were returned, a response rate of 53.3 percent.) The sample comprises 15,348 people. However, the number of cases differs according to the questions used.

The variables measured were levels of depression (Geriatric Depression Scale; GDS), self-rated health (four sets of questions collapsed into two sets), types of household, marital status (unmarried, married & divorced/widowed), marital satisfaction, socioeconomic status and age. For socioeconomic status, years of school-based education and equivalent income (calculated by dividing the annual household income by the square root of the number of people in the household) were used (see Box 2).

Results

Types of household, marital status & marital satisfaction

Table 10.1 shows the types of household by sex and age. Overall, two-person households were the most prevalent followed by people living with a spouse and their children. Sex differences were also observed with many women reporting they lived alone or did not have a spouse but lived with their children.

With respect to marital status, a higher proportion of men reported being married (Table 10.2). This may be due to the generally higher longevity of women compared to men.

Table 10.1: Types of household (by sex & age) (%)

	n	Live alone	2-person household with spouse	Live with spouse & children	No spouse but live with children	Other
Male						
65–69	2,803	3.6	45.9	37.1	4.0	9.4
70–74	2,264	4.1	48.7	33.0	6.5	7.8
75–79	1,459	5.2	46.4	32.2	8.1	8.1
80–84	633	4.9	34.0	37.1	13.6	10.4
85 +	256	8.2	27.0	30.1	27.3	7.4
Total	7,415	4.3	45.2	34.6	7.2	8.7
(n)		(320)	(3,350)	(2,569)	(533)	(643)
Female						
65–69	2,689	11.0	40.5	26.9	13.2	8.5
70–74	2,273	16.7	32.2	23.8	19.0	8.4
75–79	1,669	18.4	21.8	20.0	29.4	10.5
80–84	845	20.1	10.5	11.6	44.7	13.0
85 +	457	17.1	3.1	3.3	61.7	14.9
Total	7,933	15.5	28.8	21.5	24.4	9.7
(n)		(1,231)	(2,287)	(1,708)	(1,935)	(772)

Numbers in brackets represent the number of people.

Table 10.2: Marital status (by sex & age) (%)

	Male				Female			
	n	Married	Widowed/ divorced	Unmarried	n	Married	Widowed/ divorced	Unmarried
65–69	4,461	92.6	6.5	0.9	4,733	74.9	23.0	2.1
70–74	4,039	91.7	7.9	0.4	4,527	63.3	34.0	2.8
75–79	2,859	88.1	11.5	0.4	3,439	49.0	48.6	2.4
80–84	1,319	81.0	18.7	0.3	2,001	29.0	68.9	2.1
85 +	617	66.9	32.4	0.6	934	9.5	89.9	0.5
Total	13,295	89.0	10.4	0.6	15,634	56.1	41.7	2.3
(n)		(11,836)	(1,383)	(76)		(8,766)	(6,516)	(352)

The next analysis was limited to marital satisfaction (Table 10.3). Overall, the majority of responses were 'satisfied'. However, a disproportionate number of people failed to respond to this question compared to other questions, so it remains possible that people who were not satisfied simply failed to respond. Of the people who did respond,

Table 10.3: Marital satisfaction (by sex & age)[a] (%)

	Male				Female			
	n	High	Medium	Low	n	High	Medium	Low
65–69	2,048	22.9	68.8	8.3	1,865	14.9	67.9	17.3
70–74	1,869	28.0	64.2	7.8	1,479	16.0	64.2	19.8
75–79	1,261	32.4	60.7	7.0	868	15.9	65.7	18.4
80–84	555	33.3	60.2	6.5	320	14.7	65.0	20.3
85 +	239	31.0	58.6	10.5	49	16.3	71.4	12.2
Total	5,972	27.8	64.4	7.8	4581	15.4	66.1	18.5
(n)		(1661)	(3846)	(465)		(706)	(3029)	(846)

Note: The 'high' group comprised participants who responded 'very satisfied'. The 'medium' group comprised 'satisfied' and 'somewhat satisfied' responses. The 'low' group responded with 'somewhat dissatisfied', 'dissatisfied' and 'very dissatisfied'.

however, men reported high levels of marital satisfaction. For instance, while approximately 25 percent of men were 'very satisfied', only about 15 percent of women were 'very satisfied'. Conversely, women were more likely to respond that they were 'dissatisfied' than men.

Marital status, older people's depression & self-rated health

Using the general linear model on age-corrected data, the next analysis focused on how the type of household, marital status and marital satisfaction relate to depression and self-rated health (Table 10.4).

An analysis of the relationship between household types and depression revealed that, for men, the proportion of people responding with 'mildly depressed' or 'depressed' was significantly higher for those who lived alone than for other groups. In particular, when compared to other types of households, with depression rates at 5.5 percent to 9.6 percent, the proportion of men living by themselves who were depressed was comparatively high at just under 20 percent. The proportion of women reporting no depression was slightly lower in those living alone, although not to the same degree as for men.

There were, however, no significant differences with men's self-rated health. Women, however, were more likely to report higher levels of self-rated health if they did not have a spouse (either they lived alone or they did not have a spouse but lived with their children).

The relationship between marital status and older people's health was examined next. Levels of depression were lower in married people

Table 10.4: Types of household, depression & self-rated health (%)

Type of household	No depression		Mild depression		Moderate to severe depression		Self-rated health (poor)	
	Male	Female	Male	Female	Male	Female	Male	Female
Living alone	51.3	62.9	31.0	28.0	17.7	9.1	29.7	26.7
2-couple household with spouse	71.8	68.0	21.7	24.7	6.5	7.4	27.0	30.7
Living with spouse & children	73.3	68.4	21.2	24.8	5.5	6.8	26.9	30.4
No spouse but living with children	64.1	70.9	26.3	21.8	9.6	7.3	31.2	25.4
Other	70.8	67.0	22.8	22.6	6.5	10.4	30.2	27.9
p-value	***	**	**	*	***	*	ns	**

Notes.

***: $p < 0.001$; **: $p < 0.01$; *: $p < 0.05$.

Geriatric depression scale (GDS: 15-item version: "No depression" – GDS score of 4 or less; "Mild depression" – GDS score of 5 to 9; "Moderate to severe depression" – GDS score of 10 or more.

Self-rated health: Responded "fair" or "poor" with respect to their current health (low group).

and higher in people who had been widowed or who were divorced or unmarried. This was particularly evident for men.

The relationship between marital status and self-rated health (Table 10.5), however, failed to reach significance in men. Married women evaluated their self-rated health as lower compared to widowed/divorced and unmarried individuals.

We have seen thus far that the influence of the types of household and marital status on older people's health differs subtly depending upon whether the focus is on levels of depression or self-rated health.

The relationship between marital satisfaction, depression and self-rated health is examined next (Table 10.6). These were all statistically significant. As marital satisfaction increased, depression decreased and self-rated health increased. Note, however, that in the low marital satisfaction cohort, over 20 percent of men and women were classified as moderately to severely depressed. The findings on marital status suggest that married people with low marital satisfaction are more likely to be depressed/mildly depressed, and to have lower levels of self-rated health than unmarried, divorced or widowed individuals.

Table 10.5: Depression & self-rated health (by marital status)

Type of Marital status	No depression		Mild depression		Moderate to severe depression		Self-rated health (poor)	
	Male	Female	Male	Female	Male	Female	Male	Female
Married	69.5	67.4	23.4	25.0	7.0	7.6	29.1	31.1
Widowed/ divorced	57.7	66.2	28.4	25.3	13.9	8.5	28.7	26.0
Unmarried	41.5	57.5	41.2	28.9	17.3	13.6	27.6	28.3
p-value	***	**	***	ns	***	**	ns	***

Notes.
General linear model results after adjusting for age.
***: $p < 0.001$; **: $p < 0.01$; *: $p < 0.05$.

Table 10.6: Depression & self-rated health (by marital status)

Type of satisfaction	No depression		Mild depression		Moderate to severe depression		Self-rated health (poor)	
	Male	Female	Male	Female	Male	Female	Male	Female
Low	38.5	38.6	37.5	38.5	24.0	22.9	44.5	41.8
Medium	67.3	71.0	25.7	23.8	7.0	5.2	28.6	26.4
High	80.0	84.4	16.8	14.1	3.2	1.5	24.1	24.7
p-value	***	***	***	***	***	***	***	***

Notes.
General linear model results after adjusting for age.
***: $p < 0.001$; **: $p < 0.01$; *: $p < 0.05$.

Socioeconomic status

The findings thus far can be summarised as follows. With respect to the types of household, there was a higher prevalence of depression in men who lived alone. For marital status, essentially depression is elevated in both men and women without a spouse (with this more pronounced in men). The self-rated health of married women, when viewed overall, is lower compared to women without a spouse. For the group with low marital satisfaction, the proportion of people with depression or poor self-rated health was higher in both men and women who had been widowed, or were divorced or unmarried, with the value at roughly 30 percent.

An examination of the relationship between social and economic status follows. However, due to space restrictions, analyses will be limited to the following two investigations. The first examines the relationship between men who live alone and socioeconomic status. The reason for focusing on this lies in the fact that, despite the small number of cases overall, the proportion of men who live by themselves who are depressed is clearly higher at just under 20 percent than men with other living arrangements.

While no relationship was observed between men who lived alone and equivalent income, a statistically significant relationship was observed for years of education (Figure 10.2). These findings indicate that many more men with an education of six years or less lived alone.

The second investigation focused on the relationship between marital satisfaction and socioeconomic status. The focus here will be put on the results for women for whom both relationships were stronger. While no relationship was seen with years of education, the correlation with equivalent income was significant (Figure 10.3). The findings indicate that women experience lower levels of marital satisfaction the lower their level of equivalent income.

Discussion

The findings from the above analyses can be summarised as follows. First, in terms of types of household, it was demonstrated that many men who live alone are depressed. It was also shown that the likelihood of a man living alone increased as his level of education

Figure 10.2: Percentage of males living alone (by years of education)

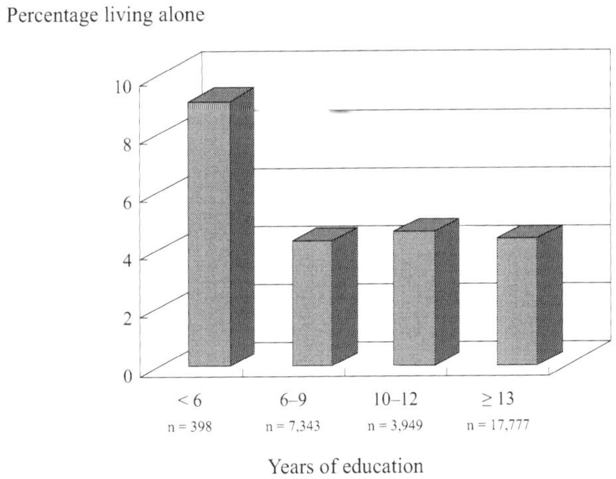

Figure 10.3: Low marital satisfaction in females (by equivalent income) (%)

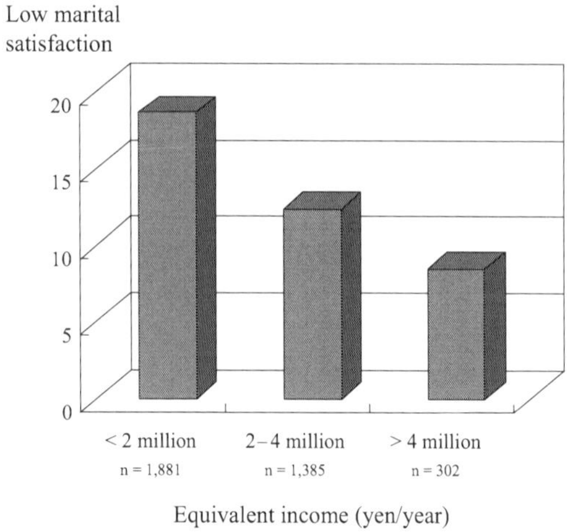

decreased. These findings hint at the importance of a person's social class when considering the relationship between family and health (Baba and Kondo 2003).

In relation to marital status, it was demonstrated that essentially a high proportion of men and women without a spouse are depressed or mildly depressed. When depression was used as the dependent variable, married people were generally shown to be healthier than those without a spouse. These findings lend support to the 'protection hypothesis'.

The relationship between self-rated health and type of household or marital status, however, was not as clear as it was for depression. For instance, when self-rated health was the dependent variable, there was no statistically significant difference found in men. This indicates that differences observed in the relationship with marital status depend upon which index is used in the analysis.

The present study used cross-sectional data and thus it is not possible to draw any conclusions about cause and effect. Accordingly, the 'selection hypothesis' remains potentially viable. Findings from research overseas suggest that married people are not necessarily healthier although the conclusions are not clear (White 1992; Williams et al. 1992). Further research is needed in this area.

Furthermore, more married women evaluated their self-rated health as low than women without a spouse. The finding that married people have lower self-rated health than those without a spouse is unique and has not been seen in previous research conducted overseas. As previously mentioned, this finding adds support to the argument that women enjoy fewer benefits from being married than men. The positive effects for married people are also stronger in men when levels of depression were considered. It would appear that, in the end, men consistently enjoy more benefits from marriage than women. The question remains, however, why this might be the case. The following interpretation may be plausible if we recall that the participants in the present study were older people. First, since men have a shorter lifespan, it is more likely that women will encounter the risks associated with nursing their spouse and more likely that their own health will deteriorate from the burden associated with caring for their spouse. An alternative explanation is that many unmarried people may be admitted to hospital or residential care, and hence it was only relatively healthy unmarried people who responded to the present survey. This would skew the results towards finding that married people had relatively poorer self-rated health.

In relation to marital satisfaction, it was found that over 20 percent of both men and women in the low satisfaction group were depressed. Comparing this to the findings for marital status, we notice that married people with low marital satisfaction have poorer self-rated health than unmarried or widowed individuals. These results suggest that, in addition to the effect of marital status, the nature of the marital relationship itself has an association with depression and self-rated health.

Analyses by regional type failed to yield any clear, region-based differences. We hope region-based differences are examined in future research.

Conclusions

The present study investigated the relationship between marital status and older people's health. More unmarried people were found to be depressed or mildly depressed than married people for both men and women. For self-rated health, while no clear relationship existed in men, women without a spouse reported higher self-rated health than married women.

The main finding relevant to home help service provision is the issue of mental health in men living alone. Previous research has found a relationship between depression and falls, meaning that such a finding cannot be ignored. The number of cases is small but this means that it could be easily targeted. The present findings on men living alone speak to the necessity of comprehensive community initiatives including suicide-prevention.

Further, the present findings also indicate that married women experience lower levels of self-rated health than those who are widowed or divorced. While there are many possible interpretations for this finding, one possible interpretation previously alluded to is that wives are shouldering the burden of caring for their husbands.

People are less likely today to expect their children to nurse them than previously, making an increase in spouse-based nursing care inevitable. Married women are faced with an increased likelihood that they will have to shoulder the burden of nursing their husbands.

Couples were one of the main household types for older people. While older couples attract less focus than single-person households, it will be important to provide home help services to men in older couples not only to preserve the men's health but also to maintain the health of older women.

Chapter 11

Membership in Community Organizations

Gōshu Yoshikawa

Introduction

This chapter discusses older people's membership in community organizations. In Japan, the organizations that older people most typically join are senior citizens' clubs (*rōjinkurabu*) (see Box 14). There are many other types of organizations that older persons can join, too, such as volunteer and hobby groups (JGSS Research Center).

Such organizations are expected not only to prevent housebound behavior by promoting the social participation of older people (see Chapter 8) but also function as social networks that provide some of the forms of social support that are believed to promote health (see Chapter 12). Social networks have also been used as an indicator of social capital (see Chapter 14), which is of increasing interest to researchers for its perceived association with health. However, a comparative study on the membership of adults (aged twenty-one years or older) in voluntary associations in fifteen countries, including Japan, has reported a relatively low membership rate in Japan (Curtis et al. 1992).

Under these circumstances, this chapter will discuss the condition of older people's membership in organizations, analyze the potential associations between older persons' membership in organizations and certain health indices (i.e. self-rated health status and depression), and assess whether there are any differences in older people's membership in organizations according to their level of income, years of education and the type of region they live in.

Older persons' social participation, social networks, social capital and health

Older persons' participation or membership in organizations has been studied for a relatively long time, both in and outside of Japan. In

Japanese studies, participation in organizations has been primarily discussed as a factor constituting part of social participation, social integration, social activities or social networks. Only a limited number of studies have dealt with participation in organizations as an independent topic. Similarly, many overseas studies have regarded participation in organizations as part of social participation or social networks. However, a number of studies have also focused on voluntary associations themselves. In recent years, there have also been an increasing number of studies discussing participation in organizations as an index of social capital.

In Japan, the organizations that have most frequently been discussed in the context of social participation (and in the other contexts as above) include local community organizations (such as neighborhood associations and senior citizens' clubs) and hobby-oriented organizations (Anme and Shimada 2000; Satō et al. 2002; Fujita et al. 2004). Other organizations that have been discussed in these contexts include religious organizations, associations of commerce and industry, volunteer groups and consumers' associations (Kishi et al. 1994; Kishi et al. 1996; Sugisawa 1994; Sugisawa, Nakatani and Maeda et al. 1994; Aoki 1997; Kim et al. 2004). One study discussed participation in sporting activities by neighborhood associations consisting of workers in their fifties (Satō and Fukuwatari 1998), rather than older persons.

In contrast, overseas studies of membership in organizations (including those targeting populations other than older people) have discussed fraternal, veterans' and nationality groups and other organizations that are not well known in Japan (Cutler 1976; Rotolo 1999; Cutler and Hendricks 2000). Churches and other religious organizations have also been frequently discussed (Cutler 1976; Rotolo 1999; Cutler and Hendricks 2000; Rietschlin 1998; Oman and Reed 1998).

Some Japanese studies have reported that persons who have higher rates of social participation or social integration, including membership in these organizations or participation in organization activities, have lower mortality rates (Anme and Shimada 2000; Sugisawa, Liang and Liu 1994) and, in men, a better life prognosis (Sugisawa 1994). Other studies have reported that persons who have higher rates of social activity participation or social integration have higher self-rated health status (Satō and Fukuwatari 1998), lower rates of depression (Aoki 1997) and, in men, better prognosis of daily living activities (Sugisawa, Nakatani and Maeda et al. 1994). Overseas studies have reported that social networks, including participation or membership in organizations, reduce mortality in older populations

(Oman and Reed 1998; Fuhrer et al. 1999) as well as middle-aged and older populations (Eng et al. 2002), and that, not only in older people but also in younger people, membership in organizations is negatively correlated with mental distress; the larger the number of memberships a person has, the stronger the alleviating effect of membership on his/her mental distress (Rietschlin 1998).

However, most of these studies from both Japan and overseas discuss participation or membership in organizations regardless of the number and/or types of organizations participated in by subjects, and few studies have focused on the types of organizations. This has made it quite unclear how, and what kind of, organization is associated with the psychosocial and economic well-being of older people. Japanese studies comparing different types of organizations have shown that: the types of organizations joined by older people are different for different ages and genders (Kishi et al. 1996); the membership rates are different in different regions (Kishi et al. 1994); and, in terms of the association between older women's membership and self-rated sense of well-being (Nobe 1999), members of religious organizations, hobby groups and sports groups have a higher self-rated sense of well-being.

Early overseas studies that discussed the types of organizations include a USA study on the potential of sixteen different types of associations with life satisfaction and happiness (Cutler 1976). The results of this study found that, out of the various organizations, only church-affiliated groups showed an association with life satisfaction and happiness. A more recent study (Baum et al. 2000) conducted on subjects aged eighteen years or older living in Adelaide, Australia discussed social participation by type of organization, including participation in several different organizations (such as social clubs, hobby groups, self-help/support groups and service groups), and certain factors related to participation in these organizations. The results showed that: participation in some types of organizations (social clubs, etc.) was associated with older age (sixty years or older), while another type of organization (school-related groups) was associated with younger ages (between eighteen and fifty-nine years); participation in some types of organizations (hobby groups, etc.) was associated with higher education levels, while another type of organization (social clubs) was associated with lower education levels; and participation in some types of organizations (political parties, campaigns and trade unions) was associated with higher household income.

In recent years, the association between social capital and health has attracted attention (Szreter and Woolcock 2004; De Silva et al.

2005; Ichida et al. 2009). One component of social capital is social networks, and various published studies have discussed organizations as a form of social network. These studies have discussed various organizations as 'voluntary associations', including: church groups, sports groups and professional societies (Kawachi et al. 1999); neighborhood associations (Lochner et al. 2003; Kim et al. 2005); and labor unions and seniors' groups (Kim et al. 2005). However, few studies have conducted an analysis by type of organization.

In short, while participation or membership in organizations has been discussed from various perspectives, only a limited number of studies have discussed it by type of organization. However, as some overseas studies have shown, there is a possibility that Japanese organizations may have different health affects depending on their types. This chapter discusses differences by type of organization in association with health indices, income, years of education and regional types.

Method

As in other chapters, the data used in this chapter were collected by the AGES (Aichi Gerontological Evaluation Study) project (see Box 2) on 32,891 subjects aged sixty-five years or older who lived at home within the areas covered by twelve long-term care insurers (corresponding to fifteen municipalities) (see Chapter 1). This chapter analyzes the associations of membership in organizations with health indices (i.e., self-rated health status [Box 6] and depression [Box 7]), years of education and income (equivalent income, see Box 3), and regional types (see Chapter 1) in the 24,405 subjects (consisting of 11,523 men and 12,882 women) who responded to all questions about their gender and their membership in eight different types of organizations. Eight different types of organizations are discussed: political organizations/groups (hereafter, 'political organizations'); industrial organizations/trade associations (hereafter, 'industrial organizations'); volunteer groups; citizens'/consumer action groups (hereafter, 'citizens' action groups'); religious organizations/groups (hereafter, 'religious organizations'); sports-oriented groups/clubs (hereafter, 'sports clubs'); neighborhood associations, senior citizens' clubs, volunteer fire corps and similar groups (hereafter, 'neighborhood associations/senior citizens' clubs'); and hobby groups. The survey asked subjects, using questions with two answer choices, whether or not they join in any of these organizations. While the eight types of organizations and groups were chosen on the basis of those used in the JGSS (JGSS Research Center), the AGES project added 'neighborhood associations, senior citizens' clubs, volunteer fire corps and similar groups' as a type of local community organization.

This chapter analyzes men and women separately, in respect of the fact that previous studies have reported gender differences in membership or participation in organizations (Curtis et al. 1992; Satō et al. 2002; Kishi et al. 1996). In the following analyses, the number of samples is different in each analysis as a result of missing values in the different variables used, such as health indices, income and years of education.

In the present analyses, ANCOVA was used and age-adjusted estimates were calculated using the SPSS General Linear Model procedure.

Results

Age distribution of membership in organizations

First, subjects' membership rates in various organizations are shown by age group (Tables 11.1 and 11.2).

In both men and women, over 60 percent of subjects joined in one or more organizations. In both genders, neighborhood associations/senior citizens' clubs had the highest proportion of memberships, followed by hobby groups and sports clubs.

Compared to women, a significantly higher proportion of men joined in one or more organizations ($p < 0.001$). Analysis by type of organization showed a significantly higher proportion of male subjects joining in all types of organizations except for citizens' action groups, hobby groups, and religious organizations ($p < 0.01$ for neighborhood associations and $p < 0.001$ for all other types of organizations). In particular, the proportion of subjects joining in industrial organizations and in volunteer groups both exceeds 10 percent in men but is considerably lower in women. In contrast, a higher proportion of women joined in hobby groups ($p < 0.001$).

No significant age-related increase or decrease in the membership rate was observed in one or more organizations, although some types of organizations (i.e., volunteer groups and sports clubs in men and political organizations, industrial organizations, citizens' action groups, sports clubs and hobby groups in women) showed decreasing membership rates with increasing age, and other types of

Table 11.1: Proportions of male subjects who are members of organizations by age group (%)

	Age (years)					
	Total	**65–69**	**70–74**	**75–79**	**80–84**	**85 +**
Number of subjects analyzed (persons)	11,523	4,030	3,422	2,359	994	469
Joined one or more organizations	66.4	66.6	67.3	66.9	66.4	57.6
Political organizations	9.3	10.3	9.4	8.3	8.1	9.4
Industrial organizations	14.6	16.1	15.1	12.6	12.3	13.2
Volunteer groups	10.1	12.2	10.9	7.8	6.5	4.5
Citizens' action groups	4.1	4.4	4.1	3.8	3.9	3.4
Religious organizations	11.1	10.1	10.3	12.5	14.4	12.8
Sports clubs	17.3	22.2	17.6	12.8	11.5	9.2
Neighborhood association/ senior citizens' clubs	48.3	43.6	50.5	52.1	53.9	45.0
Hobby groups	22.4	23.3	24.3	21.9	17.4	14.9

Table 11.2: Proportions of female subjects who are members of organizations by age group (%)

	Age (years)					
	Total	**65–69**	**70–74**	**75–79**	**80–84**	**85 +**
Number of subjects analyzed (persons)	12,882	4,182	3,673	2,621	1,452	721
Joined one or more organizations	62.7	63.7	63.3	64.3	62.1	50.1
Political organizations	3.5	4.3	3.8	3.0	2.6	1.7
Industrial organizations	4.4	6.0	4.4	3.3	3.3	1.1
Volunteer groups	8.7	12.5	9.3	6.0	4.3	1.8
Citizens' action groups	4.4	5.4	4.8	3.7	3.0	1.1
Religious organizations	11.0	9.9	11.1	12.5	11.9	10.8
Sports clubs	13.4	19.3	13.9	10.3	6.8	3.7
Neighborhood association/ senior citizens' clubs	46.3	40.3	47.0	52.1	53.0	41.9
Hobby groups	27.5	34.9	28.8	25.1	17.1	10.0

organizations (i.e., religious organizations in men and neighborhood associations and senior citizens' clubs in both men and women) showed increasing membership rates with increasing age. This trend, however, was reversed in subjects aged eighty-five years or older.

Associations between membership in organizations and health indices

Table 11.3 shows the associations between subjects' membership in organizations and health indices (the self-rated health status and depression). The figures in the table indicate the age-adjusted proportions of subjects with poor health status or depression, separately for subjects who do and do not join in each type of organization.

First, for both men and women, a significantly lower proportion of subjects who join in organizations than those who do not had a poor self-rated health status in all types of organization, except for women in religious organizations. Of all the subjects who do join in organizations, members in sports clubs were the least likely to report poor self-rated health status in both men and women. Hobby groups had the second lowest proportion of male subjects reporting poor self-rated health status, while volunteer groups had the second lowest proportion of women.

The proportions of subjects reporting depression showed trends similar to those in poor health status, and there is a significant difference between members and non-members in the proportion of subjects with depression.

Associations between membership in organizations and years of education/income

Tables 11.4 and 11.5 show the associations between subjects' membership in organizations and income/years of education. Subjects with more years of education generally tended to have higher membership rates, except that the membership rate was somewhat lower for the group with the most years of education (thirteen years or longer) in political organizations for men and in neighborhood associations/senior citizens' clubs for both men and women. In contrast, there were no significant differences observed between the groups with different years of education in citizens' action groups in men and in religious organizations in women.

Many types of organizations showed a general tendency for membership rates to increase with increasing income. However, some types of organizations showed no significant association between membership and income, including citizens' action groups for both men and women and religious organizations for men.

In sum, in all types of organization other than citizens' and religious organizations, people with higher socioeconomic status,

Table 11.3: Membership in organizations and health indices (%)

Organization membership	Self-rated health status (poor)						Depression (GDS score, ≥ 10 points)					
	Men			Women			Men			Women		
	Yes	No	p-value	Yes	No	p-value	Yes	No	p-value	Yes	No	p-value
Number of subjects analyzed (persons)	Men = 11,062			Women = 12,374			Men = 10,018			Women = 10,469		
Joined one or more organizations	25.5	37.0	***	25.2	34.6	***	5.6	13.0	***	5.1	13.7	***
Political organizations	24.2	29.9	***	24.3	28.9	*	4.9	8.3	***	3.8	8.4	**
Industrial organizations	24.2	30.2	***	21.7	29.0	***	3.7	8.7	***	2.5	8.5	***
Volunteer groups	20.6	30.3	***	16.8	29.8	***	3.5	8.5	***	2.1	8.8	***
Citizens' action groups	23.5	29.6	**	20.5	29.1	***	3.9	8.1	**	3.0	8.5	***
Religious organizations	26.5	29.7	*	29.5	28.6	n.s.	6.2	8.2	*	6.5	8.4	*
Sports clubs	17.8	31.8	***	16.0	30.7	***	2.5	9.2	***	2.4	9.2	***
Neighborhood association/ senior citizens' clubs	26.1	32.4	***	25.3	31.6	***	5.5	10.4	***	4.7	11.4	***
Hobby groups	20.2	32.0	***	19.2	32.3	***	3.0	9.5	***	3.0	10.3	***

Notes.

Figures indicate results adjusted for age using a general linear model.

*: $p < 0.05$; **: $p < 0.01$; ***: $p < 0.001$; n.s.: not significant.

Table 11.4: Membership in organizations and years of education/income in men (%)

Organization Membership	Years of education					Equivalent income (in 10,000 yen/year)[a]					
	< 6	6–9	10–12	≥ 13	p-value	< 100	100–199	200–299	300–399	≥ 400	p-value
Number of subjects analyzed (persons)	285	5,867	3,411	1,594		1,200	3,230	2,754	1,785	1,054	
Joined one or more organizations	43.6	61.0	72.9	78.5	***	54.2	61.8	72.0	77.8	78.2	***
Political organizations	6.3	8.4	10.8	10.5	***	7.3	8.0	9.5	11.9	14.0	***
Industrial organizations	6.6	12.2	17.1	19.8	***	14.0	10.2	13.5	18.3	30.6	***
Volunteer groups	4.8	7.4	12.1	16.7	***	5.8	8.0	11.7	13.6	16.0	***
Citizens' action groups	5.1	4.1	3.9	4.1	n.s.	5.2	3.5	4.0	4.5	3.7	n.s.
Religious organizations	8.0	10.2	12.1	13.2	**	11.5	11.1	11.4	11.5	11.3	n.s.
Sports clubs	10.7	13.3	20.8	26.2	***	9.1	13.8	20.2	24.1	26.9	***
Neighborhood association/senior citizens' clubs	32.6	46.0	52.8	52.0	***	36.9	45.6	53.2	58.6	52.3	***
Hobby groups	8.1	17.2	27.1	35.0	***	11.5	19.3	25.8	32.5	29.0	***

Notes.

Figures indicate results adjusted for age using a general linear model.

a: Household income (in 10,000 yen/year) divided by the square root of the number of household members.

*: $p < 0.05$; **: $p < 0.01$; ***: $p < 0.001$. n.s.: not significant.

Table 11.5: Membership in organizations and years of education/income in women (%)

Organization Membership	Years of education					Equivalent income (in 10,000 yen/year)[a]					
	< 6	6–9	10–12	≥ 13	p-value	< 100	100–199	200–299	300–399	≥ 400	p-value
Number of subjects analyzed (persons)	771	6,806	4,206	696		1,853	2,841	2,261	1,490	1,039	
Joined in one or more organizations	48.7	59.1	69.9	75.9	***	54.7	61.8	69.2	74.2	71.8	***
Political organizations	3.0	3.1	4.0	6.0	***	3.5	3.3	3.0	4.7	6.0	***
Industrial organizations	2.9	3.8	5.1	7.9	***	4.7	3.8	4.3	5.5	7.3	***
Volunteer groups	5.6	6.4	11.1	20.0	***	6.8	8.6	9.9	13.0	12.8	***
Citizens' action groups	3.2	3.8	5.2	6.3	***	4.5	3.9	4.6	4.9	5.1	n.s.
Religious organizations	10.3	11.0	11.3	12.3	n.s.	12.0	12.7	11.3	10.4	9.7	*
Sports clubs	9.9	11.6	15.6	24.8	***	10.1	12.7	17.4	18.7	17.6	***
Neighborhood association/senior citizens' clubs	33.0	44.9	51.1	48.6	***	38.1	45.4	51.2	55.4	52.4	***
Hobby groups	14.2	21.8	36.3	49.7	***	19.9	26.0	34.0	38.0	38.1	***

Notes.

Figures indicate results adjusted for age using a general linear model.

a: Household income (in 10,000 yen/year) divided by the square root of the number of household members.

*: $p < 0.05$; **: $p < 0.01$; ***: $p < 0.001$; n.s.: not significant.

whether in terms of years of education or income, have higher membership rates.

Association between membership in organizations and regional types

Finally, Table 11.6 shows the proportion of subjects who join in organizations by type of region. In many types of organizations, the membership rates showed differences between regional types. While women in all types of organizations except for volunteer groups showed significant regional differences, for men there were no significant differences observed in four types of organizations, including political organizations. Rural regions had higher membership rates than the other regional types in industrial organizations for both men and women, and religious organizations for women, but had the lowest membership rates of all three regional types in sports clubs and hobby groups. The gap between membership rates of sports clubs and hobby groups in rural regions and membership rates of these organizations in other regional types is wide.

Discussion

Membership in organizations

As discussed, this study revealed that in the target regions, over 60 percent of both men and women joined in one or more organizations, and that the membership rate was different for different types of organizations. While the international comparative study mentioned above, which analyzed only membership in voluntary associations, reported a low membership rate in Japan (Curtis et al. 1992), the present study seems to indicate a relatively active level of membership in organizations by the older population living in the target regions. For both men and women, neighborhood associations/senior citizens' clubs had the highest membership rates. Since a resident is somewhat automatically required to join the neighborhood association in his/her neighborhood (Torigoe 1994), he/she may not be aware of his/her own membership (the fact that the membership of a neighborhood association is a household membership, as is the case with Buddhist temple's *danka* (patron) organizations [see Box 13], is also likely to influence the participants' awareness/lack of awareness of their own membership). Another factor that is likely to have contributed to the higher membership rate in neighborhood associations/senior citizens' clubs than other types of organizations is that in the survey sheet used,

Table 11.6: Membership in organizations and type of region

Organization Membership	Men				Women			
	Rural	Semi-urban	Urban	p-value	Rural	Semi-urban	Urban	p-value
Number of subjects analyzed (persons)	6,279	1,762	3,233		7,838	1,861	2,950	
Joined in one or more organizations	63.0	75.5	68.2	***	59.5	71.8	65.6	***
Political organizations	9.6	9.7	8.8	n.s.	3.3	3.5	4.3	*
Industrial organizations	16.4	14.3	11.4	***	4.9	2.8	4.1	***
Volunteer groups	10.1	9.3	10.5	n.s.	9.0	7.8	8.4	n.s.
Citizens' action groups	4.0	3.4	4.7	n.s.	4.1	3.8	5.3	*
Religious organizations	11.3	10.4	11.3	n.s.	11.6	9.2	10.8	*
Sports clubs	13.9	21.1	21.9	***	11.1	16.1	18.4	***
Neighborhood association/senior citizens' clubs	43.7	62.5	50.0	***	42.7	59.6	47.1	***
Hobby groups	19.1	28.4	25.7	***	24.4	34.0	32.2	***

Notes.

Figures indicate results adjusted for age using a general linear model.

a: Household income (in 10,000 yen/year) divided by the square root of the number of household members.

*: $p < 0.05$; **: $p < 0.01$; ***: $p < 0.001$; n.s.: not significant.

the relevant choice included senior citizens' clubs with which older persons are often asked to be nominally registered even though they do not actually participate in the club/group activities, because these organizations are often entitled to subsidies according to the size of their membership.

Membership in religious organization

While the proportion of subjects joining in religious organizations was approximately 11 percent for both men and women, another survey targeting Japan's older people has reported that over 60 percent of older people regularly pray and offer water, incense, and rice to their ancestors (Krause et al. 1999; this study focused on personal religious activities only, since many Japanese people do not regularly attend formal religious services). Considering the religious population in Japan and Japanese people's sense of participation in religious practices (see Box 13), the proportion cited in the present study seems to represent those older people who conduct religious activities mainly through their affiliation with religious organizations or groups (i.e., persons who are aware of their membership in religious organizations). Some previous overseas studies distinguish people's affiliation with their church from that with other community organizations (Berkman and Syme 1979; Kawachi et al. 1996), suggesting that church affiliation is understood as an important factor constituting part of their social networks. Further studies in this regard will require the development of methods to accurately assess people's religious activities in both personal and organizational aspects.

Association with age

An earlier study has reported that some types of organizations have a higher membership rate of early older persons (e.g., women's membership in hobby groups), while other types of organizations have the opposite tendency (e.g., men's membership in senior citizens' clubs) (Kishi et al. 1996). Although that study cannot be directly compared with this one, due to the differences in target regions, this study confirmed that some types of organizations have increasing membership rates with increasing age of members, while other types have a decreasing membership rate with increasing age. The previously mentioned increasing membership rate in neighborhood associations/senior citizens' clubs with increasing age, seems to indicate that although membership in senior citizens' clubs is open

Box 13: Religious Organizations in Japan

Gōshu Yoshikawa

There are various types of religious organizations in Japan, with a total number of 226,060. The Japanese religious population is also very large and has been reported to be over 213 million persons, partly because individuals often practice more than one religion (Agency for Cultural Affairs 2005).

The majority of Japanese religious organizations are Shinto (39.3 percent) or Buddhist (38.6 percent). Other religious organizations include Christian and other faith communities (22.1 percent). In terms of proportions in the total religious population, Shinto account for the largest proportion (50.3 percent), followed by Buddhists (44.0 percent), with the remainder being represented by Christians and other religions (Agency for Cultural Affairs 2005).

As a matter of fact, many Japanese people are involved in various religious practices throughout their lives, as they say, "Japanese are born Shinto, marry as Christians, and die Buddhists" (Kisala 2006). Other people participate in annual events of various religions by: joining community Shinto shrine festivals, such as the Summer and Autumn festivals; participating in Buddhist events, such as the Buddha's birthday festival (also known as the Flower Festival) and the *Jizō-bon* festival (a local festival for children held in late August); and celebrating Christmas in December. At the household and individual levels, some families observe Buddhist customs by visiting their ancestors' graves, maintaining a Buddhist altar at home and holding memorial services for their ancestors during the *Bon* festival and the *Higan* (equinoctial) weeks, while maintaining a Shinto home altar as well. Thus, Japanese people are involved in religious practices in various settings.

However, it appears that many Japanese people are not very conscious of their own participation in religious practices (or organizations). The world value survey conducted during 2005 and 2006 has reported that approximately 85 percent of Japanese people do not join in church or any religious organizations, which is one of the higher figures among those of the countries surveyed (Dentsu Communication Institute 2008). This might be attributable to some unique features of religious practices in Japan, such as: that "conventional religions in Japan typically do not require official organizational affiliation or weekly meetings" (Miller 1992); that various religious events are often regarded as folklore or common practice (Ama 1996); and that Buddhism has become an inseparable part of Japanese culture (Gorai

1980). Other factors attributed to Japanese people's weak awareness of their own participation in religious practices include that, Buddhism is a 'family's' faith; a person who was born to the family becomes a believer of it upon his/her birth (Uryū 2008). In Shinto, a believer is not 'family' but a parishioner of the 'community', and a person becomes a believer of the community shrine as a result of his/her birth in the community rather than in his/her capacity as an individual (Uryū 2008). Furthermore unlike Christianity, Shinto does not always require personal initiation into the faith (Uryū 2008). These circumstances have resulted in the lack of awareness of personal religious affiliations. For the same reasons, the proportion of people who regard themselves as practicing a religion by personally belonging to a specific religious organization or group is low (this seems to be the reason for the lower membership rate of older persons in religious organizations than in the other organizations discussed in Chapter 11).

A Buddhist community has a *danka* (patron) organization (Kōmoto 1980; Marcure 1985), while a Shinto community has an *ujiko* (parishioner) organization (Okada 1977; Chiba 1980). *Danka* of a temple refers to a family which has appointed the temple as *bodai ji* (the temple which holds services for the family's ancestors). A *danka* organization consists of these families. In contrast, the *ujiko* organization of a shrine is a group of families which are located in the neighborhood of the shrine and believe in the shrine as *ujigami* (ancestors whom they worship as God). However, both types are seldom referred to as formal 'religious organizations.' Therefore, people who belong to these organizations seldom think that they belong to a religious organization.

to persons aged sixty-five or older, sixty-five-year-olds today do not regard themselves as older persons, as previous generations did, and thus often do not participate in these clubs until later in life.

Association with health indices

In most organizations, a lower proportion of the members reported poor health indices. From the perspective of preventing conditions requiring long-term care, it is notable that sports-related organizations, which have been discussed by few studies in Japan, showed a low proportion of subjects with poor health indices. Future cohort studies should aim to clarify whether joining in sports-oriented organizations improves health indices or people who are more confident in their health are more likely to participate in sports and other organizational activities. Religious organizations showed no significant difference between members and non-members in the proportion of women in poor self-rated health status and, compared to other types of organizations, showed smaller differences between participants and non-participants in the proportion of men in poor self-rated health status and in the proportions of both men and women reporting depression. Like sports clubs, it is possible that joining in a religious organization may improve the health indices or the other way around. However, overseas cohort studies have reported that religious activities have positive effects on health (Oman and Reed 1998; Kinney et al. 2003). A Japanese study has also reported that personal religious practices have a 'modest direct effect' on self-rated health status (Krause et al. 1999). We cannot draw any definitive conclusions about this issue because: levels of religious activity are likely to reflect differences between countries as well as different meanings of religion for different peoples; and the data used in the present study is problematic in that subjects' reporting of membership in 'religious organizations' may not always be accurate (i.e., there may be cases where a subject who participated in religious activities or practices responded that he/she did not join in any religious organization, and cases where the subject whose family belonged to a Buddhist temple's *danka* (patron) organization or Shintō shrine's *ujiko* (parishioner) organization, both of which are more like a local community organization, did not regard himself/herself as conducting religious activities; see Box 13). However, it may be that religious organizations more readily accept persons with poor health indices. While a previous Japanese study has reported, in men only, a better life prognosis for those who joined in a larger number of organizations or participated in organizational activities at a higher frequency (Sugisawa 1994), the analysis of the health indices by type of organization conducted in the present study revealed that in both men and women, subjects who join in organizations had better health indices. In addition, while an earlier overseas study, which targeted subjects aged eighteen years or older, has reported a negative association between the number of organizations participated in by subjects and their health as well as negative health effects of conflicts and other negative experiences within organizations (Ziersch and Baum 2004), the analysis by type of organization conducted in this study found no negative associations. Nevertheless, the potential negative effects of membership in organizations on older people are an issue that must be elucidated through interviews and other qualitative survey methods.

Using the same data as used in the present study, Aida et al. (2009) have reported an association between oral health and participation in organizations by dividing the organizations into two different types: (i) vertical organizations with hierarchical structures (e.g., political organizations and associations, industrial and professional groups, religious groups and associations, local community associations, senior citizens' clubs, and volunteer fire-fighting groups); and (ii) horizontal organizations (e.g., volunteer groups, citizens' and consumer action groups, sports groups and clubs, and hobby clubs). Their analysis found that a higher proportion of subjects participating in a larger number of horizontal organizations had twenty or more teeth remaining. Their multi-level analysis also found that, even after individual-level variables have been taken into account, a higher proportion of subjects living in areas with higher participation rates in local horizontal organizations had twenty or more teeth remaining. Thus, another future issue is to analyze the health effects of different types of organizations.

Association with socioeconomic status (SES)

Our analysis of the association between membership in organizations and income/years of education revealed that, generally, more years of education and higher incomes were associated with higher membership rates. However, in the highest income group and the lowest income group, this trend was reversed for some types of organizations. Whether this is an error due to the relatively small numbers of subjects in these groups or has some significance is an issue requiring further research. The present study also revealed that the association between membership in organizations and SES is different in different types of organizations. The fact that more years of education and higher incomes were associated with higher membership rates in political organizations and hobby groups indicates that the trends observed in the Adelaide study are seen in Japan as well (Baum et al. 2000). In citizens' action groups, no significant association with membership was observed for men's years of education and income and women's income. In religious organizations, no significant association with membership was observed for men's income. These can be interpreted as indicating that citizens' and religious organizations accept older people regardless of their income or years of education. Furthermore, the types of organizations whose membership rate increased with increasing income and years of education overlap with those types of organizations whose participants showed a lower proportion of subjects with poor health indices. This indicates that the different associations of the different types of organizations with the health indices demonstrated in this chapter might have been caused by differences in the members' income and years of education instead of the different types of organizations. Further, more detailed studies that take these confounding factors into account are warranted.

Differences between different regional types

Finally, regional differences in rates of membership in organizations have been reported by previous studies, including, for instance: a report from Hokkaido, Japan, which found that urban regions have higher membership rates in functional groups, such as hobby groups, while depopulated regions have higher membership rates in neighborhood associations (Kishi et al. 1994); and another report from Saitama prefecture, which observed regional differences between new towns and old areas (Kim et al. 2004). The analysis conducted in the present study produced similar results, such as the regional differences in the rate of membership in organizations and the urban regions' higher membership rates in sports clubs and hobby groups. However, whether these regional differences are caused by differences in individual-level conditions or organizational-level conditions (e.g., the difficulty of joining, the operation of the organization, etc.) must be clarified through qualitative analyses.

Summary

This chapter analyzed associations between membership in eight different types of organization (i.e., local community organizations and hobby-oriented organizations, which have been discussed by previous Japanese studies, plus political and citizens' organizations, sports club, etc.) and three factors, including certain health indices.

The results can be summarized as follows.

i. Over 60 percent of subjects in the target regions joined in one or more organizations. Neighborhood associations/senior citizens' clubs showed the highest membership rate (46.3 percent–48.3 percent), followed by hobby groups (22.4 percent–27.5 percent) and sports clubs (13.4 percent–17.3 percent). In many types of organizations, men showed a higher membership rate than women, with the proportion of subjects joining in one or more organizations being 66.4 percent and 62.7 percent in men and women, respectively.

Box 14: Senior Citizens' Clubs

Chiyoe Murata

Japanese senior citizens' clubs are independent organizations first established voluntarily by older people soon after World War Two, around 1950, for the purpose of promoting the welfare of community-dwelling older people. Under the Elderly Welfare Law enacted in 1963 and the so-called New Gold Plan (formally known as the New Ten-Year Strategy to Promote Health Care and Welfare for the Elderly) established in 1994, these senior citizens' clubs have been positioned as organizations for promoting older people's social participation and measures to give more meaning to their lives. Under these circumstances, these clubs have conducted their activities in cooperation with local government welfare departments and/or similar public agencies.

Japanese senior citizens' clubs conduct wide-ranging activities, including: group activities, such as sports, hobbies, cultural activities and performing arts; traveling; volunteer activities at welfare facilities, etc.; activities for handing down local culture, traditional performing arts, folk arts, handicrafts, local history, life documents, etc; and exchanges with children, youths and adults. Their activities may vary in nature depending on locality.

While senior citizens' clubs receive funding subsidies from local government, their revenue sources also include proceeds from the sale of used goods collected during their recycling activities and from bazaars and other community events. Since the amount of funding granted to a senior citizens' club by the local government is often determined by the size of its membership, there are reportedly a number of nominal members who do not actually participate in club activities.

In 2002, there were a total of 131,116 senior citizens' clubs in Japan, with 8,541,549 members. Since peaking in 1997, the numbers of clubs and their members have both been on the decline. According to the most recent statistics, as of 2006 the number of senior citizens' clubs and their members are 124,120 clubs and 7,807,716 persons, respectively.

ii. Some types of organizations showed decreasing membership rates with increasing age (i.e., volunteer groups and sports clubs for men, and political organizations, industrial organizations, volunteer groups, citizens' action groups, sports clubs and hobby groups for women), while other types of organizations showed increasing membership rates with increasing age, except for subjects aged eighty-five years or older (i.e., religious organizations for men and neighborhood associations/senior citizens' clubs for both men and women).

iii. For both men and women, a lower proportion of subjects joining in one or more organizations had poor health indices.

iv. With the exception of citizens' action groups and religious organizations, in general, the membership rate increased with increasing income and years of education.

v. Membership in the various types of organizations differed between the three regional types, with rural areas showing a higher membership rate in industrial organizations and lower membership rates in sports clubs and hobby groups.

The associations observed between membership in organizations and health indices and the differences observed between the different types of organizations seem to indicate a need for further analyses of the association between membership in organizations and health from a wider perspective by taking types of organizations into account.

This chapter has discussed eight different types of organizations, including those types used as survey items in the JGSS plus local community groups and organizations. However, as pointed out by another report on the JGSS (Iwai and Satō 2002), some of these types of organizations may overlap in terms of the nature of their activities, even though they are defined as different organizations (e.g., sports clubs and hobby groups). In addition, local community organizations that have been added specifically to the present study, namely, senior citizens' clubs, neighborhood associations and volunteer fire corps, would differ from each other in terms of the factors associated with membership in them. Furthermore, the frequency of (Kishi et al. 1996; Sugisawa 1994), and positive attitude towards, participation in organizations are likely to be associated with life prognosis, which has already been pointed out, and are also likely to have different associations in different types of organizations. For these reasons, a further sophisticated discussion of older people's membership in organizations and groups seems to require deeper investigations and analyses of these points.

Chapter 12

Social Support

Yoshitaka Saitō

Introduction

The health condition of an older person is, generally, positively related to the quality of interpersonal relationships he or she has, i.e., healthier people tend to have better interpersonal relationships. However, there are various types of interpersonal relationships. Among them, the term 'social support' has been mentioned frequently by researchers, policy-makers and front-line staff in the fields of health, medicine and welfare in recent years. This chapter examines how this 'social support' is related to the health of older people (see Chapter 1).

Social support refers to the support exchanged between persons. When a person interacts with another person, something is exchanged. The focus of what is called social support is on the function and quality of this exchange. Daily assistance, long-term care, financial assistance, gift giving, counseling and emotional connection can be regarded as examples of social support. Since one party 'gives' goods and services and the other party 'receives' them, it is possible to look at the functions of 'giving' and 'receiving' separately.

At the same time, social support is supported by what is called 'social network' (Noguchi 1991; Kondō 2004; Okado et al. 2004). A social network is an association of people focused on the quantity of interpersonal relationships more than the quality and the structure more than the function. It deals with the objective aspects more than subjective aspects of interpersonal relationships.

This chapter focuses on social support, which is a more subjective and functional aspect of interpersonal relationships. As in other chapters, it uses the AGES (Aichi Gerontological Evaluation Study, see Box 2) data to examine the role of interpersonal relationships of older people, policy intervention based on it, and the possibility of practical applications for welfare provision.

Aspects of social support

Some may think of social support for older people as the 'receipt' of support and care by older people as in: 'older people are cared for by family and welfare workers', for example (Okado et al. 2004). However, there are two sides to social support: the party receiving support and the party 'giving' support and care. These two components of social support are referred to as 'received support' and 'given support' respectively (Noguchi 1991; Kondō 2004).

As in the case of aged care, received support alone tends to attract attention in relation to the health of older people and many people may think that 'it is necessary to give support to older people in order to maintain their health'. Yet, that is only one aspect of social support (Kondō 2004; Noguchi and Sugisawa 1998; Kishi and Horikawa 2004). It has been pointed out that 'receiving support' has negatives as well as positives (Seeman et al. 1996; Mendes de Leon et al. 2001). Moreover, it has been suggested that 'giving support' may be beneficial for health. Accordingly, this chapter analyzes both aspects of social support on the assumption that both 'received support' and 'given support' are relevant to health.

Method

While social support can be categorized into many types, this chapter will look at two major types of social support. One is 'support in the emotional aspects' of daily living ('emotional support') and the other is what is called 'support in the instrumental aspects' ('instrumental support'), including nursing for the sick and daily living support for those having difficulties (Kondō 2004; Seeman et al. 1996; Mendes de Leon et al. 2001). Table 12.1 shows the specific questions used in the survey. The act of 'listening to concerns and complaints' was regarded as emotional support and 'nursing and looking after one who is sick in bed' as instrumental support.

This survey adopted a technique previously used in several studies (Seeman et al. 1996; Mendes de Leon et al. 2001) which involved asking the respondents whom they gave support to and received support from in order to determine the presence or absence of support and the levels of support. This survey asked whether they gave to or received support from three categories of people: family members living in the same house, family members or relatives not living in the same house, and acquaintances (including friends) (support in each category was recognized when at least one person in that category

Table 12.1: Survey questions on received and given support in the emotional and instrumental aspects

Support	Question	Response
Emotional aspect		
Received	Do you have anyone who listens to you about your concerns and complaints?	Yes/No
Given	Do you listen to another person about his/her concerns and complaints?	Yes/No
Instrumental aspect		
Received	Do you have anyone who looks after you when you are sick in bed for several days?	Yes/No
Given	Do you have anyone whom you are willing to look after when he/she is sick in bed for several days?	Yes/No

Table 12.2: Patterns of support receiving and giving

	Given support	
	Yes	**No**
Received support		
Yes	(a) Received & given	(b) Received only
No	(c) Given only	(d) None

was giving/receiving support). Table 12.2 depicts four patterns of the presence or absence of received support and given support. In pattern (a) both received and given support are present, pattern (b) is only received support, pattern (c) is only given support, and in pattern (d) neither type of support is present.

Two assessment items that are predictors of death – self-rated health and depression (GDS-15) – were adopted as indicators of mental health status (see Boxes 6 and 7). Table 12.4 indicates that the larger the scores for these two items, the higher the number of people with poor mental health status.

Socio-economic status based on the length of education and the income (equivalent income calculated by dividing the annual household income (in million yen/year) by the square root of the number of household members) was used as a variable (see Box 3). Three regional types – urban, semi-urban and rural – were used (see Chapter 1).

Analysis was carried out using the above variables based on the General Linear Model of SPSS adjusted for age. Data for this analysis came from the AGES of older people not certified for long-term nursing care living in fifteen municipalities in three prefectures (32,891 persons, 55.2 percent response rate). However, the number of cases for individual components of the analysis varies depending on the missing data for each variable.

Findings

Descriptive statistics: State of social support

First, let us look at how much support older people receive and/or give. Table 12.3 shows a distribution of social support by gender and age group in the emotional and instrumental aspects shown in Table 12.2, divided into the four patterns of receiving and giving support shown in Table 12.1. The figures from rows (a) to (b) in each column are percentage figures and add up to a total of 100. The overall result shows that the percentage of the respondents who belonged to group (a) (who reported both received and given support) was 79.3 percent in terms of emotional support and 88.8 percent in terms of instrumental support. This was followed by group (b) (received support only, 11.0 percent emotional and 5.2 percent instrumental) and group (c) (given support only, 4.0 percent emotional and 3.3 percent instrumental). The number of people in group (d) who had neither received nor given support was small (5.7 percent emotional and 2.7 percent instrumental).

Second, what is notable in the support distribution by gender is the gender difference in the aspect of emotional support ($p < 0.001$). The number of respondents in group (a) who reported both received and given support was almost 10 percent higher among women (83.5 percent) than men (74.8 percent). Conversely, the number in group (d) who reported no support was higher among men (8.1 percent) than women (3.6 percent).

The support distribution by age group shows that the ratios of group (a), receiving and giving support, and group (c), giving only, decrease as they become older (e.g., the ratio of those who were receiving and giving (group (a)) emotional support in the 65–69 age group was 83.3 percent, which decreases to 63.3 percent in the 85 and over age group). Instead, the ratios of group (b), receiving only, and group (d), neither receiving nor giving, increase (e.g., the ratio of those who were receiving (group (b)) emotional support in the 65–69 age group was 7.9 percent, which increases to 26.3 percent in the 85 and over age group). This suggests that it becomes more difficult to 'give' support than to 'receive' support as people get older.

Table 12.3: Distribution of social support by gender and age (%)

	Total	Gender		Age				
		Male	Female	65–69	70–74	75–79	80–84	85+
Emotional (concerns & complaints)								
Sample size (persons)	29,479	12,843	14,996	9,021	8,353	5,973	3,041	1,456
(a) Received & given	79.3	74.8	83.5	83.3	81.0	78.5	73.0	63.3
(b) Received only	11.0	11.3	10.5	7.9	9.1	11.4	16.6	26.3
(c) Given only	4.0	5.9	2.5	4.0	4.2	3.9	3.9	3.3
(d) None	5.7	8.1	3.6	4.8	5.7	6.2	6.4	7.1
Instrumental (nursing & care)								
Sample size (persons)	29,954	13,108	15,129	9,077	8,437	6,113	3,147	1,476
(a) Received & given	88.8	91.0	87.2	91.4	90.4	88.3	85.3	75.3
(b) Received only	5.2	5.0	5.2	2.6	3.2	5.7	9.0	20.3
(c) Given only	3.3	1.7	4.7	3.9	3.6	3.1	2.4	1.4
(d) None	2.7	2.4	2.9	2.1	2.7	2.9	3.3	2.9

Association with mental health

Let us look at how social support relates to the mental state of older people. Table 12.4 shows that people in group (a) having received and given support have the best mental state both in terms of self-rated health and depression ($p < 0.001$, adjusted for age). Take the relationship between depression and instrumental support for example, the ratio of depressive people in group (a), receiving and giving instrumental support, was 6.3 percent in contrast with 15.0 percent in group (b), receiving only, 22.4 percent in group (c), giving only, and 28.0 percent in group (d) having no support. Similar patterns can be observed with the relationship between emotional support and self-rated health. This result points to the possibility that it is more desirable for the health of older people that there are both given support and received support in their interpersonal relationships rather than 'giving only' or 'receiving only', not to mention 'no support at all'.

Although space limitations do not permit us to go into details, the following additional analysis was also carried out. First, the trend remained the same when data was statistically adjusted for gender and family structure (living alone or otherwise). Then, data was analyzed for each of the categories of the counterpart in support, namely, 'family members living in the same house', 'children or relatives not living in the same house' and 'acquaintances, friends and neighbors'. This was due to the possibility that the mental health state of older people

Table 12.4: Social support and mental health (%)

	Self-rated health		Depression	
	(poor)	p-value	(≥10 points)	p-value
Emotional (concerns & complaints)				
Sample size (persons)	27,218		23,011	
(a) Received & given	27.7	***	6.4	***
(b) Received only	31.9		9.7	
(c) Given only	34.2		14.7	
(d) None	33.1		18.2	
Instrumental (nursing & care)				
Sample size (persons)	27,602		23,252	
(a) Received & given	27.6	***	6.3	***
(b) Received only	35.3		15.0	
(c) Given only	41.4		22.4	
(d) None	38.9		28.0	

After adjustment for age by the general linear model. The values under 'self-rated health' are the ratios of 'poor' and 'fair' combined. The values under 'depression' are the ratios of the 'moderate to severe depression' group who scored 10 points or more in the GDS-15.

*** $p < 0.001$. The significance probability is based on F-values measuring significant differences between the four groups (a)–(d).

might vary depending on who is giving or receiving nursing or other types of care. However, there was no significant interpretable difference notwithstanding some minor variations. No matter who was the counterpart in support, a better mental health status was associated with the presence of both received and given support and a poor mental health status was associated with the absence of both received and given support or the existence of received support alone.

Association with income and education

Let us look at how social support relates to the level of education. Table 12.5 shows the ratios of people with the four patterns of received and given support (adjusted for age) in relation to the length of education and the level of income, divided into four and five levels respectively. Despite minor exceptions, it is possible to find a common tendency both with the length of education and the level of income: the higher they are, the higher the ratios of respondents who are giving support. For example, the ratio of people who were giving and receiving support (group (a)) in emotional aspects is 74.7 percent among the group with up to six years of education against 80.6 percent among the group with thirteen or more years of education. The ratio of people who were giving support only (group (c)) was 3.8 percent among the former and 5.6 percent among the latter. In contrast, the ratios of people with given support only (group (b)) and no support at all (group (d)) were higher at lower education and income levels. For example, the ratio of group (b) was 15.1 percent among the group with up to six years of education and 5.6 percent among the group with thirteen or more years of education with regard to emotional support. Similarly, the ratio of group (d) was 6.4 percent against 5.3 percent. This trend was applicable to support in both the emotional and instrumental aspects. It may suggest that people need to have some kind of resources to be able to afford to give support to others and that the giving of support is difficult for those who are lacking them. It appears that giving support is more difficult than receiving support for those who have a lower level of education (possibly due to insufficient knowledge or other resources).

Association with regional types

The final part of the analysis of social support was based on regional differences (rural, semi-urban and urban regions, Chapter 1) (Table 12.6). Variations by regional type are statistically significant but differences of up to 2 percentage points are not substantial in real terms.

When the data were analyzed based on the categories of the counterpart in support, however, some variations were noticed in the results. First, there were no regional differences when the counterpart in support were 'family members living in the same house'. Some regional differences were observed in the 'children or relatives not living in the same house' and 'acquaintances, friends and neighbors' categories. The ratio of group (a) with received and given support was higher in the rural regions and the ratio of group (d) with no support at all was higher in the semi-urban and urban regions. For example, the ratio of people who were giving and receiving emotional support to and from children and relatives not living in the same house (group (a)) was 24.7 percent in the rural regions, 21.9 percent in the semi-urban regions, and 22.2 percent in the urban regions ($p < 0.001$). The ratio of people with no emotional support (group (d)) was 53.6 percent in the rural regions, 58.6 percent in the semi-urban regions, and 57.8 percent in the urban regions ($p < 0.001$). Although real point differences are not substantial, it can be interpreted that the result reflects the current situation in which relationships with children and relatives not living in the same

Table 12.5: Social support, education and income (%)

	Years of education					Equivalent income (million yen/year)[a]					
	–6	**6–9**	**10–12**	**13+**	**p-value**	**< 1**	**1.01–2**	**2.01–3**	**3.01–4**	**4+**	**p-value**
Emotional (concerns & complaints)											
Sample size (persons)	1,274	15,006	8,644	2,506		3,615	6,754	5,659	3,641	2,324	
(a) Received & given	74.7	78.1	82.4	80.6	***	75.3	78.8	81.4	83.3	83.8	***
(b) Received only	15.1	11.8	9.1	8.5	***	12.9	10.1	9.3	9.7	9.0	***
(c) Given only	3.8	3.9	3.7	5.6	***	4.5	4.7	3.7	3.3	3.7	***
(d) None	6.4	6.1	4.7	5.3	***	7.3	6.4	5.4	3.7	3.6	***
Instrumental (nursing & care)											
Sample size (persons)	1,297	15,294	8,694	2,518		3,691	6,829	5,690	3,670	2,336	
(a) Received & given	79.8	88.8	90.3	90.2	***	85.5	89.1	91.8	92.4	91.5	***
(b) Received only	11.5	5.4	3.9	4.1	***	5.5	4.6	4.0	4.3	4.9	*
(c) Given only	4.8	3.2	3.4	3.2	*	5.1	3.7	2.3	2.0	2.5	***
(d) None	3.9	2.6	2.4	2.6	*	4.0	2.6	1.9	1.3	1.1	***

Notes.

After adjustment for age by the general linear model.

a: Household income (million yen/year) divided by the square root of the number of household members.

*: $p < 0.05$, ***: $p < 0.001$. Analysis by category.

Table 12.6: Social support and regional type (%)

	Rural	Semi-urban	Urban	p-value
Emotional (concerns & complaints)				
Sample size (persons)	16,772	4,126	6,946	
(a) Received & given	79.8	77.8	79.6	*
(b) Received only	11.0	11.3	10.6	n.s.
(c) Given only	3.8	4.6	4.1	*
(d) None	5.4	6.3	5.9	*
Instrumental (nursing & care)				
Sample size (persons)	17,114	4,156	6,980	
(a) Received & given	89.2	88.0	88.8	n.s.
(b) Received only	4.8	6.0	5.4	**
(c) Given only	3.3	3.4	3.3	n.s.
(d) None	2.7	2.7	2.5	n.s.

After adjustment for age by the general linear model.

*: $p<0.05$, **: $p<0.01$, n.s.: no significant difference. Analysis by category.

house or acquaintances, friends and neighbors are still strong in rural regions whereas they are weakening in cities and suburbs. However, regional differences do not appear to affect relationships with family members living in the same house as yet. Looking from another angle, the results may suggest the availability of support not dependent on family members, relatives or neighbors in the urban regions.

Discussion

Gender difference

Women had more social support than did men. It has been reported in some case studies (Akiyama 1997; Okushima 1997) that older Japanese men were not so good at conversation or small talk. In the past the problems of older people in Japan were sometimes considered to be particular to women because they received smaller pensions and tended to outlive their husbands (Tsutsui 1998; Inoue 1998; Itō and Itō 2002) but it appears that the proportion of those who are lacking received support or given support in emotional aspects is higher among men.

Causal association

Since this was a cross-section analysis, it was impossible to confirm whether abundance of social support caused mental health or vice versa. However, there are cohort studies controlled for the effects of the opposite causal association that have confirmed that the abundance of social support has a positive impact on health (Noguchi and Sugisawa 1998; Yoshii et al. 2005) and therefore it is highly likely that the giving and receiving of social support is beneficial for health.

Implications for long-term care prevention

What do these findings mean to long-term care prevention? They appear to suggest at least two things.

One is to create more opportunities for older people to have a role to play. This study has found that the bilateral relationship involving both giving and receiving support has a stronger association with improved health in older people than receiving support alone. As argued in a previous study, it is possible to hypothesize the existence of multiple health benefits from the subjective and psychological effects of one's interaction with others and social participation by way of support giving and receiving (Berkman et al. 2000).

In Japan, the focus of interest has historically been on the support measures to 'do/give something' for the benefit of older people. However, the findings of this analysis indicate that such support measures are not always sufficient. The giving of support by older people to people around them also has a potential to improve their health and lead to the prevention of long-term care. When older people are only receiving support, they may feel the psychological burden of 'being a nuisance' and eventually withdraw from society. It may mean that the family, relatives and friends of older people and various service providers need to try to provide older people with more opportunities to play the role of social support giver instead of simply trying to do something for them.

In fact, there have been some volunteer organizations formed by older people themselves for the purpose of providing support to others in recent years (Miyata and Nozawa 2002). Social participation by way of support giving perhaps deserves more recognition in policy making.

In the context of health inequalities, however, it can be pointed out that more attention should be paid to older people in the lower education and income categories as has been argued in preceding studies (Berkman et al. 2000). While support giving may be beneficial for health, the benefit may be skewed toward the people in higher social strata who can afford to give support to others. Proper attention needs to be given to social stratification for this reason.

The other implication for long-term care prevention is that the provision of support (received support) to older people still appears to be necessary. Even though support giving may be beneficial for health, the ratio of healthy people is much higher in the group with both given and received support than the group with given support only. It has also been suggested in this chapter that giving support requires youth, resources and/or skills. This means that the act of giving support becomes more difficult for older people with depleting resources or skills due to aging. While handouts of help in order to simply 'do something for older people' are not desirable, any measures to force older people to give support are not appropriate either. What appears to be needed are support programs to create opportunities and environments for older people to play a part in one way or another within the support system while receiving support at the same time.

The focus of aged care policies is shifting toward long-term care prevention as demonstrated by new restrictions imposed on housekeeping support and care equipment rentals under long-term care insurance for the relatively independent older people at the required assistance levels 1 and 2. Consequently, the need for informal support in the area of domestic assistance service is expected to grow from now on. This is exactly the type of support addressed in this chapter, the importance of which is likely to increase in the future.

Pending issues

The scope of analysis in this chapter was limited to social support. The results might have been somewhat different if quantitative association indicators such as social network had been applied. Furthermore, dependent variables were limited to self-rated health and depression as measures of health status. Life expectancy (Okado et al. 2004), for example, could be used for future analysis

The question of causal relationship, as mentioned, could not be solved in this study since it was a cross-sectional data analysis. Addressing this question will require further attempts, including cohort studies, in the future.

Conclusion

This chapter has attempted to understand the state of social support for older people and how it relates to the state of mental health by analyzing the relationships between social support and income, education and regional characteristics. Consideration was given to giving support as well as receiving support in view of existing arguments.

It was found that the ratio of the older people in group (a) who were giving and receiving support was around 80 percent, followed by group (b) who only received support and group (c) who only give support. Only a small percentage of older people belonged to group (d) with no support at all.

Statistically significant links were found between social support and the state of mental health of older people in terms of self-rated health and depression in that a high proportion of the people with both received and given support had a better health status and a high proportion of the people with no support at all had a poorer health status. This tendency was common to both emotional support and instrumental support, including nursing and other types of care in times of need. In other words, giving social support showed a positive association with the state of mental health, as did receiving social support.

Age, income and years of education were also found to be relevant to social support. The people who were younger, more educated and had higher income tended to have more abundant social support. In particular, the possibility that giving support requires youth, resources and/or skills has been highlighted.

The result appears to suggest that long-term care prevention requires not only giving support to older people but also an approach which provides older people with more opportunities to play a part in giving support to others and participate in society.

Chapter 13

Employment Status and Financial Insecurity

Hideki Endō

Introduction

Japan's policy makers have been pushing to expand employment opportunities for older people in recent years against a backdrop of a rapidly aging population and the high rate of employment among older people, both of which are higher in Japan than any other country (OECD 2004).

This raises the question: how willing are older people to work? According to Kōnenreisha Shūgyō Jittai Chōsa (Survey on Employment Conditions of Older Persons) by the Ministry of Health, Labour and Welfare (2004), 30.6 percent of men and 25.2 percent of women from 65 to 69 years of age wish to 'work forever regardless of age'. When combined with those who 'wish to work even after the age of 70', the figures rise to 41.8 percent in men and 29.8 percent in women.

Why do Japan's older people want to keep working? As explained in Box 15: 'International comparison of motives to work', the main motive is income (Cabinet Office 2005). While older people earn lower incomes than they used to, however, not all of them face financial pressures in day-to-day living because, on average, they have over ten million yen more in assets such as savings and real estate than the pre-retirement generations.

'Maintenance of good health' ranks high in the list of motives to work, which is considered to be peculiar to the Japanese. The proportion of older workers who wish to keep working for the purpose of maintaining their health is 25.9 percent in contrast to around 10–15 percent in other countries (Cabinet Office 2005). The proportion increases to 31.3 percent among older non-workers who wish to work. The 2003 edition of Kōsei Rōdō Hakusho (Annual Health, Labour and Welfare Report) describes old age as 'the second phase of active service' and states that employment is important for lively participation of older people in social activities. Let us consider how the employment of older people relates to their health.

Preceding studies and the topic of discussion

How does employment relate to the health of older people? First, employment enables them to secure stable income other than pensions. Income in old age is used for purchasing services for health promotion such as gym usage and paying medical expenses, which increase with age, as well as purchasing other goods and services. In other words, change in the objective level of income from employment tends to impact on physical health.

Second, recent studies have reported that a sense of financial insecurity in daily life has an adverse effect on depression and life satisfaction levels (Meyer and Lobao 2003; Wildman 2004; Angel et al. 2003; Hamashima 1994; Demura et al. 2003; Cabinet Office 2004). If employment can provide income stability and alleviate financial concerns, it may be able to exert a positive influence on depression and other problems through the alleviation of financial insecurity.

If the association between employment and health can be explained by income or subjective measures such as financial insecurity, then it follows that working is good for health because financial stability and high income keep the mental and physical health of older people in a good state.

However, some people appear to suffer from severe misgivings or anxiety about their jobs due to difficulties in adapting to changes in duties or interpersonal relations in the workplace. According to *Rōdōsha Kenkō Jōkyō Chōsa (Heisei 14 nen)* (Survey on State of Employee's Health (2002)) by the Ministry of Health, Labour and Welfare, the proportion of workers who are experiencing difficulty in coping with information technology and other technological innovations or interpersonal relations in the workplace is highest in the 60+ age-group. At the same time, employment is a desirable condition for older people who find in work a reason for living, or see it as a form of social participation. In any case, employment may be associated with psychological factors.

For this reason, in this chapter, using depression and self-rated health as health indices, we will discuss the following two issues:

Associations between income, financial insecurity and health indicators

While there have been advanced studies of the association between objective measures such as income levels and depression and the subjective measure of self-rated health (see Chapter 2), studies of the association between a sense of financial insecurity or other subjective measures and depression and life satisfaction are still in progress (Meyer and Lobao 2003; Wildman 2004; Angel et al. 2003; Hamashima 1994; Demura et al. 2003; Cabinet Office 2004). For example, in England, an analysis by Wildman (2004) indicated that the severer the subjective financial condition, the poorer the mental health state. In Japan, Demura et al. (2003) suggest that older people who feel insecure about their financial condition tend to have lower levels of life satisfaction. A survey about the daily life of older people by the Cabinet Office of the Japanese Government (Cabinet Office 2004) has found that there are higher proportions of older people who have lower levels of life satisfaction among those whose subjective financial condition is poor. This chapter will attempt to verify this point.

Does employment of older people still relate to health indicators after adjusting for income and financial insecurity?

Many USA studies have found that one's sense of well-being increases and depression decreases after retirement (Mindank et al. 1995; Charles 2004; Reitzes et al. 1996; Van Doorslaer and Jones 2003; Wagstaff 2002). However, it has been suggested that the situation may be different in Japan since more workers tend to report 'good' self-rated health than non-workers (in the 61–64 age group) and retirement or job loss in old age tends to increase depression (Nakazato et al. 2000; Sugisawa 1997; Shibata 2001). However, to our knowledge, while many previous studies have shown their results to be adjusted for income, they have not taken account of financial insecurity. We will take it into consideration.

In addition to the above, the length of education is associated with employment status. Also, differences in employment structures between rural and urban areas may help to explain regional differences in health indicators that are discussed elsewhere in this book. This chapter will touch on these points as well.

This analysis is based on the survey data from AGES (Aichi Gerontological Evaluation Study, Box 2) 2003.

Method

The AGES surveyed 32,891 people aged 65 and older who do not receive long-term care benefits from the long-term care insurers in fifteen municipalities (see Chapter 1, Table 1.1). Those who reported a history of serious illnesses in the past 12 months (553 subjects) are excluded from the sample population in order to exclude any who might have left their jobs due to deteriorating health. Additionally, we exclude those who did not respond to the following questions about their employment status; 'Do you have any paid work at the moment?' and 'Have you retired from work in the past 12 months?' As a result, the sample size for this study is 20,434 persons (9,550 men, 10,884 women).

Depression and self-rated health are the indices which are the objective variables of this study. For depression, the GDS-15 (Geriatric Depression Scale, Box 7) scores are divided into three levels (4 points or lower: 'depression-free', 5–9 points: 'mild depression', 10 points or higher: 'moderate to severe depression'). For self-rated health (Box 6), subjects assess their own health condition by choosing one of four-point scales ('Excellent', 'good', 'fair', 'poor' (see Box 3)). In this study, those who reported 'fair' or 'poor' are regarded as 'poor' in self-rated health.

We use equivalent income (household income (million yen/year) divided by the square root of the number of household members) (Box 3) as the surrogate variable of personal income. For financial insecurity, the subjective scales of concern about their ability to pay unexpected expenses ('not concerned at all', 'slightly concerned', 'moderately concerned', 'very concerned') are used.

We divide employment status into three categories: persons engaged in work (persons who did not change jobs or had changed jobs in the past 12 months), persons who had quit a job (in the past 12 months) and persons not working continuously (persons who did not do any work for more than 12 months).

The variables of employment status categories (persons engaged in work, persons who had quit a job, persons not working continuously) are prepared by combining questions about their employment status ('Do you have any paid work at the moment?' and 'Have you retired from your job in the past 12 months?') and dividing the change of labor force status in the past 12 months into three types by reference to *Shūgyō Kōzō Kihon Chōsa (Heisei 14 nen)* (Employment Status Survey (2002)) by the Bureau of Statistics, the Ministry of Internal Affairs and Communications (Table 13.1).

In this case, persons engaged in work includes those who are 'in work 12 months ago and now (persons who did not change jobs or had changed jobs in the past 12 months)' and 'out of work 12 months ago but in work now (newly employed)'. However, only 1.6 percent of the workers aged 65 or older were newly employed according to the above survey (2002) and therefore a majority of the people in this category is 'in work 12 months ago and now'.

Table 13.1: Categories and definitions of employment status in this study

Paid work	Retired in the past 12 months	Category	Definition
Yes	No	Persons engaged in work	Persons who did not change jobs or changed jobs in the past 12 months.
	Yes		
No	Yes	Persons who had quit a job	Persons who had quit a job in the past 12 months.
	No	Persons not working continuously	Persons who did not do any work for more than 12 months.

Other variables include the length of education and the regional type (urban, semi-urban and rural regions: see Chapter 1).

The possible associations suggested in the previous section are analyzed using the above variables under the general linear model (GLM). We used SPSS version 12.0 for this analysis.

Findings

Employment status

Table 13.2 shows the employment status by age and gender. Thirty-six and a half percent of all men and 21.9 percent of all women were in employment and in the 65–69 age group, one in two men and one in three women were working. Although the numbers decreased with age, 11.4 percent of men and 4.8 percent of women aged 85 and older were still working.

Employment status and income, financial insecurity and education

Let us begin with an analysis of the associations between income and financial insecurity and the employment status under the GLM adjusted for age. The association with the years of education is also checked for any affect on employment status.

Association between income and employment status

The proportion of persons engaged in work was high in the upper-income group (53.2 percent of men and 28.7 percent of women) and the

Table 13.2: Distribution of employment status categories by age (5 year intervals)

Employment status	Age					Total
	65–69	70–74	75–79	80–84	85+	
Men						
Persons engaged in work (%)	48.5	36.1	26.1	19.6	11.4	36.5
Persons who had quit a job (%)	8.5	9.3	6.5	8.6	9.3	8.4
Persons not working continuously (%)	43.0	54.6	67.3	71.9	79.3	55.1
Total men (persons)	3,571	2,938	1,867	807	367	9,550
Women						
Persons engaged in work (%)	33.1	22.6	13.3	8.8	4.8	21.9
Persons who had quit a job (%)	4.8	4.9	5.4	6.4	5.4	5.2
Persons not working continuously (%)	62.1	72.5	81.3	84.8	89.8	73.0
Total women (persons)	3,755	3,170	2,181	1,168	610	10,884

proportion of persons not working continuously was high in the lower-income group (60.7 percent of men and 68.1 percent of women).

Association between financial insecurity and employment status

The proportion of men engaged in work was 40.2 percent in the 'not concerned at all' group and 28.8 percent in the 'very concerned' group. The proportion of men not working continuously was 52.3 percent in the 'not concerned at all' group and 61.6 percent in the 'very concerned' group. The same trend occurred among women.

Association between education and employment status

The proportion of men engaged in work was slightly lower at 25.3 percent among those who had less than 6 years of education but it was around 34 percent for all other groups (6–9 years, 10–12 years and 13+ years) with no significant difference between the education levels. The proportions of the women engaged in work all fell within the 20.7–22.4 percent range with no significant difference.

Financial insecurity, equivalent income and health indicators

It was shown in Chapter 2 that the lower the income, the poorer the self-rated health and the higher the incidence of severe depression.

Table 13.3: Association between financial insecurity and depression

	Men		Women	
	Sample (persons)	Severe depression (%)	Sample (persons)	Severe depression (%)
Not concerned at all	766	1.3	914	1.7
Slightly concerned	3,041	2.9	3,198	3.4
Moderately concerned	1,743	7.8	1,548	8.5
Very concerned	878	15.8	1,004	18.5
p-value		***		***

Adjusted for age and equivalent income (household income (million yen/year) divided by the square root of the number of household members) by the general linear model.

Depression scales (GDS scores): depression-free (up to 4 points), mild depression (5–9 points), moderate to severe depression (10+ points).

p-value ***: $p < 0.001$.

Table 13.3 shows the association between financial insecurity and depression scales. It is clear that the proportion of people suffering moderate to severe depression was significantly higher as a sense of financial insecurity increased in both men and women. Although the proportion of people suffering moderate to severe depression was slightly higher in women than men, the trend was shared by men and women. The result is similar with regard to self-rated health.

Is there a significant relationship, though, between financial insecurity and health indicators adjusted for equivalent income? If the relationship becomes insignificant after adjustment for equivalent income, we can infer that the income level is a more important factor than financial insecurity. Figure 13.1 shows the relationship between the level of financial insecurity and depression scales in men by equivalent income levels. It demonstrates that the proportion of people suffering severe depression was higher among those who had a stronger sense of financial insecurity at all income levels. In other words, the level of financial insecurity is considered to be a factor independent of income level. Similar trends were found among women and in the association with self-rated health.

Employment status and health indicators

Table 13.4 shows how employment status relates to self-rated health and depression. The proportion of people with poor self-rated health was higher among persons not engaged in work

Figure 13.1: Association between financial insecurity and depression (men, by equivalent income level)

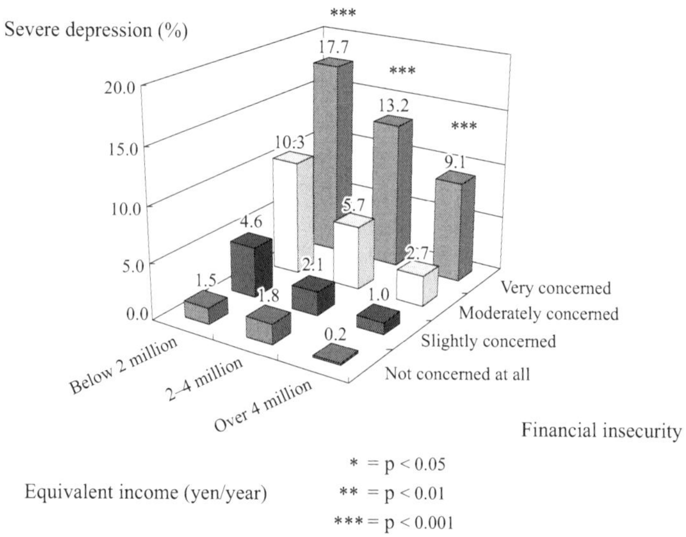

Notes.
Severe depression: 10+ points in the GDS scores.
After adjustment for age by the general linear model.

(persons who had quit a job or were not working continuously) than workers in both men and women. The persons who had quit a job appeared to be in worse health than the persons who were not working continuously. Similar trends were found with depression scales.

Figure 13.2 is the result of analysis of the relationship between financial insecurity and depression scales in men by employment status. It is clear that the proportion of people suffering moderate to severe depression was higher among persons not engaged in work than those engaged in work regardless of the level of financial insecurity and that it was also higher among the people with a stronger sense of financial insecurity than the group with less financial insecurity in all employment status categories. For example, the proportion of people suffering moderate to severe depression among persons not working continuously who were 'not concerned at all' about their financial security was 3.2

Table 13.4: Associations between employment status, self-rated health and depression (%)

	Self-rated health		Depression			
Employment status	**Sample (persons)**	**Poor**	**Sample (persons)**	**Depression-free**	**Mild depression**	**Moderate to severe depression**
Men						
Persons engaged in work	2,397	15.3	2,207	78.2	18.5	3.4
Persons who had quit a job	585	26.1	541	65.5	25.7	8.7
Persons not working continuously	3,971	25.7	3,605	70.5	22.6	6.8
p-value		***		***	***	***
Women						
Persons engaged in work	1,608	16.9	1,390	75.8	19.7	4.5
Persons who had quit a job	371	28.5	309	62.5	28.4	9.0
Persons not working continuously	5,630	25.5	4,793	69.6	23.6	6.9
p-value		***		***	**	**

After adjustment for age by the general linear model.

'Not good' in self-rated health (%): The proportion of persons who reported 'fair' or 'poor' as their own health condition by choosing one of four-point scales.

Depression scales (GDS scores): depression-free (4 points or lower), mild depression (5–9 points), moderate to severe depression (10+ points).

p-value ***: $p < 0.001$; **: $p < 0.01$; *: $p < 0.05$.

percent, which was almost the same proportion of people suffering moderate to severe depression among persons engaged in work who were 'moderately concerned' (3.3 percent). This was confirmed by the analysis of the relationship between employment status and depression by levels of financial insecurity.

Since the same trend was observed when equivalent income was used instead of financial insecurity, this result suggests that the relationship between employment status and depression still stands whether the financial condition parameter that is taken into account is objective or subjective. These trends were also found among women and when self-rated health was used.

A further analysis allowing for home ownership has been conducted because subjective financial insecurity is not only associated with income but also with ownership of assets such as real estate. The results indicated the same trends.

Figure 13.2: Association between financial insecurity and depression (men, by employment status)

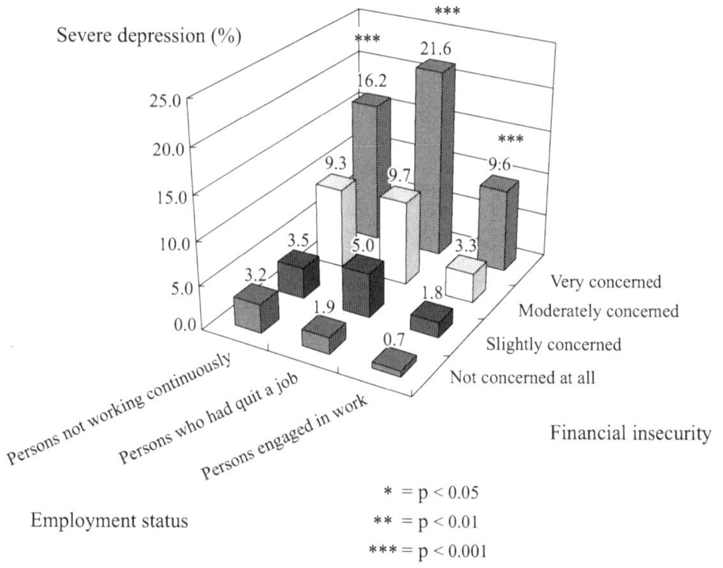

Notes.
Severe depression: 10+ points in the GDS scores.
After adjustment for age and equivalent income by the general linear model.

Comparison by regional type

Other chapters of this book have shown that the health status of older people is worse in rural regions. Can this situation be explained by variations in employment status in different types of region?

As Figure 13.3 (adjusted for age) shows, the proportion of persons engaged in work was higher in the rural regions at all income levels. When the association between employment status and self-rated health was examined for each regional type (Figure 13.4, adjusted for age), the self-rated health of persons not working continuously was significantly poorer in all regional types. This trend was also found, more or less, among women and in the association with depression scales. However, the proportion of those reporting 'poor in self-rated health' was higher in the rural regions in all employment status categories. In other words, the high proportion of rural people in poor health cannot be explained by differences in employment status.

Figure 13.3: Proportion of persons engaged in work by regional type (men, by equivalent income level)

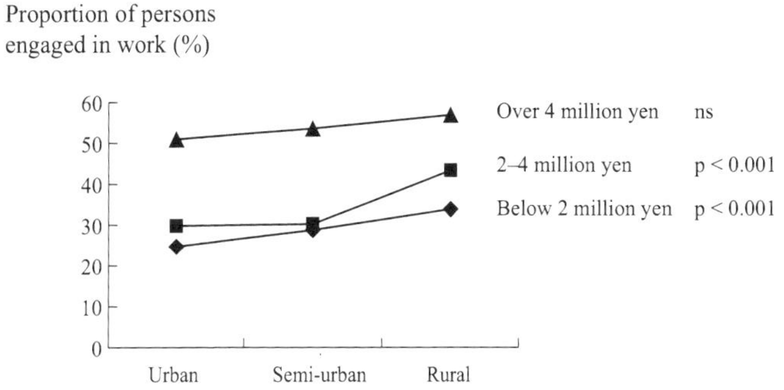

Note. After adjustment for age by the general linear model.

Figure 13.4: Proportion of persons reporting 'poor' in self-rated health by employment status (men, by regional type)

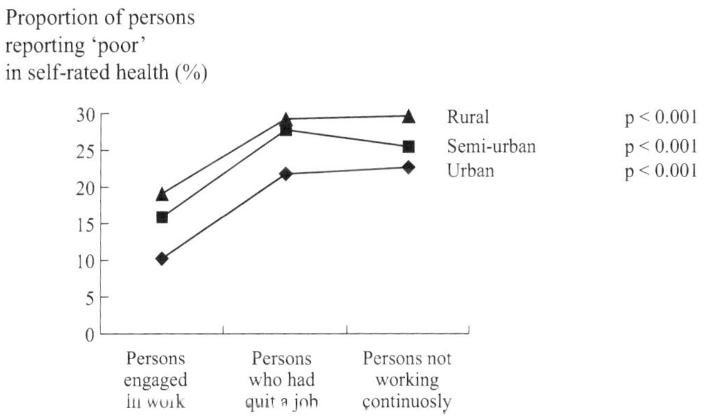

Note. After adjustment for age by the general linear model.

Discussion

The findings in this chapter can be summarized as follows. The proportion of older persons engaged in work was higher in the upper-income group and the proportion of those who were 'very concerned' about unexpected expenses tended to be smaller in this group. The

Box 15: International Comparison of Motives to Work – Peculiarity of Japan's Older People

Hideki Endō

The rate of employment among older people is reportedly higher in Japan than most other countries (OECD 2004). According to the OECD, the rate of employment in Japan's population aged 65 and older is 28.7 percent for men, third highest among thirty OECD countries, and 12.6 percent for women, which is fourth highest.

There are various reasons for older people to seek employment and work. According to a comparison survey conducted in five countries (Japan, USA, Korea, Germany and France) by the Cabinet Office of the Japanese Government (2005), the main motive for Japanese people over the age of 60 to wish to work is 'to earn income'. The situation appears to be similar in the other countries (see Table 13.5).

However, a considerable proportion of them wish to work in order to maintain good health. According to the survey, the proportion of workers aged 60 and older who wish to work continuously because 'work is good for health or preventing senility' is 25.9 percent in Japan which is much higher than 15.8 percent in Korea, 14.8 percent in France, 11.5 percent in the USA and 11.3 percent in Germany. The proportion of those who wish to work for health maintenance purposes is even higher at 31.3 percent among the non-workers aged 60 and older who wish to work (17.0 percent in Korea, 16.1 percent in France, 27.2 percent in the USA and 8.5 percent in Germany).

In Japan, about the same proportion (24.6 percent) of them wish to keep working because their work is 'interesting' or 'energizing'. In the other countries, however, there are more people who wish to work in order to keep themselves interested or energized than those who work for health, a tendency that is particularly marked in Germany and France where there are differences of more than 30 percentage points between these two groups.

health indicators were poorer in persons not engaged in work than those engaged in work. There was no significant association with the years of education.

The associations between financial insecurity and health indicators were considered based on the above findings. As a result, it was shown that the proportions of those who rated poorly in the health indicators were higher among the people with a stronger sense of financial insecurity. This tendency was also confirmed when equivalent income

Table 13.5: International comparison of motives to work (%)

	Japan	USA	Korea	Germany	France
To earn income	42.7	60.0	63.4	43.7	35.2
Work is interesting or energizing	24.6	27.7	20.1	42.3	48.1
To make friends and get to know people through work	4.7	0.0	0.0	0.0	1.9
Work is good for health or preventing senility	25.9	11.5	15.8	11.3	14.8
Other	2.2	0.4	0.8	2.1	0.0

From the 2005 survey of the people (aged 60 or older) who currently have income-generating jobs and wish to keep working.

Prepared from Cabinet Office, *Dai 6 kai kōreisha no seikatsu to ishiki ni kansuru kokusai hikaku chōsa* (The 6th International Comparison Survey of the Daily Life and Attitudes of Elderly Persons).

was taken into account. It has been pointed out in recent years that it is important to consider not only the level of absolute income but also the level of relative income by comparison in any analysis of health status or sense of well-being (Frey and Stutzer 2002). It is likely that the self-rated financial status will increase its importance as a parameter in such studies.

The next point of discussion was whether persons not working continuously were more depressive and in poorer self-rated health than persons engaged in work regardless of their financial status. It was found that persons not working continuously were in poorer health than persons engaged in work regardless of the level of financial insecurity. The result was the same when financial insecurity was substituted with equivalent income.

However, regional differences in health status could not be explained by differences in employment status.

In this chapter, we obtained these results using cross section data. For further study, the causal relationship between employment and health has to be analyzed using panel (or cohort) data which include temporal changes in individual subjects. However, it has been reported by Blau and Gilleskie (2001) in their detailed study of the change of labor force status of the middle-to-old-age people in the USA that self-rated health does not have a significant effect on the change of labor force status. In Germany, a panel data study by Winkelmann and Winkelmann (1998) has demonstrated that unemployment in old age reduces life satisfaction even allowing for household income and the state of physical health. In Japan, Nakazato et al. (2000) point out that the state of mental health of older unemployed persons may temporarily improve immediately after leaving their jobs and deteriorate from then on. According to a study of the causal relationship using the instrumental variable method based on the AGES cohort data, employment in old age extends healthy life expectancy (Endō 2009).

In view of these findings, being in work may keep depression away and maintain levels of self-rated health for older people. This remains a question for further study.

Conclusion

This chapter analyzed the relationships between the employment status of older people, financial insecurity and health indicators.

First, the subjective sense of financial insecurity was associated with poor health indicators regardless of the objective income level. This result suggests the importance of using self-rated financial condition indicators when analyzing the relationship between financial status and health.

Second, self-rated health was poorer and depressive tendency was stronger among older people in the order of persons who had quit a job in the past 12 months, not working continuously and engaged in work even allowing for age, equivalent income and financial insecurity. While this is a cross-section analysis, this finding, together with the findings of preceding studies, points to the possibility that health indicators can be maintained at good levels by employing older people and that they may be aggravated by job loss. These points require further study.

Although the proportion of older people who were employed was higher in the rural regions, the proportion of older people in poor health was also higher there. Regional differences in health indicators could not be explained by differences in employment status.

In the future, it would be necessary to consider the 'significance of the employment of older people' from the viewpoint of not only its impact on the economy but also the maintenance of good health.

Chapter 14

Social Capital and Health: A Community Perspective

Yukinobu Ichida

What is social capital?

Many of the people working in the field of public health may notice that health promotion and other activities involving residents or personnel can be more easily implemented in some local communities or workplaces than in others. While there are many possible determining factors for this, cohesiveness is an important one. Community members tend to behave in a more cooperative manner when they have relationships of trust and mutual help and actively socialize with one another on a routine basis. Roughly, such relationships are called social capital (see Box 16) and are attracting attention in a number of areas. It has been hypothesized that where there is more abundant social capital, there is a higher likelihood of producing favorable outcomes in various aspects of society (Halpern 2005).

Kawachi et al. (1997) conducted a pioneering quantitative study of the relationship between social capital and health based on data collected in thirty-nine states in the USA They demonstrated correlations between social capital indicators and mortality – the mortality rate was lower in the states with more social capital. According to a review of quantitative studies up to 2006 (Islam et al. 2006), seventeen out of the twenty-four quantitative studies which analyzed the relationship between social capital and health at the community level using the more appropriate multilevel analysis (see Box 18) demonstrated a favorable relationship. The relationship between social capital and the Gini coefficient, a measure of inequality of income distribution, has also been analyzed and has shown that social capital is more abundant in communities with less income disparities (Kawachi et al. 1997).

Theme and aims

In this chapter, we shall treat social capital as a variable of the community (see Box 16). While previous chapters discussed the relationship between 'individual variables' and the 'health of the individual', this chapter focuses on the relationship between a 'community variable' called social capital and 'the health of the individual'. First, it aims to demonstrate the existence of contextual community differences in health even allowing for compositional individual factors of community members (see Box 17). Second, it aims to examine whether the remaining community differences in health can be explained by social capital.

Method

The data for analysis in this chapter were collected as part of the AGES by self-administered postal questionnaire in 2003 (Kondō and Hirai 2005). The sample included 15,225 persons aged 65 and older not certified for long-term care and living in their own homes in ten municipalities on the Chita Peninsula, Aichi, with no missing data in the questions about self-rated health, age and gender (44 percent of the distributed forms). In this analysis, the sample in the ten municipalities were divided into twenty-five villages according to the old municipality boundaries used in the census of agriculture and forestry by the Ministry of Agriculture, Forestry and Fisheries (boundaries as at 01 February 1950).[1] The 'communities' in this chapter refer to these twenty-five villages.

Self-rated health (Box 6) was used as an indicator of the health of the individual. The responses to the question 'How do you rate your health?' were 'excellent', 'good', 'fair' and 'poor'. 'Excellent' and 'good' were counted as 0 and 'fair' and 'poor' (collectively described as 'poor') were counted as 1.

Age, gender, equivalent income, years of education and marital status were used as explanatory variables at the individual level and average equivalent income and social capital were used as explanatory variables at the community level. The equivalent income was derived by dividing the household income by the square root of the number of household members (see Box 3). The average equivalent income (hereafter referred to as 'average income') is the mean equivalent income of the sample in each community. Following the example of a previous study, a general sense of trust was used as the parameter of social capital. The responses to the question 'Generally speaking, would you say that most people can be trusted?' were 'yes', 'no' and 'it depends'. The proportions of 'yes' and 'it depends' were obtained for each community.

Box 16: Definition and Measurement of Social Capital

Yukinobu Ichida

While social capital is variously defined by different people, American political scientist Robert Putnam (1993) defines it as 'features of social organization, such as trust, norms, and networks that can improve the efficiency of society by facilitating coordinated actions'. In the field of public health there is a widely used concept of social network whose difference from social capital is the subject of continuing debate, but for present purposes we can consider social capital as a more macroscopic view of the concept of social network. Since the difference between the two concepts stems from a difference in perspectives, it is more accurate to attribute the novelty of the concept to the perspective and analytical approach towards the object in question rather than to the object itself. Metaphorically speaking, the question is whether one perceives the trees growing on a mountain as a collection of trees (i.e., networks between individuals) or a forest (social capital).

Although the term social capital was proposed in the field of sociology during the 1980s (Portes 1998), i.e., prior to Putnam, it was qualitatively transformed in the process of its 'importation' into the field of political science by Putnam (Kage 2002). In sociology, researchers regard the personal connections between individuals as social capital and have mainly studied its correlations with individual-level (microscopic) variables such as socio-economic status. In contrast, Putnam's study on the Italian states (Putnam 1993) examined correlations between social capital indicators and the performance of each state using state-level (macroscopic) variables (Kage 2002). This was new in the sense that it emphasized the idea of accumulation of social capital in areas and groups.

The idea of social capital as a macro-level perspective is becoming mainstream in the field of quantitative public health research (Hawe and Shiell 2000). Accordingly, social capital is mostly measured at the community level, generally through survey methods such as individual questionnaires to gather data about the number of community groups residents participate in, the frequency of exchange between residents, a sense of trust, norms for mutual aid and so on which are used to work out averages and proportions for each community. Major surveys include SOCAT (Social Capital Assessment Tool) by the World Bank (Krishna and Shrader 2002) and GHS (General Household Survey) by the Office for National Statistics, UK (Green and Fletcher 2003).

First, we shall work out the proportion of the people whose self-rated health was 'poor' for each community in order to confirm the existence of differences in health among the communities. Then, we shall observe whether these local differences remain after adjusting for individual factors in order to determine if there is any scope for the existence of community factors influencing health. Finally, we shall consider whether local differences can be explained by social capital even allowing for individual factors.

Analysis of community differences in health

Figure 14.1 shows the percentages of people whose self-rated health was poor in the sample communities in ascending order. They range from 21 percent to 39 percent and confirm the existence of community differences (F-test, $p < 0.01$).

Adjustment for age and gender

The age and gender of the residents may have impacted on the higher percentages in the communities on the right side of Figure 14.1 as it is conceivable, for example, that self-rated health is poorer among older residents. Figure 14.2 shows the rearranged graph after adjusting for age and gender differences (Rasbah et al. 2004).[2] Each point was obtained by deducting the overall average (28 percent) from the community average (which is the spread of community averages). The vertical axis was converted to set the maximum absolute value at 1. The line is almost symmetrical around the horizontal line in the middle and moves away from it towards each end. The variance,[3] an indicator of this spread, was 0.019 ($p = 0.027$)[4] which was significantly different from 0. This points to the existence of community differences that cannot be explained by age or gender.

Figure 14.3 shows the relationship between the spread of community averages adjusted for age and gender only and social capital. The relationship between social capital and self-rated health is observable. Pearson's correlation coefficient was -0.50.[5] However, this result was not adjusted for other individual factors, which might account for part of the correlation. The next part of the analysis shall take account of other individual factors to see: (1) if the community differences in Figure 14.2 remains, and (2) if the correlation in Figure 14.3 remains. If community differences in health cannot be explained by demographic composition alone, then it is likely that some community (contextual) factors are at work.

Figure 14.1: Ratio of residents in poor self-rated health by community

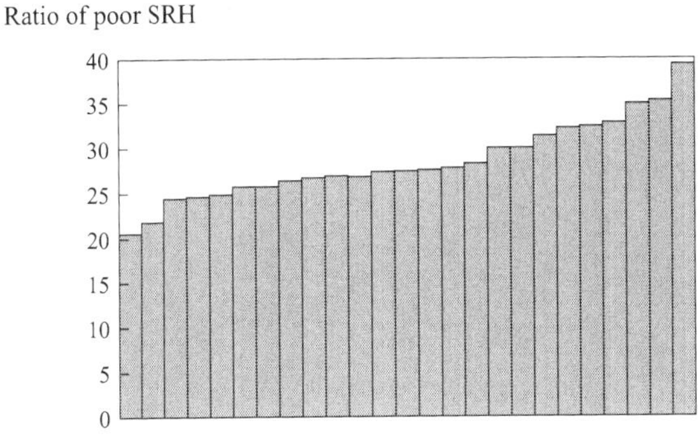

Figure 14.2: Community differences in poor self-rated health adjusted for age and gender

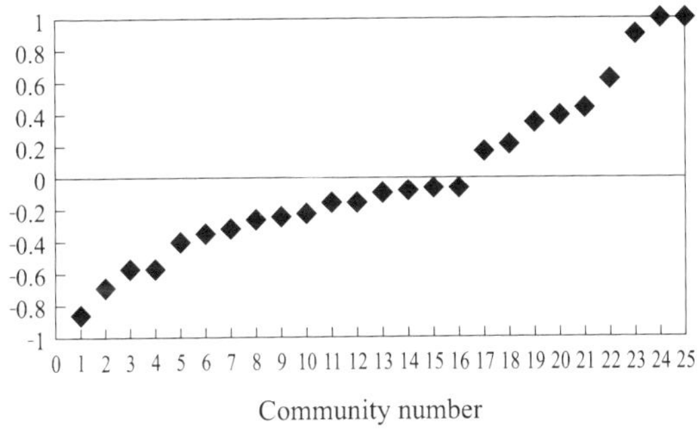

Adjustment for socio-economic factors

Figure 14.4 shows the correlation after adjustment for age and gender in Figure 14.2 (shown as a solid line) as well as the spread of community averages of self-rated health after adjustment for socio-economic variables such as equivalent income, years of education and marital status. It is clear that the spread of community averages is generally closer to the horizontal line in the middle compared with the spread in Figure 14.2 (shown as a solid line here). The variance at the community level has decreased by 0.009 points from 0.019 in Figure 14.2 to 0.010 (p = 0.077).[6] This means that community differences have decreased but the amount of change varies from one community to another.[7]

Figure 14.3: General sense of trust and self-rated health adjusted for age and gender

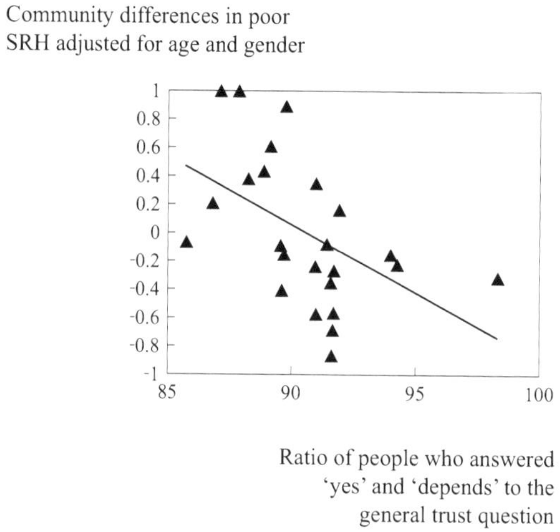

Figure 14.4: Community differences in self-rated health adjusted for age, gender, income, education and marital status

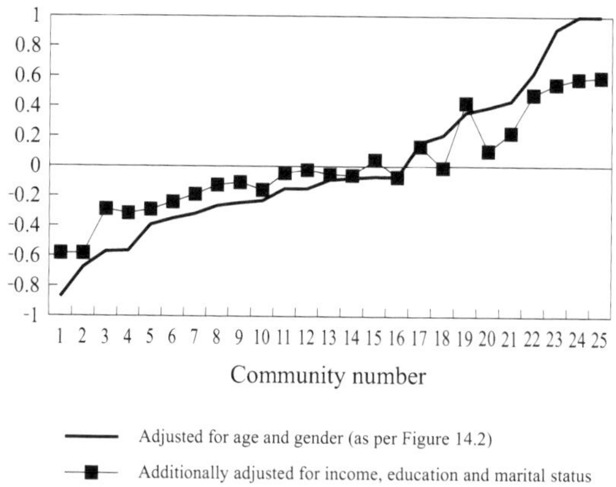

Analysis of correlation between social capital and health

Finally, Figure 14.5 shows the relationship between social capital and the spread of community averages of self-rated health after adjusting for the average equivalent income of each community and for the individual factors such as age, gender, equivalent income, education

Figure 14.5: General trust and self-rated health adjusted for individual factors and average income

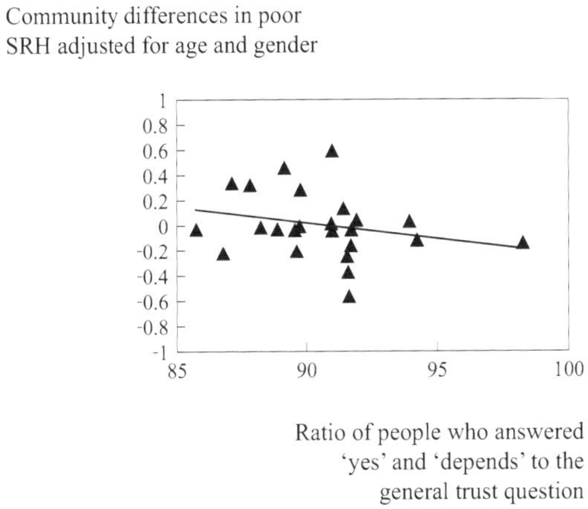

and marital status used in Figure 14.4. It is clear that the relationship is much weaker than that in Figure 14.3. Pearson's correlation coefficient has decreased from -0.50 in Figure 14.3 to -0.25 in Figure 14.5.

At the end, a model was formulated for multilevel analysis (Goldstein 2003; see Box 18), which is a more appropriate statistical method for analyzing the relationship between social capital and health, using self-rated health as the dependent variable and individual factors, and average equivalent income and social capital as the explanatory variables. It showed that the coefficient for social capital was statistically significant at $p = 0.023$ and that the probability of the respondent reporting poor self-rated health decreases by 4 percent as the value of social capital in the community increases by 1 percent.[8] The variance at the community level decreased to 0.005 ($p = 0.21$) when the social capital variable was included.

Discussion

The scatter plot representing the relationship between community differences adjusted for age and gender only and a general sense of trust shown in Figure 14.3 for the sake of comparison exhibits a stronger correlation than that in Figure 14.5. How should we interpret this?

We observed in the first half of the analysis (Figures 14.1, 14.2 and 14.4) that community differences in self-rated health adjusted for age

Box 17: A Compositional Explanation & a Contextual Explanation

Yukinobu Ichida

Is there such a thing as a 'health-enhancing community'? Differences in morbidity, mortality and health behavior between different communities have been explained by demographic composition (compositional explanation) and community context (contextual explanation). The former focuses on the demography (age, income etc.) of the community based on, for example, the reasoning that 'poorer people tend to die younger, therefore the mortality rate must be higher in communities with higher proportions of poor people'. The latter is based on, for example, the reasoning that 'communities with higher concentrations of poor people tend to have poorer infrastructure in terms of housing, hygiene and transport and expose the residents to physical and social health risks' (Macintyre and Ellaway 2003). The former uses factors relating to individual residents to explain differences in health between communities whereas the latter uses non-individual contextual factors. If a 'health-enhancing community' means that one becomes healthier when one moves into that community, the latter has to be the case. In order to find such a community, one must find community factors even after adjusting for the effects of individual factors such as a high proportion of poorer residents.

There used to be a strong tendency in epidemiology and geography to explain regional differences in health in terms of demographic compositional differences. Not enough research was done on the effects of contextual factors on the health of the individual because, first, compositional factors were more marked than contextual factors, and second, there can be an ecological fallacy (see Box 19). However, recent studies using large-scale data and progress in statistical methods such as multilevel analysis (see Box 18) are overcoming these problems and leading to more active research on the effects of contextual factors on health. As part of this trend, social capital is increasingly seen as one of the contextual factors which has positive effects on health.

and gender were partially explained by the individual socio-economic factors of the residents of each community such as equivalent income, education and marital status, and therefore the real community differences were smaller than they appeared (Figure 14.4). However, a certain amount of community differences remained after adjusting for individual socio-economic factors, which suggested the existence

Box 18: Multilevel Analysis

Yukinobu Ichida

Multilevel analysis is a statistical method used for grouped data (Goldstein 2003; Bryk and Raudenbush 1992; Subramanian 2003). For example, in studies of public health and social epidemiology, it is used in situations in which individuals are grouped on a regional or workplace basis. Statistically, it is a specific parameter estimation method that is used when no information about the variance-covariance matrix of error terms is available. More broadly, it refers to a framework of analysis based on types of the Generalized Least-Squares method. There are two reasons why this method is required.

First, and most importantly, the analysis of dependent variables exhibiting a similar tendency within the same region by a standard statistical model such as ordinary least squares method tends to produce standard errors of explanatory variable coefficients that are generally smaller than actual, resulting in falsely significant parameters. This happens because the standard statistical models perform their computations based on the assumption that no such correlations exist. In reality, people living in the same region tend to exhibit similar behavioral patterns and contract similar illnesses. The standard models are incapable of excluding this possibility. Hence, it is more appropriate to use a multilevel analysis model.

Second, analysis without regard for the structure of multiple groups of data may produce various fallacies, including an ecological fallacy (see Box 19) (Diez-Roux 2003). These fallacies can be avoided if the model contains all variables at each level. In the case of region-based groups of individual data, for example, the model should include both individual explanatory variables and regional explanatory variables. The multilevel analysis framework is useful for this.

of community-contextual factors that could not be explained by demographic composition.

In the analysis of the correlation between social capital and health (Figure 14.5) in the second half, the scatter plot of the relationship between community differences in self-rated health adjusted for individual factors (age, gender, equivalent income, education and marital status) and the average equivalent incomes of the communities and a general sense of trust, which was the indicator of social capital, exhibited a weak correlation. Yet, the result of a more rigorous multilevel analysis indicated a statistically significant correlation.

Box 19: Four Fallacies

Yukinobu Ichida

Where there are factors at the individual level and factors resulting from the grouping (by region for example) of individual factors, analysis and inference without taking account of both may lead to the four types of incorrect inference (fallacy) shown in Table 14.1 below. The following explanation assumes the grouping of individual data by region.

The first type is an ecological fallacy. It happens when one makes an incorrect inference that associations derived from an analysis of regional aggregate variables also exist in the same direction and at the same intensity at the individual level. When one finds a correlation between the proportion of residents on low incomes and the proportion of residents with illness 'α' in one region, for instance, one will be committing an ecological fallacy by inferring that a correlation between low income and illness 'α' exists in the same direction and at the same intensity at the individual level.

Table 14.2 shows a fictitious example demonstrating how a correlation found in regional aggregate data does not exist in individual data. Each of the four regions in this example has a total population of 1,000 which is grouped into low, middle and high income groups. The figures under 'ratio of low income earners' and 'ratio of people with illness α' gradually increase to the right, suggesting a positive correlation between the two values in regional aggregate data (a correlation between regional variables). However, data under each region show no difference between the ratio of residents with illness α in the low income group (b/a) and the ratio of residents with illness α in the middle- and high-income group (d/c) (a correlation between individual variables).

In other words, a positive correlation between the ratio of low income earners and the ratio of residents with illness α is found at the regional level even though no such correlation is found at the individual level in any of the regions. In this case, one may incorrectly infer that the positive correlation found in the regional level (ecological) analysis must also exist between the variables at the individual level. This is the ecological fallacy.

Large regional variation of the b/a value is uncommon in reality and a complete absence of correlation at the individual level despite the presence of a correlation among regional variables is relatively rare. Nevertheless, this possibility cannot be excluded in theory.

Table 14.1: Four fallacies

Analysis level	Inference level	Type of fallacy
Group	Individual	Ecologic
Group (excluding individual-level variables)	Group	Sociologistic
Individual	Group	Atomistic[a]
Individual (excluding group-level variables)	Individual	Psychologistic[a]

Note. a: Also called 'individualistic'.
Source: Diez-Roux (1998)1.

Table 14.2: Example of ecologic fallacy

	Region A	Region B	Region C	Region D
Total population (persons)	1,000	1,000	1,000	1,000
Ratio of low income earners (%)	20	40	60	80
Ratio of residents with illness a (%)	10	20	30	40
Total number of low income earners (a) (persons)	200	400	600	800
Low income earners with illness a (b) (persons)	20	80	180	320
Prevalence among low income earners (b/a) (%)	10	20	30	40
Total number of middle & high income earners (c) (persons)	800	600	400	200
Middle & high income earners with illness a (d) (persons)	80	120	120	80
Prevalence among middle & high income earners (d/c) (%)	10	20	30	40

Source: Prepared by the author.

The second type is a sociologistic fallacy. This happens when one makes an incorrect inference based on an association between two regional variables that a regional factor has an impact on the individual. For example, where a correlation is found between the 'ratio of drifters' and the 'ratio of people with schizophrenia' in the four regions shown in Table 14.3, one may incorrectly infer that 'a high proportion of drifters increases a sense of insecurity in the community and disrupts society, increasing the risk of schizophrenia among all residents'. Table 14.3 shows this fictitious example. The ratio of drifters and the ratio of schizophrenic patients both increase to the right in the table, indicating a positive correlation. If the abovementioned inference

Table 14.3: Example of sociologistic fallacy

	Region A	Region B	Region C	Region D
Total population (persons)	1,000	1,000	1,000	1,000
Ratio of drifters (%)	20	40	60	80
Ratio of schizophrenia (%)	1	2	3	4
Number of drifters (a) (persons)	200	400	600	800
Drifters with schizophrenia (b) (persons)	10	20	30	40
Prevalence among drifters (b/a) (%)	5	5	5	5
Number of permanent residents (c) (persons)	800	600	400	20
Permanent residents with schizophrenia (d) (persons)	0	0	0	0
Prevalence among permanent residents (d/c) (%)	0	0	0	0

Source: Prepared by the author.

that 'a high proportion of drifters increases the risk of schizophrenia among all residents' was correct, the risk of schizophrenia among residents (d/c) would increase to the right as well. It is not the case. After all, the correlation between the regional variables can be fully explained by the individual level association that 5 percent of drifters have schizophrenia.

This example demonstrates that caution should be exercised in analyzing regional-level variables derived from individual-level variables. Variables for social capital are often the regional aggregate values of individual survey responses which come to be treated as characteristics of each region. One falls into this fallacy when one infers the existence of some regional (social capital) effect (contextual effect, Box 17) based solely on some association found between regional variables (social capital and health indicators). For instance, a correlation may be found between the ratio of people who answered "yes" to the question about 'a general sense of trust' and the 'ratio of healthy people' at the regional level, this association can be fully accounted for by the individual level association that 'healthier people respond more positively to the question about a general sense of trust' (compositional explanation).

Table 14.4: Example of psychologistic fallacy

	(1) Association between individual-level variables (Region A + B)	(2) Region A with negative regional factors	(3) Region B without negative regional factors
Total population	2,000	1,000	1,000
Total number of new arrivals (a) (persons)	1,000	800	200
Number of depressive new arrivals (b) (persons)	40	40	0
Ratio of depressive new arrivals (b/a) (%)	4	5	0
Total number of permanent residents (c) (persons)	1,000	200	800
Number of depressives permanent residents (d) (persons)	10	10	0
Ratio of depressive permanent residents (d/c) (%)	1	5	0

Source: Prepared by the author.

The third type is called a psychologistic fallacy or individualistic fallacy. This occurs when one ignores the existence of the effects of regional variables on an association between individual variables and makes an incorrect inference that the association exists purely between the individual variables. Table 14.4 shows an imaginary example of this. For example, one may infer that 'relocation causes a depressive tendency' or 'new arrivals had depression genes' based on the association found between individual-level variables suggesting 'new arrivals tend to exhibit a stronger depressive tendency than permanent residents' (b/a is greater than d/c in column (1) in Table 14.4). However, there is the possibility that this was because the new arrivals could not relocate to a region other than a depression-inducing wretched region (no jobs, no medical infrastructure and so on). If so, these negative regional factors may be the real culprits rather than the experience of relocation itself (Riley 1963) (comparing column (2) and column (3) in Table 14.4, it is clear that the proportion of depressive people is also high among permanent residents in region A and that there is no difference between b/a and d/c within that region).

The fourth type is called the atomistic fallacy or individualistic fallacy. This is the opposite of an ecological fallacy and refers to making an incorrect inference about an association between group-level variables based on an association between individual-level

Table 14.5: Example of atomistic fallacy

	Country A	Country B	Country C	Country D
Total population (persons)	1,000	1,000	1,000	1,000
(1) Ratio of high income earners (%)	20	40	60	80
(2) Mortality rate of illness ß (%)	9	16	21	24
Total number of low income earners (a) (persons)	800	600	400	200
Number of deaths from illness ß among low income earners (b) (persons)	80	120	120	80
Mortality rate of illness ß among low income earners (b/a) (%)	10	20	30	40
Total number of middle & high income earners (c) (persons)	200	400	600	800
Number of deaths from illness ß among middle & high income earners (d) (persons)	10	40	90	160
Mortality rate of illness ß among middle & high income earners (d/c) (%)	5	10	15	20

Source: Prepared by the author.

variables. Table 14.5 shows a fictitious example of this. For example, an individual-level analysis of an international survey finds that the rate of mortality from myocardial infarction or angina (illness ß in Table 14.5) is lower among people with higher income (d/c is smaller than b/a in each nation). One commits an atomistic fallacy when one infers that mortality from myocardial infarction or angina is lower in countries with higher per-capita income. In reality, the rate of myocardial infarction-related death is lower in the countries with extremely low per-capita income because their people tend to die young from infectious diseases and not live long enough to develop heart complaints (Diez-Roux 1998) (association between (1) and (2) in Table 14.5).

What is common to these fallacies is the drawing of an inference based only on factors at either the individual level or the regional level despite the involvement of both individual and regional factors. In order to prevent such fallacies, it is necessary to take into account both the compositional factors and contextual factors by using a multilevel analysis technique (Box 18).

In fact, preceding studies have reported that 'people with higher income are more likely to respond positively to the question about a general sense of trust' (Subramanian, Lockner and Kawai et al. 2003; Ichida, Yoshikawa and Matsuda et al. 2005). In view of this and the relationship between 'higher income and higher self-rated health' (Kiyoko, Kondō and Hirai et al. 2005), it is obvious that the relationship shown in Figure 14.3 was an overestimation reflecting this 'compositional' relationship because the relationship between the self-rated health of each community and the social capital indicator for each community calculated from individual responses is partially explainable by the relationship between individual variables which suggests that people earning higher income are healthier and generally more trustful of others.

If all of the responses to a question designed to measure social capital (e.g., a question about a general sense of trust) can be fully explained by the individual's age, income, education and so on, the concept of social capital is of little importance. Is this really the case? A study of the residents of 343 districts in Chicago offers an answer to this question (Subramanian, Lockner and Kawai et al. 2003). The study confirmed that differences of responses to a question about a general sense of trust between districts remained after allowing for the effects of individual factors correlated with their responses (age, gender, race, marital status, income and education). Consequently, it is likely that social capital measured by individual responses in each community still reflected the community characteristics that could not be explained by the individual characteristics of community members.

Need for multilevel analysis

In any case, the health indicator and the social capital indicator collected on the basis of the community are both influenced by demographic composition factors such as age and equivalent income and therefore such influences must be excluded as much as possible before the relationship between them can be evaluated properly. One statistical method that can perform a more accurate evaluation is multilevel analysis (Subramanian 2003). The first study to examine the relationship between social capital and health using multilevel analysis was conducted by Subramanian et al. on 144,692 people in thirty-nine states in the USA (Subramanian, Kawachi and Kennedy 2001). It reported that social capital had a positive influence on self-rated health even after the influences of age, gender, race, income, health insurance membership, regular health checks, smoking and marital status were excluded. There have been fourteen overseas studies, including this USA study, of the correlation between social capital and individual health by multilevel analysis and nine of them report a favorable relationship between them (Islam, Merlo and Kawachi et al. 2009; Turrell, Kavanagh and Subramanian 2006; Kim, Subramanian and Kawachi 2006; Kavanagh, Turrell and Subramanian 2006).

The question about the ways social capital influences individual health must be examined more specifically by future studies. Kawachi (2000) suggests the following four factors: (1) close networks through which health-enhancing information is transmitted (health-related behavior), (2) provision of health-enhancing services by community organizations (provision of access to necessary services and amenities), (3) few conflicts among residents and safer neighborhoods (psychosocial factors), and (4) more egalitarian patterns of political participation (institutional performance factors). These suggestions need to be verified in the near future.

The impact of social capital on the health of the individual may vary depending on the nature of social capital, which needs to be studied. For example, Aida et al. (2009) have demonstrated using the AGES data that the number of remaining teeth is greater in communities with more social capital in the form of participation in horizontal organizations but not vertical organizations. More empirical studies focusing on different characteristics of social capital such as this are needed.

Future outlook

Although it has not yet been established as evidence, implications for those who are involved in public health will be great if the hypothesis that 'the health status of residents is better in communities with more abundant social capital' turns out to be true. They will have to take into account community development and pay attention to the community and social factors as well as the development of health based on individual factors when considering the health of the residents. For example, a Canadian study (Veenstra 2002) has found that social capital is more abundant in communities with smaller income disparities and population migration; hence these factors have some association with the residents' health. While it may be difficult to manipulate social capital itself directly through policy measures (Kawachi 2000), it should be possible to develop policies which take account of social capital.

Conclusion

Some proportion of community differences in self-rated health was found to be unexplainable by demographic composition. While they might be explained by other individual factors, this analysis was more suggestive of the existence of community-contextual factors. Social capital was considered to be one of the community contexts that could account for these community differences.

Studies using the concept of social capital attempt to provide evidence to support the claim that community development is itself conducive to residents' health. Although there are many questions that are yet to be answered, strategies involving research and application of social capital for the purpose of long-term care prevention seems promising.

Notes

1. This was used for the purpose of obtaining the required number of communities for a more accurate estimation of the impact of social capital on health by multilevel analysis. The old boundaries are still used for school zoning and organizing community events such as festivals and sports days in many cases.
2. The remaining differences at the community level estimated using MLwiN were arranged in ascending order. The remaining differences were adjusted by multiplying the average individual-level remainder of each community by a weighting factor allowing for the sample size and the individual-level variance within each community so that communities with smaller sample sizes would generate smaller absolute values.
3. The variance was calculated from the original values of the remaining differences.
4. The p-value was obtained by the Wald test.
5. The p-value was 0.22 for Figure 14.5 and 0.02 in Figure 14.3 but the result of multilevel analysis is more accurate.
6. The significance of the probability of this variance is a necessary condition but not a sufficient condition of zero variance and therefore the non-significance of the finding does not necessarily mean that the variance is zero.
7. For example, the points for communities No. 3 and No. 19 shifted upward (higher proportions of residents in poor self-rated health) after adjustment for socio-economic factors, meaning that the health condition in these communities was not as good as it looked. The appearance of good health was probably due to higher proportions of residents with relatively good socio-economic conditions in these areas. In contrast, communities No. 18, No. 20, No. 21, No. 23, No. 24 and No. 25 shifted much closer to the central horizontal line after adjusting for socio-economic factors, suggesting that much of the community differences in Figure 14.2 were explained

by individual factors and the communities were not as unhealthy as they seemed.

8. For one percentage point increase in general trust, the odds ratio was 0.96 and the confidence interval was 95 percent (from 0.931 to 0.995).

Chapter 15

Implications for Healthy Aging: Notable Findings and the Challenges of Future Research

Katsunori Kondō

Introduction

The main objectives of this study included: verifying the existence of 'inequalities in health' by presenting an accurate picture of the physical, mental and social states of Japan's older population; establishing how important a social epidemiologic approach is; and shedding light on the need to review strategies for healthy aging and long-term care prevention.

The preceding chapters have reported on the results of various analyses of large-scale data (a representative sample of residents in 15 municipalities, n = 32,891) gathered in the AGES project (see Box 2).

This final chapter will recapitulate the notable findings in each of the chapters by reference to the hypothesis (Kondō 2005) shown in Figure 1.1 and discuss the extent to which the initial hypothesis has been verified, the implications for long-term care prevention policy that have been derived from the results and challenges for future research.

Outlines of hypothesis and analytical methodology

Figure 1.1 is a diagram of the hypothesis examined in this study. In essence, the hypothesis stated that social factors (community-level characteristics and individual-level socio-economic status, such as social capital participation in community organizations and social support etc.) are related to self-rated health and depression (directly or indirectly) through psychological factors (stress management ability, sense of coherence (SOC), etc.) (Kondō 2005; Antonovsky 1987), living conditions (hobbies, withdrawal from social life, abuse etc.) or health behaviors (from left to right in the diagram).

Since this was a cross-sectional study, self-rated health (Stuck et al. 1999; Idler and Benymamini 1997) and depression (Kondō 2005; Stuck et al. 1999), which has been shown to be related to death and ill health in many cohort studies, was used as an object variable instead of healthy life expectancy (see Boxes 6 & 7). Among responses to the self-rated health question choosing from four levels, 'poor' and 'fair' were treated as 'poor' in the analysis. For depression, scores of 10 or more in the GDS-15 item questionnaire (see Box 7; Yesavage et al. 1982; Burke et al. 1999) were regarded as 'moderate to severe depression' and scores from 5 to 9 were classified as 'mild depression'.

Each of the factors shown (from right to left) in Figure 1.1 was analyzed in each chapter and considered with regard to three main points.

1. Associations between each factor and self-rated health and depression.
2. Associations between each factor and equivalent income (Box 3) and years of education.
3. Associations between these associations and three regional types (urban, semi-urban and rural; see Chapter 1)

Gender differences were also considered.

Notable findings and verification of hypothesis

Table 15.1 presents a list of notable findings in each chapter and Table 15.2 shows associations between the main factors examined in each chapter (refer to individual chapters for further detail).

Associations with self-rated health and depression

Many of the factors analyzed in the chapters were found to be associated with self-rated health and depression (Table 15.1). The ratios of people having poor self-rated health or depression were higher among those who met the key conditions of the long-term care prevention policy of the Ministry of Health, Labor, and Welfare; namely 'nutrition improvement', 'oral function improvement' and 'withdrawal prevention'. For example, the ratio of people in poor self-rated health among those with low body weight (BMI $\leq$ 18.5) was 39.0 percent, which was significantly higher than 26.8 percent among those who were not thin (BMI > 18.5) ($p < 0.001$).

Men living alone were 3.2 times more likely to suffer depression and one in three women in the low marital satisfaction group (tertile) experienced depression. The prevalence of depression was also higher among people with a sense of financial insecurity. As shown in Table 15.2, more associations were found with depression than with self-rated health in general.

Association with socio-economic status

As shown in Table 15.2, associations were found between many factors and equivalent income and education. For example, a history of falls, the rate of non-participation in health checkups, sleep disorders, hobby activities, participation in organizations, abuse, and the SOC score for stress management ability were all poor among people with low levels of equivalent income and education (see Table 15.1).

Associations with three regional types

Significant differences were found between three regional types with regard to approximately one-half of the analyzed factors (Table 15.2). For example, the ratios of people with at least twenty remaining teeth were lower in the rural regions at 19.9–29.5 percent compared with 33.9–42.0 percent in the urban regions. Some regional differences were found in housebound behavior, depending on the definition. The ratio of people with a hobby, which was found to have a favorable association with mental health, was lower in the rural regions at 62.3 percent as against 74.6 percent in the urban regions (Table 15.1).

Significance of the study – implications for long-term care prevention

The current study is considered significant, because of its large-scale, analyzing data from 32,891 samples. 'Inequalities in health' were broadly observed among older people in Japan, which in the 1980s was regarded as one of the most egalitarian societies in the world. Its life expectancy continues to be the highest in the world. From the perspective of social epidemiology – a branch of epidemiology which investigates the social determinants of health and its pathways, including psychological factors (Kondō 2005; Berkman and Kawachi 2000), we could elicit the following implications for healthy aging and long-term care prevention.

Significance of the 'bio-psycho-social model'

First, the limitations of the 'bio-medical model'-based approach to

Table 15.1: Notable findings in each chapter

Self-rated health & depression (Chapter 2)	The proportions of people in good self-rated health and depression-free were higher in the higher socio-economic status group. For example, the ratio of men in poor self-rated health was 24.2 % for people with 13 or more years of education and 44.5 % for those with less than 6 years.
Life-style choices & falls (Chapter 3)	In comparing low income earners (below 2 million yen) with those earning 4 million yen or more, the ratios of those who walked for a shorter time (e.g., 38.1 % to 31.5 % in men), had falls (e.g., 37.5% to 32.0% in women) and did not attend health checkups (e.g., 24.1 % to 16.1 % in men) were higher among the former.
Dental, oral and nutritional statuses (Chapter 4)	The proportion of people with few remaining teeth was higher among low income earners. However, there was a large difference between regional types as the rate was 6.5 % higher among high income earners (4 mil yen or more) in the rural regions than low income earners (below 2 mil yen) in the urban regions (35.9 % to 29.4 %).
Insomnia (Chapter 5)	The proportion of older people who complained of some kind of sleep disorder was higher in the lower socio-economic status group. For example, the proportion of insomniac (sleep initiation disorder) women was 36.9 % among low income earners (below 2 mil yen) compared with 23.0 % among high income earners (4 mil yen or more).
Sense of coherence (Chapter 6)	The SOC score for stress management was higher among those with higher socio-economic statuses (average 66.6 for 13 or more years of education versus 58.7 for less than 6 years of education). The high SOC score was associated with a good mental health state and moderated the association between a stressor and ill health.
Hobby activities (Chapter 7)	The proportion of people who had hobbies was higher in the high socio-economic status group. For example, the rate of 91.4% among those with 13 or more years of education and income of 4 mil yen or more was twice as high as 45.2 % among those with less than 6 years of education and income below 2 mil yen.
Housebound behavior (Chapter 8)	The proportion of 'housebound' older people who left the house less than once a week was 2.7 (female)–4.1 (male) times higher among those with less than 6 years of education compared to those with 13 or more years of education (11.6 % to 2.8 % in men, 9.4 % to 3.5 % in women).
Abuse (Chapter 9)	Those who were suffering abuse had a poorer mental health state than those who were not. For example, 20 % of the abused and suspected abuse group suffered depression compared with 7.2 % in the non-abused group. The rates of observed abuse for the groups below and above the equivalent income of 2 mil yen were 8.4 % versus 6.0 % for financial abuse. The occurrence of abuse, including physical and psychological abuse, was higher in the low income group.
Marital status (Chapter 10)	The proportion of people sufering depression was 3.2 times higher among solitary men than men living with spouse/ children (17.7% to 5.5 %). The ratio of solitary men was higher among the men with less than 6 years of education.
Participation in community organizations (Chapter 11)	The state of mental health was generally better among the members of community organizations. For example, the proportion of men with depression was 2.5 % among sports club participants and 9.2 % among non-participants. Different types of organization exhibited different patterns of association.

Table 15.1: continued

	For example, the equivalent income was positively associated with participation in some organizations (sports clubs among men and hobby groups among women) and negatively associated with others (religious organizations among women).
Social support (Chapter 12)	The state of mental health was better among older people who were receiving and giving support than those who were only receiving support. For example, the rate of depression was 2.5 times higher for the latter (15 %) than the former (6 %).
Employment status and financial insecurity (Chapter 13)	The proportion of people in poor self-rated health was higher among non-workers (about 26 %) than workers (15.3 %). Depression was associated more strongly with the subjective indicator of financial insecurity than the objective indicator of income (depression was 1.5 % among low income earners with no financial insecurity which was lower than 9.1 % among high income earners with financial insecurity).
Social capital (Chapter 14)	A favorable association was found between community-level social capital and community aggregate self-rated health. For example, the ratio of the people in poor self-rated health was lower in communities with higher proportions of people who generally trusted others and the correlation coefficient was -0.50.

Note. Income mentioned here means equivalent income (household income divided by the square root of the number of household members). See Box 3 and individual chapters for further details.

Table 15.2: Associations between major factors in the analysis

Chapter	Major factors analyzed	Depression	Self-rated health	Socio-economic status	Regional type
2	Years of education, income	○	○	–	–
3	Lifestyle choices & falls	△	△	△	△
4	Dental, oral and nutritional statuses	○	○	△	△
5	Insomnia	○	○	○	×
6	Sense of Coherence	○	○	○	×
7	Hobby activities	○	○	○	○
8	Housebound behavior	○	○	△	△
9	Abuse	○	○	△	△
10	Marital status	○	△	△	×
11	Participation in community organizations	○	△	△	△
12	Social support	○	○	○	△
13	Employment and financial insecurity	○	○	△	–
14	Social capital	△	–	○	–

○: Associated

△: Partially associated

×: Unlikely to be associated

–: Not analyzed

long-term care prevention were confirmed. For example, our analysis found that psychological factors such as depression were associated with under nutrition (see Chapter 4). We also found an association between a history of falls and equivalent income which suggested that 'the wealthy are less likely to fall' (see Chapter 3). Some overseas studies also report associations between falls, bone fracture and socio-economic factors (Bacon and Hadden 2000; Farahmand et al. 2000; West et al. 2004). Our analysis also found that psychological issues such as depression, with socio-economic factors in the background, are associated with elder abuse, which municipal governments in Japan can now deal with under the Elder Abuse Prevention Law. Moreover, a higher proportion of non-respondents in the low income group (Box 20) means that the tendency toward poor health among lower income strata identified in this analysis is likely to have been underestimated.

These findings disclose the limitations of a healthy aging strategy which overemphasizes visible issues such as under nutrition and a history of falls. Such a strategy relies too much on causal models that focus solely on physical conditions such as poor oral function and muscle weakness as causes of those issues. Instead a new approach is needed which takes into account psychological and social factors that lie in the background of these problems. It was particularly surprising to find that the living conditions of older people were influenced so strongly by the number of years of education they had received several decades earlier, perhaps due to the difference it had made to their subsequent life-course experience.

Public health nurses run nutrition education classes but many of the undernourished people who are the target of these classes are depressed and tend to 'withdraw' into their homes. In contrast, highly health-conscious 'regulars' repeatedly attend such classes. Our analyses have revealed that decades-old socio-psychological factors are behind this difference. Hence, it is little wonder that health promotion classes aimed at teaching older people how to change unhealthy lifestyle habits do not yield results. This is one of the reasons that the present check-list screening procedures of people who have health checkups find very few people who are eligible / targeted for long-term care prevention programs; older people with many problems tend to have lower levels of income and education and do not present for health checkups (Chapter 3). Our analyses confirmed that ecological assessment of many intertwined factors, taking into account psycho-social factors such as depression and inadequate social support which underlie risks for frailty and long-term care as well as elder abuse, should not be neglected (Kondō 2005). Health and long-term care policy makers must expand their paradigm from the 'bio-medical model' to a 'bio-psycho-social model'.

Importance of giving/receiving social support and social participation

The proportion of depressed people was lower among those who were involved in both receiving and giving social support than those who were either only receiving or only giving support (Table 15.1; see Chapter 12). Participation in volunteer, hobby or sports organizations was found to be associated with better health (see Chapter 7). The proportion of people in good self-rated health was higher among still working older people than retired or non-working people (except for 553 people who 'had serious illnesses in the last 12 months') (Chapter 13).

These findings suggest the importance of increasing opportunities for older people to have jobs and take an active part in society, rather than providing them with unilateral support measures for long-term care prevention. Increasing the involvement of older people not only in employment but also in community activities such as local festivals, neighborhood safety and other community development programs, volunteer groups and NPO activities is likely to contribute to long-term care prevention.

Importance of stress management ability, anxiety and cognitive faculty

Some psychological factors were found to have strong associations with the health indicators used in this analysis – self-rated health and depression – even allowing for the fact that these indicators themselves are psychological/subjective parameters.

For example, the people with higher levels of equivalent income and education had higher SOC scores for stress management ability. Those who scored high in the SOC scale were less likely to experience depression than those with lower SOC scores even when they encountered stressful life events such as the death of a spouse (Table 15.1; see Chapter 6). The indicator of marital satisfaction (the functional state of one's marital relationship and one's awareness of it) exhibited stronger associations with the health indicators than marital status itself (a structural and objective indicator) (Chapter 10). Furthermore, a sense of financial insecurity had a stronger association

Box 20: Tendency to Non-Response

Kei Suemori

This box reports on an analysis of people's tendency to not respond to the survey questionnaire. The data in this analysis were limited to those from the municipalities which supplied basic information about the residents to us. The sample size was 3,843 persons. Associations between the rate of response (the ratio of the number of respondents to the number of people who received survey forms) and age, gender and income level are considered below.

Regarding the effect of age, no major difference was found in the response rate from age 65 to age 80. However, the response rate decreased over the age of 80 and decreased even further over the age of 85 (56.7 percent at ages 65–69, 54.6 percent at 70–74, 57.8 percent at 75–79, 52.6 percent at 80–84, 47.8 percent at 85 and older). A significant relationship between age and response rate was confirmed ($p < 0.10$).

There was no large difference between the response rates of men and women (55.3 percent for men, 52.5 percent for women). The rate was slightly higher for men than women but the difference was not significant. Table 15.3 shows the result of cross tabulation between the response rate, gender and age.

Regarding the income level, the response rate decreased significantly ($p < 0.001$) as the income level decreased (Figure 15.1). The response rate was 65.1 percent for people whose household income was 2 million yen or more (income level 4), 62.7 percent for household income below 2 million yen (income level 3), 52.0 percent for those who did not pay municipal tax but another household member was paying municipal tax (income level 2) and 49.5 percent for people whose household income was below the municipal tax threshold (income level 1). There was a difference of approximately 15 points between the response rates of level 4 and level 1. The differences in the response rate between income levels were not negligible.

Based on the above, it is likely that the findings of this study reflect the tendencies of older people under the age of 80 and respondents with middle to high levels of household income a little more strongly.

with depression than the more objective indicator of income level did (Chapter 13).

These findings might mean that associations between subjective, cognitive and psychological factors and health are stronger than previously thought under the 'bio-medical model'.

Table 15.3: Response rate (by age and gender) (%)

Age	n	Men	Women	Total
n		1,813	2,030	
65–69	1,407	60.2	53.2	56.7
70–74	1,116	54.3	54.9	54.6
75–79	734	58.1	57.5	57.8
80–84	358	53.3	51.9	52.6
85 +	228	50.7	44.9	47.8

Figure 15.1: Income levels and response rates

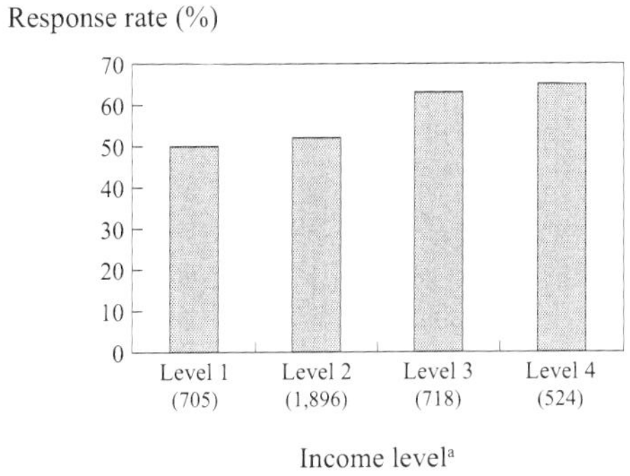

Note.
a: Income level 1 includes people whose household income is exempted from municipal tax payment (including public assistance recipients), level 2 includes respondents who are municipal tax exempted but live with a household member who is liable to pay municipal tax, level 3 includes people whose household income subject to municipal tax is below 2 million yen, and level 4 includes the people whose household income subject to municipal tax is 2 million yen or more.

Regional peculiarity and social capital

The analysis found greater than expected differences between regions. And many of the findings betrayed the common perception that 'the rural regions may be poorer economically but better off in daily living and health'. For example, the proportions of respondents with depression, few remaining teeth and no hobby activities were higher in the rural regions.

These findings imply a need for a greater focus on regional peculiarities, empirical assessment of particular regional characteristics and formulating policy according to the priorities in each region. They also imply limitations of high-risk strategies such as screening targeted individuals and providing health education programs, because differences between regions were not explained by compositional differences of individuals alone. Population strategies (Rose 1992) such as community interventions focusing on fostering social capital might be worth developing, as relationships between social capital and health have been reported in various studies (Kawachi et al. 2008) as well as being observed in the AGES project (Chapter 14; Ichida 2009, Aida 2009).

Gender differences

Finally, the analysis found that gender differences were great, not only biologically, but also psychologically and socially. For example, men tended to have less social support than women and the proportion of respondents who neither received nor gave emotional support was twice as high among men than among women (Chapter 12).

Long-term care prevention policies might need to provide separate programs for men and women. The development of programs for men is especially needed considering that the participants in the existing prevention programs are skewed to women. For example, programs can emphasize themes such as 'muscle and physical strengthening' or 'contributing to society' rather than recreational activities or chatting, which men tend to see as 'childish activities'.

Future issues

The findings reported in this book have demonstrated the importance of the social determinants of health, social epidemiology, and changing long-term care prevention strategies based on them (Kondō 2005). But we must also recognize some limitations of these findings and the future issues they have raised.

First, this study was a cross-sectional analysis limited to an age-adjusted cross-tabulation level analysis. Consequently, it could not verify the directions of the causal relationships between the factors shown in Figure 1.1; it merely established that there are, in fact, associations between them (Kondō 2005). The discovery of associations between many of the factors considered in this analysis points to the possibility that there are various confounding effects or interactions between them. In order to incorporate them into any future attempt to identify causal relationships, longitudinal studies and multivariate analyses will be essential. Cohort studies on the subjects of the loss of healthy life expectancy (death + care requirement certification; Yoshii et al. 2005; Hirai et al. 2009) and dementia (Takeda 2007) are already under way; their outcomes will be reported as they become available.

Second, cohort studies to follow up the findings of this study will not suffice. When the baby-boomer generation, who brought about a transformation of Japanese society, reaches old age, their condition may differ from what has been observed among the subjects of this study (i.e., cohort effects). As demonstrated by the strong impact of the years of education on one's condition in old age, studies have found that one's health is influenced by one's life course (a life process from birth to old age) (Kuh and Ben-Shlomo 2004). In formulating effective long-term care prevention policies, we need to understand 'why' and 'how' this process influences health. For this purpose, future longitudinal empirical studies of older people as well as children, the young and the middle-aged are desirable.

Third, we may uncover causal relationships but we cannot necessarily intervene in all of them. Even for socio-economic factors, intervention is possible with some and impossible or difficult with others. The results of this study presented a motivation for intervening in SOC and social capital. However, it did not establish whether it would be possible to nurture these characteristics in a short period of time or whether such intervention would lead to improvement in the health status of the older population. In the future, we need to develop specific intervention methods and verify their effectiveness (Kondō 2005).

We found that high-risk strategies are not enough to ensure healthy aging; additional 'population strategies' should also be pursued. Such strategies might include 'giving older people a role to play', 'social/community participation', 'networking' and 'NPOs'. They can be classified as interventions based on the bio-psycho-social model rather than solely on the bio-medical model, intervention at the community or regional level instead of at the individual level, and improving the environment rather than changing personal lifestyle habits. A community intervention study is currently underway; its interim outcome evaluations are already producing the anticipated results (Takeda et al. 2009). We need to continue to develop such interventions and application studies.

It is our task to make contributions to theoretical, empirical, basic and application studies in social epidemiology in order to carry out the mission of the Center for Well-being and Society: to foster well-being (happiness/health) in society.

Appendix

The questionnaires used in the "Survey of the Daily Lives of Older People"

1. The version of the questionnaire consisting of dementia-related and intellectual function items (hereafter called "Dementia Version")
2. The version of the questionnaire consisting of family sociological and abuse-related items (hereafter called "Family/Abuse Version")
3. The version of the questionnaire consisting of dental health and nutritional items (hereafter called "Dental/Nutritional Version")

Approximately 80 to 90 percent of the items included in the three versions of the questionnaires are common.

✶ = Items that are version-specific are denoted in the questionnaires.

Survey of the Daily Lives of Older People

Please take some time to complete this questionnaire.

We would like to express our appreciation for your understanding and support of our municipal administration.

The number of older people with care needs is expected to increase with the aging population in our municipality. Thus, more effort has to be made to minimise their care needs and prevent them from being confined to bed or developing dementia.

In order to provide you, as our citizens, with better quality of services, we decided to conduct a survey of your daily life and your opinions and requests on our municipal administration.

The survey targets the citizens over 65 years old who are currently not using any aged care services.

Information you provide us will be used as basic data to direct our efforts to minimise care needs in older people. Please understand the aims of the survey and give us your honest opinions. We may individually provide the information about potentially beneficial services to the people who return the questionnaire. The data will be statistically compiled and analysed with the collaboration of Nihon Fukushi University and your name and responses will not be disclosed publicly.

Thank you for your time and cooperation.

Notes

1. In principle, we would like the addressee to complete the questionnaire.
2. The questionnaire consists of a number of multiple-choice questions. Please circle the number next to the appropriate answer in the questions.
3. When you finish, please return the questionnaire to us in the enclosed envelope by (DATE). (No postage is necessary)

If you have any enquiries regarding this survey, please contact us on the following number.

@@Section, @@Division, @@City
Phone: @@
(Extension: @@)

Survey of the Daily Lives of Older People: Dementia Version

Question 1. First we would like to ask you about your physical status. Please circle the number next to the most appropriate answer in the following questions.

1. How do you rate your health?
    1. Excellent
    2. Good
    3. Fair
    4. Poor
2. How do you feel about your current physical functions (i.e. the abilities to walk independently and take care of yourself) compared to other people of the same age?
    1. Excellent
    2. Good
    3. Fair
    4. Poor
3. Are you currently receiving any medical treatment?
    1. I have no illnesses or disabilities
    2. I have illness(es) or disability(ies) but need no treatment at the moment
    3. I discontinued treatment of my own decision
    4. I am currently receiving some treatment

SQ. If your answer is 2, 3 or 4, what is/are your illness(es) or disability(ies)? Please circle numbers next to all applicable answers.

1. Cancer
2. Heart disease (including irregular heartbeat)

3. Stroke
4. High blood pressure
5. Diabetes (including mild type)
6. Obesity
7. Hyperlipidaemia
8. Osteoporosis
9. Joint disease / neuralgia
10. Injury / fracture
11. Respiratory disease
12. Gastrointestinal disease
13. Liver disease
14. Mental disease
15. Difficulty swallowing
16. Impaired vision
17. Impaired hearing
18. Elimination problems (including incontinence, frequent urination, difficulty in starting urination, leaking of urine, etc.)
19. Undiagnosed illness
20. Other ( )

4. How many kinds of prescribed medicine do you take daily?
   1. None
   2. 1 to 2
   3. 3 to 5
   4. 6 to 9
   5. More than 10
5. Have you ever had any check-ups at a health centre, your workplace, etc.?
   1. I had one within a year
   2. I had one within 2 to 3 years
   3. I had one more than 4 years ago
   4. I've never had one
6. Please reproduce the below figure in the space provided.
   ★This item was included in the Dementia Version only.
   Figure

Question 2. The next questions are about your daily life. Please circle the number next to the most appropriate answer in the following questions.

1. Can you walk independently?
   1. I can walk without assistance
   2. I can walk with partial assistance by hand, etc.

   3. I need full assistance in walking
2. Can you take a bath independently?
   1. I can take a bath without assistance
   2. I can take a bath with partial assistance when washing the body, etc.
   3. I need full assistance in taking a bath
3. Can you use a toilet independently?
   1. I can use a toilet without assistance
   2. I can use a toilet with partial assistance when sitting on a toilet seat, etc.
   3. I need full assistance in using a toilet
4. How is your ability to chew?
   1. I can chew anything I want.
   2. I can chew most foods with some exceptions.
   3. I can eat limited foods as I cannot chew very well.
   4. I can hardly chew anything.
   5. I have liquid foods as I cannot chew at all.
5. What are your current height and weight (Approximate values would be fine).
   Height: Approximately (   ) cm
   Weight: Approximately (   ) kg
6. Do you have any of the following problems in your dietary life?
   ① Has your intake of staple foodstuffs (e.g. rice) been decreasing?
      1. Yes
      2. No
   ② Has your intake of subsidiary foodstuffs (e.g. fish, meat, vegetables) been decreasing?
      1. Yes
      2. No
   ③ Have you lost more than 3 kg over the past six months?
      1. Yes
      2. No
7. What time do you wake up and go to bed?
   ✶ This item was included in the Dementia and the Family/Abuse Versions only.
   I wake up about ( ) am or pm
   I go to bed about ( ) am or pm
8. Do you have any of the following sleeping problems?
   ✶ This item was included in the Dementia and the Family/Abuse Versions only.
   ① Do you have any difficulty in falling asleep?

1. Yes
2. No

② Do you wake up frequently during the night?

1. Yes
2. No

③ Are you unable to feel well-rested when waking in the morning?

1. Yes
2. No

9. Do you take a daytime nap? "Daytime nap" means you lie down to sleep after lunch.
    1. Yes
    2. No

    SQ. If your answer is "1. Yes", please answer the following questions.

    ① How often do you take a daytime nap?

    1. Once or twice a week
    2. Three or four times a week
    3. More than five times a week

    ② How long is your daytime nap?

    1. Less than 30 minutes
    2. 30 to 60 minutes
    3. 60 to 120 minutes
    4. More than 120 minutes

10. How much alcohol do you drink? Note that one gō of sake (approx. 180ml) includes the same amount of alcohol as a medium-sized bottle of beer (approx. 500ml) or 2 ounces of whiskey (approx. 60ml).
    1. I don't drink any alcoholic beverages
    2. I drink alcoholic beverages but not everyday
    3. I drink up to 1½ gō of sake, or equivalent, on average, everyday
    4. I drink more than 1½ gō of sake or equivalent, on average, everyday
11. Do you smoke cigarettes?
    1. I don't smoke or rarely smoke
    2. I used to smoke
    3. I currently smoke
12. How long do you walk a day on average?
    1. Less than 30 minutes
    2. 30 to 60 minutes
    3. 60 to 90 minutes

4. More than 90 minutes

13. How often do you do housework?
    1. Always
    2. Sometimes
    3. Rarely
    4. Never
14. Do you have any roles at home apart from the housework (e.g. keeping the garden or the household vegetable garden, looking after the house, grandchildren or pets)?
    1. Yes
    2. No
15. Do you have any paid work at the moment?
    1. Yes
    2. No
16. How often do you see your family members or relatives who are living apart?
    1. Almost everyday
    2. Twice or three times a week
    3. Once a week
    4. Once or twice a month
    5. Several times a year
    6. Rarely
    7. I have no family members or relatives who are living apart
17. How often do you make contact with your family members or relatives who are living apart by letter, phone or email?
    1. Almost everyday
    2. Twice or three times a week
    3. Once a week
    4. Once or twice a month
    5. Several times a year
    6. Rarely
    7. I have no family members or relatives who are living apart
18. How often do you see your friends?
    1. Almost everyday
    2. Twice or three times a week
    3. Once a week
    4. Once or twice a month
    5. Several times a year
    6. Rarely
19. How often do you make contact with your friends by letter, phone or email?
    1. Almost everyday

2. Twice or three times a week
3. Once a week
4. Once or twice a month
5. Several times a year
6. Rarely

20. How often do you go out to see someone, go shopping, go for a walk or go to hospital, etc.?
    1. Almost everyday
    2. Twice or three times a week
    3. Once a week
    4. Rarely

Question 3. Do you engage in any leisure activities at the moment?
1. Yes
2. No

If your answer is "2. No", please go to 3) on Page 5.
If your answer is "1. Yes", please answer the following questions."

1. (For those with leisure activities) Please circle the number next to the most appropriate answer in the following questions.
   a) Sports activities (e.g. ground golf; gateball [Japanese croquet]; walking; jogging; physical exercises)
      1. I don't engage in any sports activities
      2. Almost everyday
      3. Twice or three times a week
      4. Once a week
      5. Once or twice a month
      6. Several times a year
   b) Cultural activities (e.g. reading; haiku [Japanese poetry consisting seventeen syllables]; tanka [Japanese poetry consisting thirty-one syllables]; calligraphy; language learning; using the computer; playing go [Japanese board game played with black and white stones])
      1. I don't engage in any cultural activities
      2. Almost everyday
      3. Twice or three times a week
      4. Once a week
      5. Once or twice a month
      6. Several times a year
   c) Musical activities (e.g. playing musical instruments; choral singing; folk singing; karaoke; dancing)
      1. I don't engage in any musical activities
      2. Almost everyday

   3. Twice or three times a week
   4. Once a week
   5. Once or twice a month
   6. Several times a year
- d) Creative activities (e.g. handicraft; painting; photography)
   1. I don't engage in any creative activities
   2. Almost everyday
   3. Twice or three times a week
   4. Once a week
   5. Once or twice a month
   6. Several times a year
- e) Horticulture; gardening; growing crops; rearing animals; fishing; nature hiking, etc.
   1. I don't engage in any of the above activities
   2. Almost everyday
   3. Twice or three times a week
   4. Once a week
   5. Once or twice a month
   6. Several times a year
- f) Watching TV; watching videos; listening to the radio, etc.
   1. I don't engage in any of the above activities
   2. Almost everyday
   3. Twice or three times a week
   4. Once a week
   5. Once or twice a month
   6. Several times a year
- g) Driving; travelling; visiting historical shrines and temples, etc.
   1. I don't engage in any of the above activities
   2. Almost everyday
   3. Twice or three times a week
   4. Once a week
   5. Once or twice a month
   6. Several times a year
- h) Stock investment; betting on the boat races; playing pachinko [Japanese pinball], etc.
   1. I don't engage in any of the above activities
   2. Almost everyday
   3. Twice or three times a week
   4. Once a week
   5. Once or twice a month
   6. Several times a year

2. (For those with leisure activities) What are the purposes of your leisure activities? Please circle the number next to the most appropriate answer in the following questions.
   ✶ This item was included in the Dementia Version only.
   a) To improve knowledge and skills
      1. Disagree
      2. Somewhat disagree
      3. Neither agree nor disagree
      4. Somewhat agree
      5. Agree
   b) For pleasure
      1. Disagree
      2. Somewhat disagree
      3. Neither agree nor disagree
      4. Somewhat agree
      5. Agree
   c) To communicate with other people
      1. Disagree
      2. Somewhat disagree
      3. Neither agree nor disagree
      4. Somewhat agree
      5. Agree
   d)To maintain physical fitness
      1. Disagree
      2. Somewhat disagree
      3. Neither agree nor disagree
      4. Somewhat agree
      5. Agree
   e) To prevent dementia
      1. Disagree
      2. Somewhat disagree
      3. Neither agree nor disagree
      4. Somewhat agree
      5. Agree
3. (For those without any leisure activities) What are the reasons for your nonparticipation in leisure activities. Please circle numbers next to all applicable answers.
   1. I don't have enough motivation
   2. I discontinued for some reason
   3. I cannot find anything interesting
   4. I feel it troublesome to associate with people
   5. I don't have enough money

6. I don't have enough time
7. I've had no opportunities
8. Other ( )

Question 4. Have you experienced any of the following events over the past year?

Have you retired from your job?
1. Yes
2. No

Have you lost your spouse?
1. Yes
2. No

Have you lost any close relatives, family members or friends?
1. Yes
2. No

Have you suffered from any serious illnesses?
1. Yes
2. No

Have you experienced any changes in your living environment due to moving house, etc.?
1. Yes
2. No

Have you experienced increased financial difficulties?
1. Yes
2. No

Have you started caring for any sick family members?
1. Yes
2. No

Question 5. We would like to ask you how you feel about your life. Some of the following questions may seem to be difficult to answer but please try to do so as they are very important.

Circle 1 if your feeling in the given situation would be exactly 1 or circle 7 if it would be exactly 7. If it would be neither 1 nor 7, circle the number above the answer that best describes how you would feel in the given situation.

E.g. Do you feel refreshed by exchanging morning greetings with others? Circle 4 if your feeling in the above situation would be exactly between "1. Never" and "7. Very often".

1	2	3	4	5	6	7
Never						Very often

1. Do you have the feeling that you don't really care about what goes on around you?
   1 2 3 4 5 6 7
   Very seldom or never Very often
2. Has it happened in the past that you were surprised by the behavior of people whom you thought you knew well?
   1 2 3 4 5 6 7
   Never happened Always happened
3. Has it happened that people whom you counted on disappointed you?
   1 2 3 4 5 6 7
   Never happened Always happened
4. Until now your life has had:
   1 2 3 4 5 6 7
   No clear goals or purpose at all Very clear goals and purpose
5. Do you have the feeling that you're being treated unfairly?
   1 2 3 4 5 6 7
   Very often Very seldom or never
6. Do you have the feeling that you are in an unfamiliar situation and don't know what to do?
   1 2 3 4 5 6 7
   Very often Very seldom or never
7. Doing the things you do every day is:
   1 2 3 4 5 6 7
   A source of deep pleasure and satisfaction
   A source of pain and boredom
8. Do you have very mixed-up feelings and ideas?
   1 2 3 4 5 6 7
   Very often Very seldom or never
9. Does it happen that you have feelings inside you would rather not feel?
   1 2 3 4 5 6 7
   Very often Very seldom or never
10. Many people – even those with a strong character – sometimes feel like sad sacks (losers) in certain situations. How often have you felt this way in the past?
    1 2 3 4 5 6 7
    Very often Very seldom or never
11. When something happened, have you generally found that:
    1 2 3 4 5 6 7
    You overestimated or underestimated its importance
    You saw things in the right proportion

12. How often do you have the feeling that there's little meaning in the things you do in your daily life?
    1 2 3 4 5 6 7
    Very often Very seldom or never
13. How often do you have feelings that you're not sure you can keep under control?
    1 2 3 4 5 6 7
    Very often Very seldom or never

Question 6. The next questions are about your relationships with others. If your answer is "Yes", please put circles in the square brackets next to all applicable answers in the following questions.

1. Do you have someone who listens to your concerns and complaints?
   1. Yes
   2. No
      [ ] Family members living together
      [ ] Children or relatives living apart
      [ ] Acquaintances, friends or neighbours
2. Do you listen to someone's concerns and complaints?
   1. Yes
   2. No
      [ ] Family members living together
      [ ] Children or relatives living apart
      [ ] Acquaintances, friends or neighbours
3. Do you have someone who looks after you when you are sick and stay in bed for a few days?
   1. Yes
   2. No
      [ ] Family members living together
      [ ] Children or relatives living apart
      [ ] Acquaintances, friends or neighbours
4. Do you look after someone when he/she is sick and stays in bed for a few days?
   1. Yes
   2. No
      [ ] Family members living together
      [ ] Children or relatives living apart
      [ ] Acquaintances, friends or neighbours
5. Do you have someone who acknowledges your existence and value?
   1. Yes

2. No
   [ ] Family members living together
   [ ] Children or relatives living apart
   [ ] Acquaintances, friends or neighbours

6. Is there anyone (including your family members) who embezzles your savings or pension without your consent?
   1. Yes
   2. No
      [ ] Family members living together
      [ ] Children or relatives living apart
      [ ] Acquaintances, friends or neighbours

Question 7. The next questions are about your house.

1. What is the type of your house?
   1. Owned house
   2. Privately-rented house
   3. Municipally-managed house
   4. Company-owned house
   5. Other
2. The next questions are about the conditions inside or around your house.
   Are there any steps at the toilet or bathroom doorway?
   1. Yes
   2. No

   Are there any steps or uneven surfaces between the front door and the adjacent road?
   1. Yes
   2. No

   Are there any conditions that make you feel uneasy about going out alone (e.g. busy roads, hills around the house)?
   1. Yes
   2. No
3. Have you had any falls over the past year?
   1. Many times
   2. Once
   3. None

   SQ. If your answer is "1. Many times" or "2. Once", where was/were the scene(s) of the fall(s)? Please circle numbers next to all applicable answers.
   1. Toilet
   2. Bathroom or washroom
   3. Bedroom or living room

4. Corridor
5. Stairs inside the house
6. Front door
7. Garden
8. Road
9. Stairs outside the house
10. Train or bus
11. Other ( )

Question 8. The next questions are about your daily life. Please circle the number next to the (most) appropriate answer in the following questions.

1. Can you use public transportation (bus or train) by yourself?
    1. Yes
    2. No
2. Are you able to prepare meals by yourself?
    1. Yes
    2. No
3. Are you able to pay bills?
    1. Yes
    2. No
4. Can you handle your own banking?
    1. Yes
    2. No
5. Are you able to fill out forms for your pension?
    1. Yes
    2. No
6. Do you read books or magazines?
    1. Yes
    2. No
7. Are you interested in news stories or programs dealing with health?
    1. Yes
    2. No
8. Do you visit the homes of friends?
    1. Yes
    2. No
9. Are you sometimes called on for advice?
    1. Yes
    2. No
10. Are you able to visit sick friends?
    1. Yes

    2. No

11. Do you sometimes initiate conversations with young people?
    1. Yes
    2. No
12. Are you able to shop for daily necessities?
    1. Yes
    2. No

    SQ. If your answer is "1. Yes", how often do you go shopping?
    1. Almost everyday
    2. Twice or three times a week
    3. Once a week
    4. Once or twice a month
    5. Less than several times a year
13. Do you read newspapers?
    1. Yes
    2. No

    If your answer is "1. Yes", how often do you read papers?
    1. Almost everyday
    2. Twice or three times a week
    3. Once a week
    4. Once or twice a month
    5. Less than several times a year
14. Do you often get into trouble as you leave your belongings behind somewhere?
    1. Yes
    2. No
15. Do you often get times or places confused?
    1. Yes
    2. No
16. Do you often forget things that happened recently (e.g. what you had for breakfast)?
    1. Yes
    2. No

Question 9. Please circle the number next to the most appropriate answer in the following questions.

1. Generally speaking, would you say that most people can be trusted?
    1. Yes
    2. No
    3. It depends on the situation

2. Do you think most people would try to take advantage of you if they got the chance?
   1. Yes
   2. No
   3. It depends on the situation
3. Would you say that most of the time people try to be helpful?
   1. Yes
   2. No
   3. It depends on the situation

Question 10. Imagine a big earthquake occurs in the area where you live. What kind of actions or thoughts do you expect the people living in your area are likely to have or take around that time? Please circle the number above the most appropriate answer in the following questions.

1. They will;

   1 2 3 4 5 6 7

   Successfully overcome many hardships in the wake of the earthquake

   Take long to overcome many hardships in the wake of the earthquake
2. They will;

   1 2 3 4 5 6 7

   Only be confused

   Judge what they should do calmly
3. They will find;

   1 2 3 4 5 6 7

   No meaning in this experience

   Some meaning in this experience

Question 11. Imagine a local problem (e.g. frequent crimes) occurs in the area where you live. What kind of actions or thoughts do you expect the people living in your area are likely to have or take around that time? Please circle the number above the most appropriate answer in the following questions.

1. They;

   1 2 3 4 5 6 7

   Will successfully solve the problem by collective efforts

   Won't be able to solve the problem by collective efforts
2. They will;

   1 2 3 4 5 6 7

Only be confused

Try to understand the true nature of the problem and seek a solution to it

3. The relations of trust within the area will be;

1	2	3	4	5	6	7
Damaged						Strengthened

Question 12

1. Which of the following did you regard as the "area" when answering Question 10 and 11?
   1. Neighbourhood association level
   2. Municipal level
   3. Prefectural level
   4. Regional level (e.g. Tōkai Region)
   5. National level
2. How long have you been living in the current municipality?
   1. Less than 4 years
   2. 5 to 9 years
   3. 10 to 19 years
   4. 20 to 29 years
   5. 30 to 39 years
   6. 40 to 49 years
   7. More than 50 years
3. How attached are you to the area you live?
   1. Very
   2. Moderately
   3. Neutral
   4. Slightly
   5. Not at all
4. Do you belong to the following organisations or groups?

   Political organisation or group
   1. Yes
   2. No

   Industrial or trade association
   1. Yes
   2. No

   Volunteer group
   1. Yes
   2. No

   Citizen or consumer group
   1. Yes
   2. No

Religious organisation or group
1. Yes
2. No

Sports group or club
1. Yes
2. No

Neighbourhood assoc./Senior citizens' club/Fire-fighting team
1. Yes
2. No

Hobby group
1. Yes
2. No

SQ. For those who belong to any of the above organisations or groups.

① Do you serve as the head, manager or treasurer in the organisation(s) or group(s)?
1. Yes
2. No

② How often do you participate in the activities all together?
1. Almost everyday
2. Twice or three times a week
3. Once a week
4. Once or twice a month
5. Several times a year
6. Rarely

③ Is your participation in the activities generally voluntary or obligatory?
1. Very voluntary
2. Somewhat voluntary
3. Neither voluntary nor obligatory
4. Somewhat obligatory
5. Very obligatory

④ Which of the following services or activities would you like to use or participate in? Please circle numbers next to all applicable answers.
1. Household assistance
2. Meal delivery
3. Provision or lending of emergency contact devices
4. Safety confirmation by neighbours, volunteers, etc.
5. Attendance service when going out
6. Health consultation or course conducted by physicians, public health nurses, etc.

7. Nutritional consultation or course conducted by nutritionists, etc.
8. Dental consultation or course conducted by dentists, dental hygienists, etc.
9. Fall prevention course
10. Dementia prevention course
11. Sports or leisure activity group
12. University for seniors, etc.
13. Local volunteer activities

Question 13. Please circle the number next to the appropriate answer in the following questions.

1. Are you basically satisfied with your life?
    1. Yes
    2. No
2. Do you have as much pep as you had last year?
    1. Yes
    2. No
3. Do little things bother you more this year?
    1. Yes
    2. No
4. Do you feel that as you get older you are less useful?
    1. Yes
    2. No
5. Do you sometimes worry so much that you can't sleep?
    1. Yes
    2. No
6. Do you feel pretty worthless the way you are now?
    1. Yes
    2. No
7. Are you as happy now as you were when you were younger?
    1. Yes
    2. No
8. Do you have a lot to be sad about?
    1. Yes
    2. No
9. Do things keep getting worse as you get older?
    1. Yes
    2. No
10. Do you take things hard?
    1. Yes
    2. No

11. Do you get upset easily?
    1. Yes
    2. No
12. Have you dropped many of your activities or interests?
    1. Yes
    2. No
13. Do you feel that your life is empty?
    1. Yes
    2. No
14. Do you often get bored?
    1. Yes
    2. No
15. Are you in good spirits most of the time?
    1. Yes
    2. No
16. Are you afraid that something bad is going to happen to you?
    1. Yes
    2. No
17. Do you feel happy most of the time?
    1. Yes
    2. No
18. Do you feel helpless?
    1. Yes
    2. No
19. Do you prefer to stay at home, rather than go out and do things?
    1. Yes
    2. No
20. Do you feel that you have more problems with memory than most?
    1. Yes
    2. No
21. Do you think it is wonderful to be alive now?
    1. Yes
    2. No
22. Do you feel full of energy?
    1. Yes
    2. No
23. Do you feel that your situation is hopeless?
    1. Yes
    2. No
24. Do you think that most people are better off then you are?
    1. Yes

2. No

Question 14. Please answer the following questions.
★ This item was included in the Dementia Version only.

1. Do you think dementia is a disease?
   1. Yes
   2. I think anyone can develop it as they grow older.
   3. Not certain
2. Do you practise something to prevent dementia in your daily life?
   1. Yes
   2. No

   SQ. If your answer is "1. Yes", which of the following are you practising to prevent dementia? Please circle numbers next to all applicable answers.
   1. Orderly life
   2. Balanced diet
   3. Moderate exercise
   4. Adequate sleep
   5. Going out
   6. Regular health checkups
   7. Communication with others
   8. Trying something new
   9. Other ( )

Question 15. We would like to ask you about yourself. Please circle the number next to the (most) appropriate answer in the following questions.

1. Sex
   1. Male
   2. Female
2. Date of birth
   1. Meiji
   2. Taisho
   3. Showa

   Date of birth:
   ( ) years old
3. How many years did you receive school education? Please circle the number next to the most appropriate answer.
   1. Less than 6 years
   2. 6 to 9 years

   3. 10 to 12 years
   4. More than 13 years
   5. Other
4. What is your marital status?
   1. Married
   2. Widowed or divorced
   3. Never married
   4. Other
5. Do you live with anyone in the following? Please circle numbers next to all applicable answers.
   1. I live alone
   2. Spouse
   3. Children
   4. Spouses of children
   5. Grandchildren or great-grandchildren
   6. Parents
   7. Parents-in-law
   8. Brothers or sisters
   9. Brothers/sisters-in-law
   10. Other relatives
   11. Unrelated person/people
   12. Other (   )
6. How many children do you have (excluding the deceased)?
   (   ) children
7. How many people live in your household?
   (   ) people
8. Which of the following was your pretax annual household income for 2002?
   1. Less than 500,000 yen
   2. 500,000 to 1,000,000 yen
   3. 1,000,000 to 1,500,000 yen
   4. 1,500,000 to 2,000,000 yen
   5. 2,000,000 to 2,500,000 yen
   6. 2,500,000 to 3,000,000 yen
   7. 3,000,000 to 4,000,000 yen
   8. 4,000,000 to 5,000,000 yen
   9. 5,000,000 to 6,000,000 yen
   10. 6,000,000 to 7,000,000 yen
   11. 7,000,000 to 8,000,000 yen
   12. 8,000,000 to 9,000,000 yen
   13. 9,000,000 to 10,000,000 yen
   14. More than 10,000,000 yen

9. How worried are you if you have to deal with an unexpected expense?
    1. Not at all
    2. Slightly
    3. Moderately
    4. Very
10. Can you afford leisure activities or simple luxuries?
    1. Very
    2. Moderately
    3. Slightly
    4. Not at all

✶ Please give us your opinions or requests on our municipal administration.

Thank you for your cooperation

Survey of the Daily Lives of Older People: Family/Abuse Version

Question 2

18. How often do you see your friends?

    ✶ This item was included in all the versions but an additional answer "7. I have no friends" was added to the Family/Abuse and the Dental/Nutritional Versions.
    1. Almost everyday
    2. Twice or three times a week
    3. Once a week
    4. Once or twice a month
    5. Several times a year
    6. Rarely
    7. I have no friends
19. How often do you make contacts with your friends by letter, phone or email?

    ✶ This item was included in all the versions but an additional answer "7. I have no friends" was added to the Family/Abuse and the Dental/Nutritional Versions.
    1. Almost everyday
    2. Twice or three times a week
    3. Once a week
    4. Once or twice a month
    5. Several times a year
    6. Rarely
    7. I have no friends

Question 3. Do you engage in any leisure activities at the moment?
1. Yes
2. No

If your answer is "2. No", please go to 2) on Page 4.
If your answer is "1. Yes", please answer the following questions.

Question 14. The next questions are about your family life. Please circle the number next to the most appropriate answer in the following questions.

✶ This item was included in the Family/Abuse Version only.

1. Your eldest child listens to your worries and problems.
   1. Strongly agree
   2. Agree
   3. Somewhat agree
   4. Somewhat disagree
   5. Disagree
   6. Strongly disagree
   7. I have no children
2. Your youngest child listens to your worries and problems.
   1. Strongly agree
   2. Agree
   3. Somewhat agree
   4. Somewhat disagree
   5. Disagree
   6. Strongly disagree
   7. I have no children or have only one child
3. How satisfied are you with your marital relationship?
   1. Very satisfied
   2. Satisfied
   3. Somewhat satisfied
   4. Somewhat dissatisfied
   5. Dissatisfied
   6. Very dissatisfied
   7. I have no spouse
4. How often do you have a quarrel or argument with your spouse?
   1. More than three times a week
   2. Once a week
   3. Once a month
   4. Once every six months
   5. Once a year
   6. Rarely
   7. I have no spouse

5. How often do you see your grandchildren?
    1. More than three times a week
    2. Once a week
    3. Once a month
    4. Once every six months
    5. Once a year
    6. Rarely
    7. I have no grandchildren
6. Have you ever received the following treatment from any family members?
    ✶ This item was included in the Family/Abuse Version only.
    a) Physical abuse such as punching, kicking, throwing things and confining.
        1. Never
        2. Once or twice
        3. Sometimes
        4. Often
    b) Psychological abuse such as using abusive language, making sarcastic comments and ignoring for a long time.
        1. Never
        2. Once or twice
        3. Sometimes
        4. Often
    c) For those whose answer is other than "1. Never" in the above questions, have you ever consulted with someone on this issue?
        1. Yes
        2. No

    SQ1. Who have you consulted with?
        1. Friends or acquaintances
        2. Family members or relatives
        3. The police
        4. Doctor
        5. Court
        6. Other (   )

    SQ2. Would you like to consult with someone reliable?
        1. Yes
        2. No

Survey of the Daily Lives of Older People: Dental/Nutritional Version

Question 1

5. Are you taking any of the following medications? Please circle numbers next to all applicable answers.
   ✶ This item was included in the Dental/Nutritional Version only.
   1. Sleeping pills
   2. Tranquiliser
   3. Laxative
   4. Antihypertensive (Medicine to lower blood pressure)
   5. Other (   )

Question 2

4. What are the status of your dental health and your use of dentures at mealtimes?
   ✶ This item was included in the Dental/Nutritional Version only.
   1. I have 20 or more natural teeth
   2. I have 19 or less natural teeth and use dentures (including partial dentures)
   3. I have 19 or less natural teeth but use no dentures (including partial dentures)
   4. I have few natural teeth and use dentures
   5. I have few natural teeth but use no dentures
6. Do you try to do something for your dental health (e.g. brushing teeth, rinsing out the mouth or cleaning dentures)?
   ✶ This item was included in the Dental/Nutritional Version only.
   1. Yes
   2. No
   3. Not certain
7. Do you have a regular dentist?
   ✶ This item was included in the Dental/Nutritional Version only.
   1. Yes
   2. No
8. Do you have any of the following dental health problems? Please circle numbers next to all applicable answers.
   ✶ This item was included in the Dental/Nutritional Version only.
   1. I have none of these problems
   2. Pain in teeth or gums
   3. Difficulty in eating due to sensitive / loose teeth or impaired chewing ability
   4. Dry mouth
   5. Bad breath

6. Irregular or discoloured teeth
7. Impaired taste
8. Poorly-fitted dentures
9. Other ( )

10. Eating is not enjoyable but bothersome.
✶ This item was included in the Dental/Nutritional Version only.
1. Yes
2. No

17. Do you have any family members who require nursing care because of old age, illness or disability?
✶ This item was included in the Dental/Nutritional Version only.
1. Yes
2. No

24. Do you have any important people in your life who make your life worth living or are the source of emotional support. Please circle numbers next to all applicable answers.
✶ This item was included in the Dental/Nutritional Version only.
1. I have no important people in my life
2. Spouse
3. Children
4. Grandchildren
5. Parents
6. Brothers or sisters
7. Other relatives
8. Neighbours, local acquaintances or friends
9. Work-related acquaintances or friends
10. Acquaintances or friends from childhood
11. Acquaintances or friends from school days
12. Former teachers
13. Acquaintances or friends with common interests
14. Acquaintances or friends from volunteer activities
15. Great religious figures or acquaintances or friends from religious activities
16. Fictional characters or historical figures
17. Show business or cultural figures
18. Other acquaintances or friends
19. Other ( )

Question 3. Do you engage in any leisure activities at the moment?
1. Yes
2. No
If your answer is “2. No”, please go to 2) on Page 5.

If your answer is "1. Yes", please answer the following questions.

2. (For those without any leisure activities) What are the reasons of your nonparticipation in leisure activities. Please circle numbers next to all applicable answers.
   1. I discontinued

Question 6

7. What is the ratio of the amount of support you provide to others (including family members) to the amount of support you receive from others?
   ✶ This item was included in the Dental/Nutritional Version only.
   1. I receive much more support from others
   2. I receive a little more support from others
   3. I provide and receive about the same amount of support
   4. I provide a little more support to others
   5. I provide much more support to others

Bibliography

8020 Suishin Zaidan, *80-sai ni nattemo jibun no ha o20-pon ijō motō* (How to retain at least 20 of your own teeth even when you are 80): http://www.8020zaidan.or.jp/

Agency for Cultural Affairs (2005), *Shūkyō nenkan heisei 16 nen ban* (Religion year book 2004), Tokyo: Gyōsei.

Aida, Jun, Tomoya Hanibuchi, Miyo Nakade *et al.* (2009), 'The different effects of vertical social capital and horizontal social capital on dental status: A multilevel analysis', *Social Science & Medicine*, 69(4), pp. 512–18.

Aida, Jun and Katsunori Kondō (2007), 'Shika shikkan ni okeru kenkō kakusa to sono taisaku (Inequalities in oral health and countermeasures)', *Hokenshi jinrui* (Japanese journal of public health nursing), 63(11), pp. 1038–43.

Akerstedt, T., A. Knutsson, P. Westerholm, T. Theorell, L. Alfredsson and G. Kecklund (2002), 'Sleep disturbances, work stress and work hours: A cross-sectional study', *Journal of Psychosomatic Research*, 53(3), pp. 741–8.

Akihusa S., I. Soh, T. Ansai *et al.* (2005), 'Relationship of number of remaining teeth to health-related quality of life in community-dwelling elderly', *Gerodontology* 22(2), pp. 91–7.

Akiyama, Toyoko (1997), 'Media no ukete ga kawaru (Change in the receiver of the media)' in Hiroshi Oyama and Haruo Sudō (eds), *Fureai no nettowāku* (Communal networks), Tokyo: NHK Books, pp. 161–88.

Ama, T. (1996), *Nihonjin wa naze mushūkyō nanoka* (Why do Japanese people have no religion?), Tokyo: Chikuma Shobō.

American Geriatrics Society, British Geriatrics Society, and American Academy of Orthopedic Surgeons Panel on Falls Prevention (2001), 'Guideline for the prevention of falls in older persons', *Journal of the American Geriatric Society*, 49, pp. 664–72.

American Psychiatric Association (2000), *Diagnostic and Statistical Manual of Mental Disorders, Fourth Edition*, Washington, D.C.: American Psychiatric Publishing, Inc.

Andō, Yūichi (2000), '8020-sha no dēta banku kōchiku (The creation of an 8020 persons data bank)', in *Kōreisha no kenkō chōsa ni okeru kōkū jōtai no hyōka, denshō kara kagaku he: Kōkū hoken to zenshinteki na kenkō jōtai no kankei ni tsuite, sasshi 1* (Oral health status assessment in the health survey of the aged: From myth to science II: Relationship between oral health and general health, volume 1), Tokyo: Kōkū Hoken Kyōkai, pp. 12–43.

Angel, R. J. *et al.* (2003), 'Financial strain and health among elderly Mexican-origin individuals', *Journal of Health and Social Behavior*, 44, pp. 536–51.

Anme, T. and C. Shimada (2000), 'Kōreisha no shakai kanren-sei to seimei yogo: Shakai kanren-sei shihyō to 5-nen go no shibō-ritsu no kankei (Social interaction and mortality: A five-year longitudinal study of the elderly)', *Nippon kōshū eisei zasshi* (Japanese journal of public health), 47, pp. 127–33.

Anme, T., R. Shinohara, Y. Sugisawa *et al.* (2006), 'Kōreisha no shakai kanren-sei to seimei yogo: Shakai kanren-sei shihyō to 7-nenkan no shibō-ritsu no kankei (Social interaction and mortality: A seven-year longitudinal study of elderly people)', *Nippon kōshū eisei zasshi* (Japanese journal of public health), 53, pp. 681–7.

Antonovsky, A. (1987), *Unraveling the Mystery of Health: How People Manage Stress and Stay Well*, Jossey Bass Social and Behavioral Science Series. San Francisco: Jossey Bass (Translated by Hoshihiko Yamazaki and Kiyoko Yoshii and published as *Kenkō no nazo o nozoku: Sutoresu tasho to kenkō hojino mekanizumu*, Tokyo: Yūshindō).

Antonovsky, A. (1993), 'The structure and prosperities of the sense of coherence scale', *Social Science & Medicine*, 36(6), pp. 725–33.

Anzai, Y., T. Ohkubo, Y. Nishino *et al.* (2000), 'Relationship between health practices and education level in the rural Japanese population', *Journal of Epidemiology*, 10, pp. 149–56.

Aoki, K. (1997), 'Kōreisha no yokuutsu jōtai to kanren yōin (Depressive state of the elderly and its correlates)', *Rōnen seishin igaku zasshi* (Japanese journal of geriatric psychiatry), 8, pp. 401–10.

Asahi Shimbun Sha (ed.) (2004), *Minryoku (2004 Nenban)* (A picture of the people: 2004 Edition), Tokyo: Asahi Shimbun Sha.

Aseltine, R. H. and R. C. Kessler (1993), 'Marital disruption and depression in a community sample', *Journal of Health and Social Behavior* 34, pp. 237–51.

Avlund, K, M. Vass and C. Hendriksen (2003), 'Onset of mobility disability among community-dwelling old men and women: The role of tiredness in daily activities', *Age and Ageing*, 32(6), pp. 579–84.

Baba, M. and H. Une (2005), 'An epidemiological study of the relationship between the number of remaining teeth and the disabled elderly receiving long-term care', *Nihon rōnen igakkai zasshi* (Japanese journal of geriatrics) 42(3), pp. 353–9.

Baba, Y., Katsunori Kondō, *et al.* (2003), 'Marriage and psychological health: Socioeconomic status in the background', *The Institute for Research on Household Economics*, 58, pp. 77–85.

Bacon, W. E. and W. C. Hadden (2000), 'Occurrence of hip fractures and socioeconomic position', *Journal of Aging and Health*, 12, pp. 193–203.

Baldwin, R. C., E. Chiu, C. Katona *et al.* (2002), *Guideline on Depression in Older People: Practising the Evidence*, United Kingdom: Martin Dunitz Ltd.

Bandura, A. (1997), *Self-efficacy: The exercise of control*, New York: Freeman.

Barmes, D. E. and M-H. Leclercq (1994), 'Intercountry application of standard epidemiology tools in oral health', *World Health Statistics Quarterly* (Rapport trimestriel de statistiques saritaries mordiales), 47(2), pp. 83–94.

Barnett, S., P. Roderick, D. Martin, *et al.* (2001), 'A multilevel analysis of the effects of rurality and social deprivation on premature limiting long term illness', *Journal of Epidemiology and Community Health,* 55, pp. 44–51.

Bartley, M. (2004), *Health inequality: An introduction to theories, concepts and methods*, Cambridge: Polity.

Baum, F. E., R. A. Bush, C. C. Modra, *et al.* (2000), 'Epidemiology of participation: An Australian community study', *Journal of Epidemiology and Community Health*, 54, pp. 414–23.

Berkman, C. and B. J. Gurland (1998), 'The relationship among income, other socioeconomic indicators, and functional level in older persons', *Journal of Aging and Health*, 10(1), pp. 81–98.

Berkman, L. F. and I. Kawachi (2000), *Social Epidemiology*, New York: Oxford University Press

Berkman, L. F. and L. Syme (1979), 'Social networks, host resistance, and mortality: A nine-year follow-up study of Alameda County residents,' *American Journal of Epidemiology*, 109(2), pp. 186–204.

Berkman, L. F., T. Glass, I. Brissette *et al.* (2000), 'From social integration to health', *Social Science & Medicine*, 51, pp. 843–57.

Blau, D. M. and D. B. Gilleskie (2001), 'The effect of health on employment transitions of older men' in S. W. Polachek (ed.), *Worker Wellbeing in a Changing Labor Market* (Research in Labor Economics; vol. 20), Amsterdam: JAI Press, pp. 35–65.

Brownwell, P., S. Carl, E. Podnieks *et al.* (2004), *Sekai no kōreisha gyakutai bōshi puroguramu* (Elder abuse prevention programs around the world), T. Tatara and N. Tsukada (tr.), Akashi Shoten.

Bryk, A. and S. Raudenbush (1992), *Hierarchical Linear Models: Applications and Data Analysis Methods*, London: Sage.

Bureau of Statistics (2002) *Shūgyō kōzō kihon chōsa: Heisei 14 nen* (Employment Status Survey), Tokyo: Japan Statistical Association.

Burke, W. J., W. H. Roccaforte and S. P. Wengel (1991), 'The short form of the geriatric depression scale: A comparison with the 30-item form', *Journal of Psychiatry and Neurology*, 4, pp. 173–8.

Cabinet Office (ed.) (2002), *Dai 5-kai kōreisha no seikatsu to ishiki ni kansuru kokusai hikaku chōsa kekka no gaiyō* (A summary of the Fifth International Comparison Survey of Daily Living and Awareness of Elderly Persons), http://www8.cao.go.jp/kourei/ishiki/h12_kiso/gaiyou.html (accessed 30 June 2009).

Cabinet Office (2004), *Kōreisha no jutaku to seikatsu kankyō ni kansuru ishiki chōsa kekka* (Findings from the survey on housing and life environment of the elderly 2001), http://www8.cao.go.jp/kourei/ishiki/h12_sougou/html/0-1.html (accessed 21 December 2004).

Cabinet Office (2004), *Kōreisha no nichijō seikatsu ni kansuru ishiki chōsa* (Attitude Survey on the Daily Life of the Elderly): http://www8.cao.go.jp/kourei/ishiki/h16_nitizyou/index2.html

Cabinet Office (2004), *Annual Report on the Aging Society: 2004 (Summary)*, http://www8.cao.go.jp/kourei/english/annualreport/2004/04wp-e.html, accessed on 26 June 2009.

Cabinet Office (2005), *Annual Report on the Aging Society: 2005 (Summary)*, http://www8.cao.go.jp/kourei/english/annualreport/2005/05wp-e.html, accessed on 30 June 2009.

Cabinet Office (2005), *Kōreisha no seikatsu to ishiki ni kansuru kokusai hikaku chōsa* (International Comparison Survey of the Daily Life and Attitudes of Elderly Persons): http://www8.cao.go.jp/kourei/ishiki/h17_kiso/index2.html

Cabinet Office (ed.) (2005), *Dai 6-kai kōreisha no seikatsu to ishiki ni kansuru kokusai hikaku chōsa kekka nit suite (yōyaku)* (A summary of the Sixth International Comparison Survey of Daily Living and Awareness of Elderly Persons), http://www8.cao.go.jp/kourei/ishiki/h17_kiso/pdf/youyaku.pdf (accessed 30 June 2009).

Cabinet Office Director-general for Policies on Cohesive Society (2002), 'Kōreisha no kenkō nikansuru ishiki chōsa kekka no gaiyō (Result of consciousness investigation about the health of elderly), pp. 29–30.

Cabinet Office (2007), *White Paper on the Aging Society (Summary) FY 2007*, http://www8.cao.go.jp/kourei/english/annualreport/2007/2007.pdf, accessed on 26 June 2009.
Center for Well-being and Society (CWS) http://cws.umin.jp/
Chaix, B. and P. Chauvin (2003), 'Tobacco and alcohol consumption, sedentary lifestyle and overweightness in France', *European Journal of Epidemiology*, 18, pp. 531–8.
Charles, K. K. (2004), 'Is retirement depressing? Labor force inactivity and psychological well-being in later life' in S. W. Polachek (ed.), *Accounting for Worker Well-Being* (Research in Labor Economics; vol. 23), Amsterdam: JAI Press, pp. 269–300.
Chen, Y. Y., I. Kawachi, S. V. Subramanian, D. Acevedo-Garcia and Y. Lee (2005), 'Can social factors explain sex differences in insomnia? Findings from a national survey in Taiwan', *Journal of Epidemiology and Community Health*, 59(6), pp. 488–94.
Chiba, M. (1980), 'Chiiki jinja to ujiko ken (Community Shinto shrine and *ujiko* sphere)', in S. Gorai, T. Sakurai, T. Ōshima *et al.* (eds) *Kōza Nihon no minzoku shūkyō 5 Minzoku shūkyō to shakai* (Seminar Japanese folk religions 5 Folk religions and society), Tokyo: Kōbundō, pp. 32–56.
Colette, F., L. Luc, F. D. Jean *et al.* (1995), 'Social and leisure activities and risk of dementia: A prospective longitudinal study', *Journal of the American Geriatrics Society*, 43, pp. 485–90.
Comijs, H. C., A. M. Pot, J. H. Smit *et al.* (1998) 'Elder abuse in the community; prevalence and consequences', *Journal of the American Geriatric Society* 7, pp. 885–8.
Curtis, J. E., E. G. Grabb and D. E. Baer (1992), 'Voluntary association membership in fifteen countries: A comparative analysis', *American Sociological Review*, 57, pp. 139–52.
Cutler, S. J. (1976), 'Membership in different types of voluntary associations and psychological well-being', *The Gerontologist*, 16, pp. 335–9.
Cutler, S. J. and J. Hendricks (2000), 'Age differences in voluntary association memberships: Fact or artifact', *The Journals of Gerontology Series B: Psychological Sciences and Social Sciences*, 55, pp. S98–107.
Dalstra, J. A. A., A. E. Kunst, J. P. Mackenbach *et al.* (2006), 'A Comparative appraisal of the relationship of education, income and housing tenure with less than good health among the elderly in Europe', *Social Science & Medicine*, 62, pp. 2046–60.
Davey-Smith, G. (2003), *Health inequalities: Lifecourse approaches*, Bristol: The Policy Press.
De Silva, M. J., K. Mackenzie, T. Harpham *et al.* (2005), 'Social capital and mental illness: A systematic review', *Journal of Epidemiology and Community Health*, 59, pp. 619–27.
De Vogli, R., R. Gnesotto, M. Goldstein *et al.* (2005), 'The lack of social gradient of health behaviors and psychosocial factors in Northern Italy', *Sozial- und Präventivmedizin/Social and Preventive Medicine*, 50, pp. 197–205.
Decalmer, P. and F. Glendenning, (eds) (1998) *Kōreisha gyakuta hakken / yobō no tame ni* (Elder abuse: Identification and prevention), M. Tabata and N. Sugioka (tr.), Minerva Shobo.
Demura, Shinichi *et al.* (2003), 'Chihō toshi zaijū no zaitaku kōreisha ni okeru yokuutsu to seikatsu yōin no kankei (Association between depression

and lifestyle factors of stay-at-home elderly people in regional cities), *Nihon seirijinrui gakkaishi* (Journal of Japan Society of Physiological Anthropology), 8, pp. 45–9.

Dentsu Communication Institute, Nihon Research Center (eds) (2008), *Sekai shuyōkoku kachikan data book* (Values of world's leading countries data book), Tokyo: Dōyūkan.

Diez-Roux, A. V. (1998), 'Bringing context back into epidemiology: Variables and fallacies in multilevel analysis', *American Journal of Public Health*, 88(2), pp. 216–22.

Diez-Roux, A. V. (2003), 'The examination of neighborhood effects on health: Conceptual and methodological issues related to the presence of multiple levels of organization' in I. Kawachi and L. F. Berkman (eds), *Neighborhoods and Health*. New York: Oxford University Press, pp. 65–111.

Doi, Y., M. Minowa, M. Okawa and M. Uchiyama (2000), 'Prevalence of sleep disturbance and hypnotic medication use in relation to sociodemographic factors in the general Japanese adult population', *Journal of Epidemiology*, 10, pp. 79–86.

Dore, Ronald P. (1997) *The Diploma Disease: Education, Qualification and Development*, 2nd edition, Institute of Education University of London.

Editorial Committee on the Rights of the Elderly and the Disabled, Japan Federation of Bar Associations (2006), *Kōreisha gyakutai bōshihō katsuyō handobukku* (Handbook to the law for the prevention of elder abuse), Minjihō Kenkyūkai Co., Ltd.

Elderly Treatment Workgroup (*Kōreisha shogū kenkyūkai*) (1994), 'Kōreisha no fukushi shisetu ni okeru ningenkankei no chōsei ni kakawaru sōgōteki kenkyū (sono 2) – wagakuni ni okeru kōreisha gyakutai no kisokenkyū (Comprehensive research relating to the adjustment of interpersonal relations in welfare facilities for elderly people (No. 2): Basic research on elder abuse in Japan)', *Gekkan chi'iki fukushi jōhō* (Monthly community welfare bulletin), 32, pp. 200–24.

Elderly Treatment Workgroup (*Kōreisha shogū kenkyūkai*) (1997), *Kōreisha no anzen kakuho ni kansuru chōsa kenkyū jigyō hōkokusho – Kōreisha gyakutai no jittai ni kansuru chōsa kenkyū* (Research project report on ensuring the safety of the elderly: Research on elder abuse), Tokyo: International Longevity Center.

Elderly Treatment Workgroup (*Kōreisha shogū kenkyūkai*) (1998), *Zaitaku / shisetu ni okeru kōreisha oyobi shōgaisha no gyakutai ni kansuru ishiki to jittai chōsa* (Awareness and fact-finding research on abuse of the elderly and disabled at home and in facilities), Tokyo: International Longevity Center.

Elderly Treatment Workgroup (*Kōreisha shogū kenkyūkai*) (2000), *Tokubetsu yōgo rōjin hōmu ni okeru kōreisha gyakutai ni kansuru jittai to ishiki chōsa kenkyū hōkokusho* (Report on research concerning the nature and perception of elder abuse in nursing homes), Tokyo: International Longevity Center.

Endō, Hideki (2009), 'Hataraku kōreisha wa kenkō ni nagaiki dekirunoka? AGES kohōto dēta ni yoru bunseki (Can the aged in work live a longer, healthier life? An analysis using AGES cohort data)', Unpublished mansucript.

Eng, P. M., E. B. Rimm, G. Fitzmaurice *et al.* (2002), 'Social ties and change in social ties in relation to subsequent total and cause-specific mortality and coronary heart disease incidence in men', *American Journal of Epidemiology*, 155, pp. 700–9.

Eriksson, M. and B. Lindstrom (2005), 'Validity of Antonovsky's sense of coherence scale: A systematic review', *Journal of Epidemiology and Community Health*, 59(6), pp. 460–6.

Farahmand, B. Y., P. G. Persson *et al.* (2000), 'Socioeconomic status, marital status and hip fracture risk: A population-based case-control study', *Osteoporosis International*, 11, pp. 803–8.

Federation Dentaire Internationale (1982), 'Global goals for oral health in the year 2000', *International Dental Journal*, 32, pp. 74–7.

Ford, D. E. and D. B. Kamerow (1989), 'Epidemiologic study of sleep disturbances and psychiatric disorders: An opportunity for prevention?' *Journal of American Medical Association*, 262, pp. 479–84.

Frey, B. S. and A. Stutzer (2002), *Happiness and Economics: How the Economy and Institutions Affect Human Well-Being*, Princeton: Princeton University Press.

Fuhrer, R., C. Dufouil, T. C. Antonucci *et al.* (1999), 'Psychological disorder and mortality in French older adults: Do social relations modify the association?', *American Journal of Epidemiology*, 149, pp. 116–26.

Fujimoto K., K. Okada, T. Izumi *et al.* (2004), 'Chiiki zaijū kōreisha no ikigai o kitei suru yōin ni tsuite no kenkyū (Factors defining the purpose in life in community-dwelling elderly people)', *Journal of Health and Welfare Statistics* 51(4), pp. 24–32.

Fujita, K., Y. Fujiwara, S. Kumagai *et al.* (2004), 'Chiiki zaitaku kōreisha no gaishutsu hindo betsu ni mita shintai, shinri, shakai-teki tokuchō (The frequency of going outdoors and physical, psychological and social functioning among community-dwelling older adults)', *Nippon kōshū eisei zasshi* (Japanese journal of public health), 51, pp. 169–80.

Fujita, Toshiharu and Shu-ichi Hatano (1990), 'Chiiki rōjin no kenkōdo jiko hyōka no kanren yōin to sono go ninenkan no shibō (Factors related to self-rated health among the elderly in regional Japan and the prevalence of death two years later)', *Shakai rōnengaku* (Journal of socio-gerontology), 31, pp. 43–51.

Fukai, K. (2003), 'The relevance of behavioral science in oral health promotion', *Journal of the National Institute of Public Health*, 52(1), pp. 46–54.

Fukuda, Y., K. Nakamura and T. Takano (2005a), 'Socioeconomic pattern of smoking in Japan: Income inequality and gender and age differences', *Annals of Epidemiology*, 15, pp. 363–72.

Fukuda, Y., K. Nakamura and T. Takano (2005b), 'Accumulation of health risk behaviours associated with lower socioeconomic status and women's urban residence: A multilevel analysis in Japan', *BMC Public Health*, 5(53), doi:10.1186/1471-2458-5-53.

Gallo, J. J., W. Reichel and L. Anderson (eds) (1995), *Handbook of Geriatric Assessment*, Aspen: Gaithersburg.

Ganguly, M., H. H. Dodge, and B. H. Mulsant (2002), 'Rates and predictors of mortality in an aging, rural, community-based cohort: The role of depression', *Archives of General Psychiatry*, 59, pp. 1046–52.

Ganguly, M, A. Fox, J. Gilby, and S. Belle (1996), 'Characteristics of rural homebound older adults: A community-based study,' *Journal of the American Geriatric Society*, 44(4), pp. 363–70.

Geroldi, C., G. B. Frisoni, R. Rozzini and M. Trabucchi (1996), 'Principal lifetime occupation and sleep quality in the elderly', *Gerontology*, 42(3), pp. 163–9.

Geyer, S. (1997), 'Some conceptual considerations on the sense of coherence', *Social Science & Medicine*, 44(12), pp. 1771–9.

Gilbert G. H., L. G. Branch, and E. J. Orav (1992), 'An operational definition of the homebound,' *Health Services Research*, Feb. 26(6), pp. 787–800.

Gill, T., A. W. Taylor and A. Pengelly (2005), 'A population-based survey of factors relating to the prevalence of falls in older people', *Gerontology*, 51, pp. 340–5.

Glass, T. A., C. M. De Leon, R. A. Marottoli *et al.* (1999), 'Population based study of social and productive activities as predictors of survival among elderly Americans', *British Medical Association Journal*, 319, pp. 478–82.

Goldstein, H. (2003), *Multilevel Statistical Models*, 3rd edition, London: Arnold.

Gorai, S. (1980), 'Shushōe, shunie to minzoku (Buddhist services *shushōe* and *shunie* and folklore)', in S. Gorai, T. Sakurai, T. Ōshima *et al.* (eds), *Kōza Nihon no minzoku shūkyō 2 Bukkyō minzokugaku* (Seminar Japanese folk religions 2 Buddhist folklore), Tokyo: Kōbundō, pp. 84–98.

Gove, W. R. (1973), 'Sex, marital status, and mortality', *American Journal of Sociology*, 79(1), pp. 45–67.

Green, H. and L. Fletcher (2003), *The Development of Harmonised Questions on Social Capital*, http://www.statistics.gov.uk/socialcapital/downloads/Draft UserGuide v3.pdf

Grootaert, C. and T. Bastelaer (2001), 'Understanding and measuring social capital: A synthesis of findings and recommendations from the social capital initiative', *Social Capital Initiative Working Paper No. 24*: The World Bank, http://web.worldbank.org/WBSITE/EXTERNAL/TOPICS/EXTSOCIALDEVELOPMENT/EXTTSOCIALCAPITAL/0,contentMDK:20194767~menuPK:401035~pagePK:148956~piPK:216618~theSitePK:401015,00.html

Grundy, E. and G. Holt (2000), 'Adult life experiences and health in early old age in Great Britain', *Social Science & Medicine* 51(7), pp. 1061–74.

Grundy, E. and G. Holt (2001), 'The socioeconomic status of older adults: How should we measure it in studies of health inequalities?' *Journal of Epidemiology and Community Health*, 55, pp. 895–904.

Grundy, F., and K. Glaser (2000), 'Demographic differences in the onset and progression of disability in early old age: A longitudinal study', *Age and Ageing*, 29, pp. 149–57.

Hajat, S., A. Haines, C. Bulpitt *et al.* (2004), 'Patterns and determinants of alcohol consumption in people aged 75 years and older: Results from the MRC trial of assessment and management of older people in the community', *Age and Ageing*, 33, pp. 170–7.

Halpern, D. (2005), *Social Capital*, Cambridge: Polity Press.

Hamashima, Chisato (1994), 'Kōreisha no kuoriti obu raifu (Quality of life of the aged)', *Nihon eiseigaku zasshi* (Japanese journal of hygiene), 49, pp. 533–42.

Hanada, N., M. Morimoto, K. Miyatake, *et al.* (2004), 'WHO dai 2 kai kokusai kyōdō kenkyū (ICS II) hōkoku-sho no gaiyō. Shakai gurūpu-betsu no kōkō hoken yōkyō (sono 2) (Outline of report on the WHO 2nd International Collaborative Study (ICS II)). Oral health status by social group (No. 2))', *Dental Review*, 64(8), pp. 178–82.

Hanibuchi, Tomoya, Jun Aida, Miyo Nakade, Hiroshi Hirai, and Katsunori Kondō (in press), 'Geographical accessibility to dental care in the Japanese elderly', *Community Dental Health*.

Hanibuchi, Tomoya, Yukinobu Ichida, Hiroshi Hirai, and Katsunori Kondō (2007), 'Soshiaru kyapitaru to chiiki komyuniti no rekishi (Does the history of local community affect social capital? Analyzing a large-scale questionnaire survey by using old topographical maps)', *GIS–Riron to ōyō* (Theory and applications of GIS), 15, pp.11–22.

Harada, K., H. Sugisawa, Y. Sugihara *et al.* (2005), 'Daitoshibu ni okeru kōki kōreisha no tojikomori ni kanren suru yōin (Related factors of old-old housebound in metropolitan areas)', *Kōsei no shihyō* (Journal of health and welfare statistics), 52, pp. 28–33.

Haraldsson, K., B. Fridlund, A. Baigi *et al.* (2005), 'The self-reported health conditions of women after their participation in a stress management programme: A pilot study', *Health and Social Care in the Community*, 13(3), pp. 224–30.

Hashimoto, S., R. Aoki, A. Tamakoshi *et al.* (1997), 'Kōreisha ni okeru shakai katsudō jōkyō no shihyō no kaihatsu (Development of index of social activities for the elderly)', *Nippon kōshū eisei zasshi* (Japanese journal of public health), 44, pp. 760–8.

Hatono, Y. (2000), 'Kōreisha no tojikomori ni kansuru kenkyū no jōkyō: Kaigai no housebound no teigi shutsugenritsu o chūsin ni (Present status of research on housebound elderly: Definition and incidence of housebound behavior around the world)', *Hokenfu zasshi* (The Japanese journal for public health nursing), 56, pp. 28–33.

Hatono, Y., H. Tanaka, K. Furukawa *et al.* (2001), 'Chiiki kōreisha no tojikomori no jōkyō to sono haikei yōin no bunseki (Actual conditon of community-dwelling housebound elderly and background factors)', *Nihon chiiki kangogaku zasshi* (Journal of the Japan Academy of Community Health Nursing), 3, pp. 26–31.

Hawe, P. and A. Shiell (2000), 'Social capital and health promotion: A review', *Social Science & Medicine*, 51(6), pp. 871–85.

Hayasaka S., Y. Gotō, Y. Nakamura *et al.* (2005), 'Nichijō no kanshin no shikō-sei to shukan-teki seikatsu no shitsu ga kōreisha no shukan-teki kenkō-kan ni oyobosu eikyō: Chiiki, sei, nennrei-betsu no kentō (The effects of interest orientation in daily life and subjective quality of life on self-rated health in elderly people: Comparison by area, gender and age)', *Journal of Health and Welfare Statistics* 52(7), pp. 32–8.

Herzog, A. R., M. M. Franks, H. R. Markus *et al.* (1998), 'Activities and well-being in old age: Effects of self-concept and educational attainment', *Psychology and Aging*, 13, pp. 179–85.

Hirai, Hiroshi and Katsunori Kondō (2008), 'Kōreisha no machi shisetsu riyō no kanren yōin bunseki: Kaigo yobō jigyō shinka sokushin ni muketa kisoteki kenkyū (Related factors in the elderly's use of municipal institutions: Basic study for promoting participation in a care prevention program)', *Nippon kōshū eisei zasshi* (Japanese journal of public health), 55(1), pp. 37–44.

Hirai, Hiroshi, Katsunori Kondō and Tomoya Hanibuchi (2008), 'Kōreisya no "Tojikomori" wariai to kyojūchi no jinkō mitudo no kanren no kentō (An examination of correlation between rate of "Tojikomori" elderly and population density of residential area)', *Rōnen shakai kagaku* (Japanese journal of gerontology), 30, pp. 69–78.

Hirai, Hiroshi, Katsunori Kondō, Toshiyuki Ojima and Chiyoe Murata (2009), 'Chiiki zaijū kōreisha no yōkaigo nintei no risuku yōin no kentō: AGES purojekuto 3-nenkan no tsuiseki kenkyū (Risk factors for the long-term care requirement of community-living elderly people: AGES project 3-year follow-up study), *Nippon kōshū eisei zasshi* (Japanese journal of public health), 56, pp. 501–12.

Hiramatsu, Makoto, Katsunori Kondō, Ken-ichi Umehara *et al.* (2006), 'Kazoku kaigosha no kaigo futankan to kanren suru yōin no kenkyū (dai 1ho): Kihon zokusei to kainyū kon-nan na yōin no kentō (Research on factors related to the burden felt by family carers: Part 1, An investigation of demographic variables and variables which are difficult to intervene)', *Kōsei no shihyō* (Journal of health and welfare statistics), 53(3), pp. 8–24.

Hiramatsu, M., Katsunori Kondō, and Hiroshi Hirai (2009), 'Kaigo yobō shisaku no taishosha ga kenshin o jushin shinai haikei yōin: Shakai keizaiteki inshi ni chakumoku shite (The background factors that explain why those targeted for preventive measures do not have physical check-ups)', *Kōsei no shihyō* (Journal of health and welfare statistics), 56, pp. 1–8.

House, J. S., J. M. Lepkowski, A. M. Kinney *et al.* (1994), 'The social stratification of aging and health', *Journal of Health and Social Behavior*, 35, pp. 213–34.

House, J. S., K. R. Landis and D. Umberson (1982), 'Social relationships and health', *Science*, 241(4865), pp. 540–4.

Huisman, M., A. E. Kunst, and J. P. Mackenbach (2005), 'Inequalities in the prevalence of smoking in the European Union: Comparing education and income', *Preventative Medicine*, 40, pp. 756–64.

Ichida, Yukinobu, Katsunori Kondō, Hiroshi Hirai, Tomoya Hanibuchi, Goshuu Yoshikawa and Chiyoe Murata (2009), 'Social capital, income inequality and self-rated health in Chita peninsula, Japan: A multilevel analysis of older people in 25 communities', *Social Science & Medicine*, 69(4), pp. 489–99.

Ichida, Yukinobu, Gōshu Yoshikawa, Ryōzō Matsuda *et al.* (2005), 'Nihon no kōreisha: Kaigo yobō ni muketa shakai ekigakuteki daikibo chōsa (11) sōsharu capitaru to kenkō (Japan's elderly people: A large-scale social epidemiologic survey towards long-term care prevention (11) social capital and health), *Kōshū eisei* (Public health), 69(11), pp. 914–19.

Ide R., A. Tsutsui, T. Mizoue, *et al.* (2000), 'Evaluation of subjective oral health status in the general population perceived dental health and disability by oral problems', *Journal of Dental Health*, 50(2), pp. 247–53.

Idler, E. L. and Y. Benyamini (1997), 'Self-rated health and mortality: A review of twenty-seven community studies', *Journal of Health Social Behavior*, 38, pp. 2–37.

Idler, E. L., S. V. Kasl, and J. H. Lemke (1990), 'Self-evaluated health and mortality among the elderly in New Haven', *American Journal of Epidemiology*, 131, pp. 91–103.

Imuta, H., S. Yasumura, M. Fujita *et al.* (1998), 'Chiiki zaijū kōreisha no tojikomori yūbyōritsu narabini shintai shinri shakaiteki tokuchō to idō-nōryoku no henka (Homebound elderly in a Japanese community: Related factors and change of mobility)', *Nippon kōshū eisei zasshi* (Japanese journal of public health), 45, pp. 883–92.

Ing, J. D. and L. Rutter (2003), 'Socioeconomic status, sense of coherence and health in Canadian women', *Canadian Journal of Public Health*, 94(3), pp. 224–8.

Inoue, Haruyo (1998), 'Kōrei josei no shakai sanka (Social participation by elderly women)' in Yasuo Konishi (ed.), *Rōjin no shakai sanka* (Social participation by the elderly), Tokyo: Chūō Hōki Shuppan, pp. 161–97.

Islam, M. K., J. Merlo, I. Kawachi *et al.* (2006), 'Social capital and health: Does egalitarianism matter? A literature review', *International Journal for Equity in Health*, 5(1), p. 3.

Itō, Jun and Setsu Itō (2002), 'Jendā ni kubunshita kōreisha no keizai jōkyō no haaku (Economic status of the aged by gender)', *Gakuen* (Education and welfare magazine), 740, pp. 75–92.

Iwai, N. and H. Satō (eds) (2002), *Nihonjin no sugata – JGSS ni miru ishiki to kōdō* (Japanese values and behavioral patterns seen in the Japanese General Social Survey), Tokyo: Yūhikaku.

Japan Federation of Senior Citizens Clubs website, http://www4.ocn.ne.jp/~zenrou/

Japan Health Promotion and Fitness Foundation (2000), *Healthy Japan 21* (21 seiki ni okeru kokumin kenkō zukuri undō ni tsuite: National Health Promotion in the 21st Century), pp. 127–36.

Japanese Ministry of Health, Labour and Welfare (2002), *Heisei 14-nendo shakai fukushi gyōsei gyōmu hōkoku no gaiyō, 4: Rōjin fukushi kankei* (An outline report on social welfare administrative services, 4: Senior citizens' welfare), http://www.mhlw.go.jp/toukei/saikin/hw/gyousei/02/kekka4.html (accessed 26 June 2009).

Japanese Ministry of Health, Labour and Welfare (2004), *Chiiki ni okeru utsu taisaku kentōkai manyuaru – Hoken iryō jūjisha no tame ni* (The Local Depression Study Group depression treatment manual: For healthcare professionals), http://www.mhlw.go.jp/shingi/2004/0/s026-5f.html

Japanese Ministry of Health, Labour and Welfare, *2008 Vital Statistics*. http://www.mhlw.go.jp/toukei/saikin/hw/jinkou/kakutei08/index.html

Jarvis, M. J., and J. Wardle (1999), 'Social patterning of individual health behaviours: The case of cigarette smoking', in M. Marmot and R. G. Wilkinson (eds), *Social Determinants of Health*, Oxford: Oxford University Press, pp. 240–55.

JGSS Research Center, Japanese General Social Surveys Website, http://jgss.daishodai.ac.jp/english/eframe/englishtop.html (last accessed at 3.51 pm, 25 February 2010).

Jingu S., Y. Egami, N. Kinukawa *et al.* (2003), 'Factors related to functional capacity in community-dwelling elderly people', *Nippon kōshū eisei zasshi* (Japanese journal of public health), 50(2), pp. 92–105.

Jorm, A. F. (2000), 'Is depression a risk factor for dementia or cognitive decline?' *Gerontology*, 46, pp. 219–27.

Joung, I. M., H. D. van de Mheen, K. Stronks, F. W. van Poppel and J. P. Mackenbach (1998), 'A longitudinal study of health selection in marital transitions', *Social Science & Medicine* 46(3), pp. 425–35.

Kagamimori, S., A. Gaina and A. Nasermoaddeli (2009), 'Socioeconomic status and health in the Japanese population', *Social Science & Medicine*, 68(12), pp. 2152–60.

Kage, Rieko (2002), 'Sōsharu kyapitaru omeguru kenkyū dōkō (1) (A review of studies on social capital (1))', *Hōgaku ronsō* (Kyoto law review), 151, pp. 101–19.

Kaigo Yobō Manyuaru no Kaitei ni kansuru Kenkyūhan (2009) *Kaigo yobō manyuaru* (Long-term care prevention manual), http://www.mhlw.go.jp/topics/2009/05/tp0501-1.html (accessed on 30 June 2009).

Kaplan, G. A., D. E. Goldberg, S. A. Everson *et al.* (1996), 'Perceived health status and morbidity and mortality: Evidence from the Kuopio ischaemic heart disease risk factor study', *International Journal of Epidemiology*, 2(2), pp. 259–65.

Kaplan, G. A., V. Barell and A. Lusky (1988), 'Subjective state of health and survival in elderly adults', *Journal of Gerontology: Social Sciences*, 43, pp. S114–S120.

Katō, Etsuko, Katsunori Kondō, Yoshii Kiyoko (2006), 'Kaigo hoken saabisu o riyō shite inai kōreisha ni okeru gyakutai no jittai (The actual circumstance of abuse among elderly people who have not used Long-term Care Insurance Services)', *Kōreisha gyakutai boshi kenkyū* (Journal of the Japan Academy for the Prevention of Elder Abuse), 2, pp. 73–83.

Katō, Etsuko (2004), 'Kōreisha gyakutai no hassei wariai to risku taipu betsu tokuchō (Prevalence of elder abuse and characteristics by risk type)', *Gekkan sōgō kea* (Comprehensive care monthly), 14(11), pp. 57–62.

Katō, Etsuko, Katsunori Kondō, Kiyoko Higuchi, *et al.* (2004) 'Gyakutai ga utagawareta kōreisha no jōkyō kaizen ni kansuru yōin (Factors relating to improved circumstances for elderly people who are suspected of being abused)', *Rōnen shakai kagaku* (Japanese journal of gerontology), 25(4), pp. 482–93.

Katō, Etsuko and Katsunori Kondō, (2008), 'AGES purojekuto: Kaigosha/kaigo jōkyō/ippan kōreisha chōsa no gaiyō (An overview of Aichi Gerontological Evaluation Study [AGES] project), *Shakai seisaku kenkyū* (Journal of social policy studies), 8, pp. 216–29 (with English abstract p. 341).

Kavanagh, A. M., G. Turrell and S. V. Subramanian (2006), 'Does area-based social capital matter for the health of Australians? A multilevel analysis of self-rated health in Tasmania', *International Journal of Epidemiology*, 35(3), pp. 607–13.

Kawachi, I. (2000), 'Social cohesion, social capital, and health' in L. F. Berkman and I. Kawachi (eds), *Social Epidemiology*, New York: Oxford University Press, pp. 174–90.

Kawachi, I., B. P. Kennedy, K. Lochner *et al.* (1997), 'Social capital, income inequality, and mortality', *American Journal of Public Health*, 87(9), pp. 1491–8.

Kawachi, I., B. P. Kennedy and R. Glass (1999), 'Social capital and self-rated health: A contextual analysis', *American Journal of Public Health*, 89, pp. 1187–93.

Kawachi, I., G. A. Colditz, A. Ascherio *et al.* (1996), 'A prospective study of social networks in relation to total mortality and cardiovascular disease in men in the USA', *Journal of Epidemiology and Community Health*, 50, pp. 245–51.

Kawachi, I., S. V. Subramanian and D. Kim (2008), *Social Capital and Health*, New York: Springer Science + Business Media, LLC.

Kawakami, Norito (2007), 'Utsubyō no ekigaku to kōkusai hikaku (Epidemiology of depression and international comparison)'. *Nihon rinshō* (Japanese journal of clinical medicine), 65(9), pp. 1578–84.

Kelly, J. R. and M. W. Steinkamp (1987), 'Later-life satisfaction: Does leisure contribute?', *Leisure Sciences*, 9, pp. 189–200.

Kenkō Nippon 21 (Healthy Japan 21), http://www.kenkōnippon21.gr.jp/

Kim, D., S. V. Subramanian and I. Kawachi (2006), 'Bonding versus bridging social capital and their associations with self-rated health: A multilevel analysis of 40 U.S. communities', *Journal of Epidemiology & Community Health*, 60(2), pp. 116–122.

Kim, J., S. Shinkai, S. Kumagai *et al.* (2004), 'Chiiki chūkōnen sha no shakai sanka no genjō to sono kanren yōin: Saitama-ken Hatoyama-machi no chōsa kara (Present state of social participation and associated factors among middle-aged and older people: A survey in Hatoyama town, Saitama prefecture)', *Nippon kōshū eisei zasshi* (Japanese journal of public health), 51, pp. 323–34.

Kim, S., M. Symons and B. M. Popkin (2004), 'Contrasting socioeconomic profiles related to healthier lifestyles in China and the United States', *American Journal of Epidemiology*, 159, pp. 184–91.

Kimura, C., Y. Yamazaki, H. Ishikawa *et al.* (2001), 'Daigakusei no sense of coherence (shubi ikkan kankaku, SOC) to sono kanren yōin no kentō (An analysis of sense of coherence (SOC) and related factors in college students)', *Nippon kenkō kyōiku gakkaishi* (Japanese journal of health education and promotion), 9(1&2), pp. 37–48.

Kimura, Eri, Aya Gotō, Masashi Tsunoda *et al.* (2003), 'Kōreisiha no zenshibōritsu o kitei suru shakai keizai yōin: Shogaikoku no hōkoku to Okinawa ken Ogimi-son kōreisha deno kento (The socio-economic factors contributing to the overall mortality rate among the elderly: Looking at reports from several overseas countries and considering the aged in Ogimi village, Okinawa prefecture)', *Fukushima igaku zasshi* (The Journal of Fukushima Society of Medical Science), 53(4), pp. 345–54.

Kinney, A. Y., L. E. Bloor, W. N. Dudley *et al.* (2003), 'Roles of religious involvement and social support in the risk of colon cancer among blacks and whites', *American Journal of Epidemiology*, 158, pp. 1097–107.

Kisala, Reiko (2006), 'Japanese religions', in P. L. Swanson and C. Chilson (eds), *Nanzan guide to Japanese religions*, Honolulu: University of Hawaii Press, pp. 3–13.

Kishi, Reiko, T. Eguchi and N. Maeda (1996), 'Zenki kōreisha to kōki kōreisha no kenkō jōtai to sōsharu sapōto nettowāku: Nōson chiiki ni okeru kōreisha (69–80 sai) no hikaku kenkyū (Health status, social networks and support systems of so called old old in a population-based comparative study of residents ages 69–74 and 75–80)', *Nippon kōshū eisei zasshi* (Japanese journal of public health), 43, pp. 1009–23.

Kishi, Reiko, T. Eguchi, H. Sasatani *et al.* (1994), 'Kōreisha no shakai-teki sapōto oyobi nettowāku no genjō to kenkō jōtai: Kyū santan-chi Yūbari to dai-toshi Sapporo no jittai (Health status, social networks and support system of elderly men and women in a large city and in former coal-mining areas: A population-based comparative study of 70-year-old residents of Sapporo and Yūbari)', *Nippon kōshū eisei zasshi* (Japanese journal of public health), 41, pp. 474–88.

Kishi, Reiko and Naoko Horikawa (2004), 'Kōreisha no sōki narabini shintai kinō ni oyobosu shakai sapōto nettowāku no yakuwari (The role of social support networks in relation to the early-stage and physical functions of the aged)', *Nippon kōshū eisei zasshi* (Japanese journal of public health), 51, pp. 79–93.

Kohut, M. L., W. Lee, A. Martin *et al.* (2005), 'The exercise-induced enhancement of influenza immunity is mediated in part by improvements in psychosocial factors in older adults', *Brain, Behavior and Immunity*, 19(4), pp. 357–66.

Kōmoto, M. (1980), 'Jiin to danka no soshiki (Temples and supporter *danka* organizations)', in S. Gorai, T. Sakurai, T. Ōshima *et al.* (eds), *Kōza Nihon no minzoku shūkyō 5: Minzoku shūkyō to shakai* (Seminar Japanese folk religions 5: Folk religions and society), Tokyo: Kōbundō, pp. 100–23.

Kondō, Katsunori (2000), 'Kaigo hoken seisaku no rinshōteki hyōka kenkyū no kihon kōso zukuri (Building the fundamentals for clinical evaluation of policies for long-term care insurance)', in *Kōsei kagaku kenkyūhi hojokin (Seisaku kagaku suishin kenkyu jigyo) 1999 nendo hōkoku* (The 1999 report on defraying the cost of research on health and welfare science [Research activities to support policy science]) Compiled under the direction of Sadahisa Noguchi. Tokyo: Ministry of Health and Welfare, pp. 92–4.

Kondō, Katsunori (2002), 'Kaigo hoken wa kaigosha no futan o keigen shitaka: Kaigosha no shūkanteki kōfukukan-yokuutsu-kaigosha futan e no inpakuto (Has care insurance lowered the burden of carers? The impact on the sense of burden felt by carers, depression, and the overall sense of well-being)', *Shakai hoken junpō* (Social insurance journal), 235, pp. 25–9.

Kondō, Katsunori (2004), 'Kaigo hoken kaikaku o megutte: Rihabiriteeshon iryō no kadai (Some considerations concerning the reform of Long-term Care Insurance: Challenges for rehabilitation medicine)', *Sōgō rihabiriteishon* (Comprehensive rehabilitation), 33, pp. 7–23.

Kondō, Katsunori (2004), 'Kaigo hoken seido to sono mondaiten (The system of care insurance and some problems it faces)', *Riumachika* (Rheumatology), 32, pp. 85–93.

Kondō, Katsunori (2004), 'Ikinuku chikara: Shakai to shintai teki kenkō o tsunagu mono (3) (Survival power: A link between society and physical health [3])', *Kōshū eisei* (Public health), 68, pp. 562–8.

Kondō, Katsunori (2004), 'Naze shakai keizai inshi ga kenkō ni eikyō suru noka' (Why are health outcomes affected by socio-economic factors?), *Kōshū eisei* (Public health), 68, pp. 306–10.

Kondō, Katsunori (2004), 'New Public Health no paradaimu: Shakai ekigaku eno sasoi (9) shakai no ariyō to kenkō (2) sōsharu kyapitaru (New public health paradigm: An invitation to social epidemiology (9) the state of society and health (2) social capital)', *Kōshū eisei* (Public health), 68(9), pp. 721–7.

Kondō, Katsunori (2004), 'Ningen kankei to kenkō (Interpersonal relationships and health)', *Kōshū eisei* (Public health), 67(3), pp. 224–8.

Kondō, Katsunori (2005), *Kenkō kakusa shakai: Nani ga kokoro to kenkō o mushibamu no ka* (The health-gap society: What is harming our minds and our health?), Tokyo: Igaku Shoin.

Kondō, Katsunori (2009), 'Social relationship and health', in N. Kawakami *et al.* (eds), *Health and Social Disparity: Japan and Beyond*, Melbourne: Trans Pacific Press, pp. 182–207.

Kondō, Katsunori, Hiroshi Hirai, Kiyoko Yoshii *et al.* (2005), 'Nihon no kōreisha – Kaigo yobō ni muketa shakai ekigaku teki daikibo chōsa (1): Chōsa mokuteki to chōsa taishō sha, chiiki no tokusei (The AGES Project on the Health of Older People in Japan)', *Kōshū eisei* (Public health), 69, pp. 69–72 (reproduced as Chapter 1 of this book).

Kondō, Katsunori and Hiroshi Hirai (2005), 'Chōsa mokuteki to chōsa taishōsha, chiiki no tokuchō, rensai "Nihon no kōreisha: Kaigo yobō ni muketa shakai ekigakuteki daikibo chōsa" (Survey objectives, survey sample and area characteristics: Serialized articles "Japan's older people: A large-scale social epidemiologic survey towards long-term care prevention")', *Kōshū eisei* (Public health), 69(1), pp. 69–72.

Kondō, Katsunori, K. Niino and K. Shidō (1994), 'A case-control study of Alzheimer's disease in Japan: Significance of life-style', *Dementia*, 5, pp. 314–26.

Kondō, Katsunori, Hiroshi Hirai, Tokunori Takeda, Yukinobu Ichida and Jun Aida (in press), 'Social capital and health', *Kodo keiryogaku* (Japanese journal of behaviormetrics).

Kondō, Naoki, Ichiro Kawachi, Hiroshi Hirai, Katsunori Kondō, S.V. Subramanian, Tomoya Hanibiuchi and Zentaro Yamagata (2009), 'Relative deprivation and incident functional disability among older Japanese women and men: Prospective cohort study', *Journal of Epidemiology and Community Health*, 63, pp. 461–9.

Kono, A. (2000), 'Zaitaku shōgai rōjin ni okeru tojikomori to tojikomerare no tokuchō (Characteristics of "Tojikomori" and "Tojikomerare" among home disabled elderly: Daily life of the housebound elderly)', *Nippon kōshū eisei zasshi* (Japanese journal of public health), 47, pp. 216–29.

Kōreisha Kaigo Kenkyūkai (The Study Group on Research on Aged Care) (2003), *2005 Nen no kōreisiha kaigo* (Aged care in 2005), Tokyo: Kōsei Rōdō Shō homepage: http//www.mhlw.go.jp/topics/kaigo/kentou/5kourei/3.html (accessed in 2003).

Kōreisha Rihabiriteeshon Kenkyūkai (The Study Group on Rehabilitation for the Aged) (2004), *Kōreisiha rihabireteeshon no arubeki hōkō* (The direction in which rehabilitation for the aged ought to be going), Tokyo: Kōsei Rōdō Shō homepage: http//www.mhlw.go.jp/ahingi/2004/3/s033-3.html (accessed in 2004).

Koskinen, S., and T. Martelin, (1994), 'Why are socioeconomic mortality differences smaller among women than men?' *Social Science & Medicine*, 38(1), pp. 1385–96.

Kosteniuk, J. G. and H. D. Dickinson (2003), 'Tracing the social gradient in the health of Canadians: Primary and secondary determinants', *Social Science & Medicine*, 57(2), pp. 263–76.

Krantz, G. and P. Ostergren (2004), 'Does it make sense in a coherence way? Determinants of sense of coherence in Swedish women 40 to 50 years of age', *International Journal of Behavioral Medicine*, 11(1), pp. 18–26.

Krause, N., B. Ingersoll-Dayton, J. Liang and H. Sugisawa (1999), 'Religion, social support, and health among the Japanese elderly', *Journal of Health and Social Behavior,* 40, pp. 405–21.

Krishna, A. and E. Shrader (2002), 'The social capital assessment tool: Design and implementation' in C. Crootaert and T. V. Bastelaer (eds), *Understanding and Measuring Social Capital*, Washington D.C.: World Bank, pp. 17–40.

Kuh, D. and Y. Ben-Shlomo (2004), *A Life Course Approach to Chronic Disease Epidemiology*, 2nd edition, Oxford: Oxford University Press.

Kumagai S., H. Shibata, H. Yukawa *et al.* (2005), 'Predictors of nutritional decline in well-nourished community-living elderly people', *Japanese Journal of Nutrition and Dietetics*, 63(2), pp. 83–8.

Kurihara, R. and K. Katsura (2003), 'Hitorigurashi kōreisha no tojikomori yobō oyobi shakai katsudō eno sanka ni kansuru yōin (Factors affecting the lifestyle of the elderly who live alone)', *Nihon Nouson Igakukai zasshi* (Journal of the Japanese Association of Rural Medicine), 52, pp. 65–79.

Lantz, P. M., J. S. House, J. M. Lepkowski *et al.* (1998), 'Socioeconomic factors, health behaviors, and mortality: Results from a nationally representative prospective study of US adults', *Journal of the American Medical Association,* 279, pp. 1703–8.

Lawton, M. P. (1975), 'The Philadelphia Geriatric Center Morale Scale: A revision', *Journal of Gerontology,* 30(1), pp. 85–9.

Lawton, M. P. (1982), 'Environment and other determinants of well-being in older people', *Gerontologist*, 23, pp. 349–55.

Levin, K. A. and A. H. Leyland (2005), 'Urban/rural inequalities in suicide in Scotland, 1981–1999', *Social Science & Medicine*, 60, pp. 2877–90.

Lochner, K. A., I. Kawachi, R. T. Brennan *et al.* (2003), 'Social capital and neighborhood mortality rates in Chicago', *Social Science & Medicine*, 56, pp. 1797–1805.

Lorant, V., D. Deliège, W. Eaton, A. Robert, P. Philippot and M. Ansseau (2003), 'Socioeconomic inequalities in depression: A meta-analysis', *American Journal of Epidemiology*, 57, pp. 98–102.

Lundberg, O. (1997), 'Childhood conditions, sense of coherence, social class and adult ill health: Exploring their theoretical and empirical relations', *Social Science & Medicine*, 44(6), pp. 821–31.

Lynch J., and G. Kaplan (2000), 'Socioeconomic position', in L. F. Berkman and I. Kawachi (eds), *Social Epidemiology*, Oxford: Oxford University Press, pp. 13–35.

Macintyre, S. and A. Ellaway (2000), 'Ecological approaches: Rediscovering the role of the physical and social environment', in L. F. Berkman and I. Kawachi (eds), *Social Epidemiology*, Oxford: Oxford University Press, pp. 332–48.

Macintyre, S. and A. Ellaway (2003), 'Neighborhoods and health: An overview' in I. Kawachi and L. F. Berkman (eds), *Neighborhoods and Health*, New York: Oxford University Press, pp. 65–111.

Mackenbach, J. P. (2006), *Health inequalities: Europe in profile. An independent, expert report commissioned by the UK Presidency of the EU*, London: Department of Health.

Marcenes, W., J. G. Steele, A. Sheiham *et al.* (2003), 'The relationship between dental status, food selection, nutrient intake, nutritional status, and body mass index in older people', *Cadernos de Saúde Pública*, 19(3), pp. 809–16.

Marcure, A. M. (1985), 'The danka system', *Monumenta Nipponica*, 40, pp. 39–67.

Marmot, M. (1997), 'Inequality, deprivation and alcohol use', *Addiction*, 92 (supplement 1), pp. S13–S20.

Mendes de Leon, C. F., D. T. Gold, T. A. Glass *et al.* (2001), 'Disability as a function of social network and support in elderly African Americans and Whites', *Journal of Gerontology*, 56B(3), pp. S179–90.

Meyer, K. and L. Lobao (2003), 'Economic hardship, religion and mental health during the Midwestern farm crisis', *Journal of Rural Studies*, 19, pp. 139–55.

Middelkoop, H. A., D. A. Smilde-van del Doel, A. K. Neven, H. A. Kamphuisen and C. P. Springer (1996), 'Subjective sleep characteristics of 1,485 males and females aged 50–93: Effects of sex and age, and factors related to self-evaluated quality of sleep', *Journal of Gerontology Series A: Biological Sciences and Medical Sciences*, 51, pp. 108–15.

Miller, S. M. (1992), 'Conventional religious behavior in modern Japan: A service industry perspective', *Journal for Scientific Study of Religion*, 31, pp. 207–14.

Mindanik, L. T. *et al.* (1995), 'The effect of retirement on mental health and health behaviors: The Kaiser Permanente Retirement Study', *Journal of Gerontology*, Series B, 50B, S59–S61.

Ministry of Education (1959) *Wagakuni no kyōiku suijun* (The standard of education in Japan).

Ministry of Education (1962) *Nihon no seichō to kyōiku* (Education and growth in Japan). An abridged translation is available as *Japan's Growth and Education* at http://www.mext.go.jp/b_menu/hakusho/html/hpae196301/index/html (accessed 17 July 2009).

Ministry of Education (1972), *Gakusei hyakunen-shi* (A history of 100 years of Japan's education system). *Shiryō-hen* (Statistics and charts). An abridged translation is available as *Japan's Modern Educational System: A History of the First Hundred Years* at http://www.mext.go.jp/b_menu/hakusho/html/hpbz1981031/index/html (accessed 17 July 2009).

Ministry of Health and Welfare (2000), *Kenkō Nihon nijyū-ichi* (Healthy Japan 21), Tokyo: Kōsei Shō.

Ministry of Health and Welfare, Health Policy Bureau, Dental Health Division (ed.) (1999), *Heisei 11-nen shikaikan jittai chōsa hōkoku* (Report on the national survey of dental diseases in 1999), Tokyo: Oral Health Association of Japan.

Ministry of Health, Labour and Welfare (2002), *Long-term Care Insurance in Japan*, http://www.mhlw.go.jp/english/topics/elderly/care/index.html (accessed on 30 June 2009).

Ministry of Health, Labour and Welfare (2005), *Heisei 17-nen shika shikkan jittai chōsa no gaiyō* (Summary report on the 2005 national dental health survey), http://www.mhlw.go.jp/topics/2007/01/tp0129-1.html

Ministry of Health, Labour and Welfare (2008) *Kōsei rōdō hakusho* (Annual health, labour and welfare report). Tokyo: Gyōsei.

Ministry of Health, Labour and Welfare (2008), *Average life expectancy in Japan*, http://www.mhlw.go.jp/toukei/saikin/hw/life/life07/index.html (accessed on 30 June 2009).

Ministry of Health, Labour and Welfare, Health and Welfare Bureau for the Elderly (2005), *Dai 4 kai kaigo yobō saabisu hyōka kenkyū iinkai July 20 shiryō* (Material for the 4th conference of the Evaluation and Research Committee on Long-term Care Prevention Services held on 20 July).

Ministry of Health, Labour and Welfare, Research Review Committee, Institute for Health Economics and Policy (2004), *Kateinai ni okeru kōreisha ni kansuru chōsa: Heizei 5 nendo rōjin hoken kenkō zōshin to jigyō* (Research on elder abuse in the home: FY1993 Elderly health promotion project).

Ministry of Health, Labour and Welfare, Statistics and Information Department (2003), *Heisei jūgo nendo jinkō dōtai chōsa* (Survey of population trends, 2003) (accessed on 21 December 2004 from http://www/mhlw.go.jp/toukei/saikin/hw/hinkou/kakutei03/index.html)

Ministry of Internal Affairs and Communications, Statistics Bureau (2005), *Tōkei de miru shi-ku-machi-mura no sugata 2005* (Statistical observations of *shi, ku, machi, mura* (municipalities) in 2005), http://www.stat.go.jp/data/ssds/5b.htm

Mitsuhashi Y., R. Kishi, T. Eguchi *et al.* (2003), 'Factors associated with participation in medical checkups of the elderly at home: Comparison of 3 regions with different social background', *Nippon kōshū eisei zasshi* (Japanese journal of public health), 50(1), pp. 49–61.

Miyata, Kakuko and Shinji Nozawa (2002), 'Atarashii media to sōsharu sapōto kenkyū (A study of the new media and social support)', *Kenkyūjo nenpō (Meiji Gakuin Daigaku shakai gakubu fuzoku kenkyūjo)* (Research bulletin of the Institute of Sociology and Social Work, Meiji Gakuin University), 32, pp. 87–94.

Moore, P. J., N. E. Adler, D. R. Williams and J. S. Jackson (2002), 'Socioeconomic status and health: The role of sleep', *Psychosomatic Medicine*, 64(2), pp. 337–44.

Murata, Chiyoe, Katsunori Kondō, Hiroshi Hirai, Yukinobu Ichida and Toshiyuki Ojima (2008), 'Association between depression and socio-economic status among community-dwelling elderly in Japan: The Aichi Gerontological Evaluation Study (AGES)', *Health and Place*, 14, pp. 406–14.

Murata, Chiyoe, T. Kondō, K. Tamakoshi, *et al.* (2006), 'Determinants of self-rated health: Could health status explain the association between self-rated health and mortality?' *Archives Gerontology Geriatrics*, 43(3), pp. 369–80.

Murata, Chiyoe, Tetsuji Yamada, Chia-Ching Chen, Toshiyuki Ojima, Hiroshi Hirai and Katsunori Kondō (2010), 'Barriers to Health Care among the Elderly in Japan', *International Journal of Environmental Research and Public Health,* 7, pp. 1330–41.

Naikaku Kokumin Seikatsu-kyoku (2003), *Sōsharu kyapitaru: Yutakana ningen kankei to shimin katsudō no kōjunkan omotomete* (Social capital: In search of a virtuous circle of full interpersonal relationships and civic activity), Tokyo: Kokuritsu Insatsukyoku.

Nakamura, H., Y. Ogawa, H. Nagase *et al.* (2003), 'Kitsuen kōdō ni kanren suru sutoresu to sense of coherence (SOC): Seikatsu shūkan to shinri teki yōin omochiita seijun hanbetsu kaiseki (Stress associated with smoking behavior and sense of coherence (SOC): A canonical discriminant analysis using lifestyles and psychological factors)', *Journal of Physical Fitness, Nutrition and Immunology*, 13(1), pp. 23–30.

Nakanishi N., K. Nagano, Y. Hino *et al.* (1998), 'Chiiki kōreisha no soshaku nōryoku no teika ni kanren suru yōin to seimei yogo ni kansuru kenkyū (Study of factors related to masticatory disability and life prognosis in community-dwelling elderly people)', *Journal of Health and Welfare Statistics* 45(13), pp. 19–24.

Nakata, H., K. Takasaki and M. Ohchi (2002), 'Chiiki zaitaku kōreisha ni okeru kaigo yobō katsudō ni kansuru kenkyū (Activities for the prevention of bedridden in the elderly: Focused on the factor of preliminary housebound behavior)', *Nihon zaitaku care gakkaishi* (Journal of the Japan Academy of Home Care), 6, pp. 61–9.

Nakaya, T. and D. Dorling (2005), 'Geographical inequalities of mortality by income in two developed island countries: A cross-national comparison of Britain and Japan', *Social Science & Medicine*, 60, pp. 2865–75.

Nakazato, Katsuharu *et al.* (2000), 'Chūkōnenki ni okeru shokugyō seikatsu kara no kanzenna intai to shitsugyō eno shinriteki tekiō purosesu (The process of psychological adaptation to complete retirement from working life and unemployment at middle age and old age)', *Rōnen shakai kagaku* (Japanese journal of gerontology), 22(1), pp. 37–45.

National Center for Health (1998), *Statistics: Health, United States, 1998 (With socioeconomic status and health chartbook),* Hyattsville, MD: US National Center for Health Statistics.

National Center on Sleep Disorders Research and Office of Prevention Education and Control (1998), *Insomnia: Assessment and Management in Primary Care*, National Institute of Health, Publication No.98–4088, Bethesda, MD: US National Institute of Health.

Neumark, Y. D., G. Rahav and D. H. Jaffe (2003), 'Socio-economic status and binge drinking in Israel', *Drug and Alcohol Dependence*, 69, pp. 15–21.

Newman, D. K. and D. A. Smith (1989), 'Incontinence in elderly homebound patients', *Holistic Nursing Practice*, 4, pp. 52–60.

NHK Broadcasting Culture Research Institute (2005), *2005-nen kokumin seikatsu jikan chōsa hōkokusho* (2005 Japanese people's life hours survey report), http://www.nhk.or.jp/bunken/research/life/life_20060210.pdf (accessed on 30 June 2009).

Nilsson, B., L. Holmgren, B. Stegmayr *et al.* (2003), 'Sense of coherence-stability over time and relation to health, disease, and psychosocial changes in general population: A longitudinal study', *Scandinavian Journal of Public Health*, 31, pp. 297–304.

Nishi, Nobuo (2006), 'Shakai keizai yōin no tajū reberu bunseki (Multilevel analysis of socio-economic factors)' in Norito Kawakami, Yasuki Kobayashi *et al.* (eds), *Shakai kakusa to kenkō: Shakai ekigaku kara no apurōchi* (Social inequalities and health: Socio-epidemiological approach), Tokyo: Tokyo Daigaku Shuppankai.

Nobe, M. (1999), 'Chihō toshi ni sumu kōrei josei no shukan-teki kōfuku kan (The sense of well-being of elderly women in a medium-size Japanese city)', *Riron to hōhō* (Sociological theory and methods), 14, pp. 105–23.

Noguchi, Yūji (1991), 'Kōreisha no sōsharu sapōto (Social support for the aged)', *Shakai rōnengaku* (Social gerontology), 34, pp. 37–48.

Noguchi, Yūji and Hidehiro Sugisawa (1998), 'Shakaiteki chūtai to kenkō (Social ties and health)' in Hajime Orimo (ed.), *Shin rōnengaku* (New gerontology), Tokyo: Tokyo Daigaku Shuppankai, pp. 1343–8.

Nohara, Masaru, Toshiyuki Onoda, and Akira Okayama (2003), 'Jisatsu no chiiki shuseki to sono yōin ni kansuru kenkyū (Research on factors affecting the regional record of suicide)', *Kōsei no shihyō* (Journal of health and welfare statistics), 50(6), pp. 17–23.

OECD (2003) *Ageing and employment policies: Japan*. Paris, OECD Publishing.

OECD (2004), *Ageing and Employment Policies: Japan*, Paris: OECD Publishing.

OECD (2005), *OECD in Figures 2005: Health Status table*, http://ocde.p4.siteinternet.com/publications/doifiles/012005061T003.xls

OECD (2005), *Sekai no iryō seido kaikaku: Shitsu no yoi kōritsuteki na iryō shisutemu ni mukete* (The OECD health project: Towards high-performing health systems), translated by Tetsuya Aman, Tokyo: Akashi Shoten, pp. 56–9.

Ogg, J., and G. Bennett (1992) 'Elder abuse in Britain', *British Medical Journal*, 305, pp. 998–9.

Okada, Y. (1977), *Nihon shi shō hyakka: Jinja* (Japanese history handbook: Shinto shrines), Tokyo: Tōkyōdō Shuppan.

Okado, Junichi, Gyokuren Tomoyama, Naoko Sakurai *et al.* (2004), *Kōreisha ni okeru shakaiteki nettowāku to seimei yogo tono kanrensei: Kōreisha no kenkō tokusei to sono iji yōin* (Correlation between social networks and life expectancy in the aged: Characteristics and factors of the health of the aged), Tokyo: Tokyo Toritsu Daigaku Shuppankai, pp. 163–79.

Okubo, S., T. Saitou, H. Lee *et al.* (2005), 'Kaigo yobōjigyō eno dansei sanka ni kanrensuru jigyō yōin no yobiteki kentō (Correlates to male participation in disability prevention programs for the elderly)', *Nippon kōshū eisei zasshi* (Japanese journal of public health), 52, pp. 1050–8.

Okumiya K., T. Wada, M. Ishine *et al.* (2005), 'Honpō-chiiki kōreisha no keikatsu kinō (Associated factors for activities of daily living in 3 towns in Japan)', *Nihon rōnen igakkai zasshi* (Japanese journal of geriatrics) 42, pp. 164–6.

Okushima, Shigeru (1997), 'Fukushi komyuniti saihen no tame no saron katsudō (Salon activity for reorganization of the welfare community)', *Gekkan fukushi* (Welfare monthly), 80(13), pp. 36–41.

Oman, D. and D. Reed (1998), 'Religion and mortality among the community-dwelling elderly', *American Journal of Public Health*, 88, pp. 1469–75.

Osaka Elder Abuse Prevention Workgroup (1997), *Kōreisha gyakutai no zenkoku jittai chōsa: Shu to shite hoken / fukushi kikan chōsa yori* (National fact-finding research on elder abuse: Initial main focus on health and welfare institutional research), International Longevity Center, Japan.

Pasternak, R., A. Rosenweig, B. Booth *et al.* (1999), 'Morbidity of homebound versus inpatient elderly psychiatric patients', *International Psychogeriatrics*, 11, pp. 105–6.

Pelton, L. H. (1978) 'Child abuse and neglect: The myth of classlessness', *American Journal of Orthopsychiatry*, 48, pp. 608–17.

Pillemer, K. and D. Finkelhor (1988), 'The prevalence of elder abuse: A random sample survey', *Gerontologist* 28, pp. 51–7.

Podnicks, E. (1992), 'National survey on abuse of the elderly in Canada', *Elder Abuse Neglect*, 4, pp. 5–58.

Poppius, E., L. Tenkanen, M. Hakama *et al.* (2003), 'The sense of coherence, occupation and all-cause mortality in the Helsinki Heart Study', *European Journal of Epidemiology*, 18(5), pp. 389–93.

Portes, A. (1998), 'Social Capital: Its origins and applications in modern sociology', *Annual Review of Sociology*, 24(1), pp. 1–24.

Putnam, R. (1993), *Making Democracy Work; Civic Traditions in Modern Italy*, Princeton: Princeton University Press.

Ragheb, M. G. (1993), 'Leisure and perceived wellness: A field investigation', *Leisure Sciences*, 15, pp. 13–24.

Rasbash, J., F. Steele, W. Browne *et al.* (2004), *A User's Guide to MLwiN version 2.0*: Centre for Multilevel Modeling.

Reitzes, D. C. *et al.* (1996), 'Does retirement hurt well-being? Factors influencing self-esteem and depression among retirees and workers', *The Gerontologist*, 36, pp. 649–56.

Ren, X. S. (1997), 'Marital status and quality of relationships: The impact on health perception', *Social Science & Medicine* 44(2), pp. 241–9.

Richards, K. C., C. Beck, P. S. O'Sullivan and V. M. Shue (2005), 'Effect of individualized social activity on sleep in nursing home residents with dementia', *Journal of the American Geriatrics Society*, 53, pp. 50–7.

Riemann, D. and U. Voderholzer (2003), 'Primary insomnia: A risk factor to develop depression?', *Journal of Affective Disorders*, 76, pp. 255–9.

Rietschlin, J. (1998), 'Voluntary association membership and psychological distress', *Journal of Health and Social Behavior*, 39, pp. 348–55.

Riley, M. W. (1963), *Sociological Research I: A Case Approach*, New York: Harcourt, Brace & World.

Ritchie C. S., K. L. Burgio, J. L. Locher *et al.* (1997), 'Nutritional status of urban homebound older adults', *The American Journal of Clinical Nutrition* 66(4), pp. 815–18.

Roberts, S. A. (1998), 'Community-level socioeconomic status effects on adult health', *Journal of Health and Social Behaviour*, 39, 1, pp. 18–37.

Rose, G. (1992), *The Strategy of Preventive Medicine*: Oxford, Oxford University Press. Japanese translation by K. Sota and H. Tanaka (1998), *Yobō igaku no sutoratejī: Seikatsu shūkanbyō taisaku to kenkō zōshin* (The strategy of preventive medicine: Lifestyle disease prevention and health promotion), Tokyo: Igaku Shoin.

Ross, C. E. and C. Wu (1996), 'Education, age, and the cumulative advantage in health', *Journal of Health and Social Behaviour*, 37, pp. 104–20.

Ross, C. E. and J. Mirowsky (2002), 'Family relationships, social support and subjective life expectancy', *Journal of Health and Social Behavior*, 43, pp. 469–89.

Ross,C. E., J. Mirowsky *et al.* (1990), 'The impact of the family on health: The decade in review', *Journal of Marriage and the Family*, 52(4), pp. 1059–78.

Rotolo, T. (1999), 'Trends in voluntary association participation', *Nonprofit and Voluntary Sector Quarterly*, 28, pp. 199–212.

Rotter, J. B. (1966), 'Generalized expectancies for internal versus external control of reinforcement', *Psychological Monographs*, 80(1), pp. 1–28.

Saitō, Y., Katsunori Kondō, Hiroshi Hirai *et al.* (2007), 'Kankoku ni okeru kōreisha muke chiiki fukushi seisaku keirōdō kara no shisa (A community-based welfare policy for the elderly in Korea: Suggestions from the "KyungRoDang" policy)', *Kaigai shakai hoshō kenkyū* (Review of comparative social security research), 59, pp. 76–84.

Satō, H. and Y. Fukuwatari (1998), '50-dai kinrō sha no kenkō do jiko hyōka ni kanren suru shintai, shinri, shakai-teki yōin (Physical, psychological and social factors affecting the self-rated health of company workers in their fifties)', *Nihon hoken fukushi gakkai shi* (Japanese journal of human sciences of health-social services), 5, pp. 61–70.

Satō, H., S. Satō and K. Yamashita (2002), 'Chiiki zaitaku kōreisha ni okeru katsudō nōryoku to shakai katsudō no kanren-sei (Relationship between competence level and participation in social activities by elderly people living at home)', *Nihon hoken fukushi gakkai shi* (Japanese journal of human sciences of health-social services), 8, pp. 3–15.

Scarmeas, N., G.. Levy, M. X. Tang *et al.* (2001), 'Influence of leisure activity on the incidence of Alzheimer's disease', *Neurology*, 57, 2236–42.

Seeman, T. R., M. L. Bruce and G. J. McAvay (1996), 'Social network characteristics and onset of ADL disability', *Journal of Gerontology*, 51B(4), pp. S191–200.

Seida, Y., A. Yoshihara, Y. Ando *et al.* (2002), 'Two-year cohort study on risk predictors for tooth loss in the community 70-year-old subjects', *Journal of Dentistry*, 52, pp. 663–71.

Sekine, M., T. Chandola, P. Martikainen, D. McGeogphegan, M. Marmot and S. Kagamimori (2006), 'Explaining social inequalities in health by sleep: The Japanese civil servants study', *Journal of Public Health* (Oxford), 28(1), pp. 63–70.

Senior, M., H. Williams and G. Higgs (2000), 'Urban-rural mortality differentials: Controlling for material deprivation', *Social Science & Medicine*, 51, pp. 289–305.

Shakai Hoshō Shingikai Kaigo Hoken Bukai (Committee on Long-Term Care Insurance, Social Security Council) (2004), *Kaigo hoken seido no minaoshi ni kansuru iken* (A vision for long-term care insurance reform), Tokyo: Kosei Rōdōshō.

Sheiham, A., J. G. Steele, W. Marcenes *et al.* (2002), 'The relationship between oral health status and Body Mass Index among older people: A national survey of older people in Great Britain', *British Dental Journal*, 192(12), pp. 703–6.

Sheikh, J. I. and J. A. Yesavage (1986) 'Geriatric Depression Scale (GDS): Recent evidence and development of a shorter version', in Terry L. Brink (ed.) *Clinical Gerontology: A Guide to Assessment and Intervention*, New York: The Haworth Press, pp. 165–73.

Shibata, Hiroshi (2001), *Chūkōnenreisha no shokugyō karano intai katei to kenkō keizai tono kanren ni kansuru kenkyū* (Kōsei rōdō kagaku kenkyūhi hojokin chōju kagaku sōgō kenkyū jigyō sōkatsu kenkyū hōkokusho) (A study of the association between the retirement process of the middle or advanced age people and health and economy (Study Report on Health and Labour Sciences Research Grants: Comprehensive Research on Aging and Health)), Tokyo: Ministry of Health, Labour and Welfare.

Shinkai, S. (2000), 'Kōreisha no tojikomori checklist no teian to sono katsuyō hōhō (Checklist of housebound elderly)', *Seikatsu kyōiku* (Life education), 44, pp. 12–18.

Shinkai, S., K. Fujita, Y. Fujiwara *et al.* (2005), 'Chiiki kōreisha ni okeru type betsu tojikomori no shutsugen hindo to sono tokuchō (Prevalence and characteristics of different types of homeboundness among community-living older adults)', *Nippon kōshū eisei zasshi* (Japanese journal of public health), 52, pp. 443–55.

Shinkai, S., K. Fujita, Y. Fujiwara *et al.* (2005), 'Chiiki kōreisha ni okeru taipu betsu tojikomori no yogo ni nenkan no tuiseki kenkyū (Prognosis of different types of homeboundness among community-living older adults:

Two-year prospective study)', *Nippon kōshū eisei zasshi* (Japanese journal of public health), 52, pp. 627–38.

Shinkai S., S. Watanabe, S. Kumagai *et al.* (2001), 'Incidence, prognosis and risk factors for the home-bound in a community elderly population', *Nippon kōshū eisei zasshi* (Japanese journal of public health), 48(9), pp. 741–52.

Smith, P. M., F. C. Breslin and D. E. Beaton (2003), 'Questioning the stability of sense of coherence: The impact of socio-economic status and working conditions in the Canadian population', *Social Psychiatry and Psychiatric Epidemiology*, 38, pp. 475–84.

Smits, C. H. M., D. J. H. Deeg and R. J. Bosscher (1995), 'Well-being and control in older persons: The predictions of well-being from control measures', *International Journal of Aging and Human Development*, 40(3), pp. 237–51.

Social Exclusion Unit (2006), *A Sure Start to Later Life: Ending Inequalities for Older People*, A Social Exclusion Unit Final Report, Office of the Deputy Prime Minister, London, UK.

Soini, H., P. Routasalo, H. Lagstrom *et al.* (2004), 'Characteristics of Mini-Nutritional Assessment in elderly home-care patients', *European Journal of Nutrition*, 58, pp. 64–70.

Sōmuchō, Tōkei-kyoku (Bureau of Statistics, Ministry of Internal Affairs and Communication) (2004), *Tōkei de miru shi-ku-chō-son no sugata 2004* (A statistical overview of Japan's municipalities 2004), Tokyo: Nihon Tōkei Kyōkai.

Steinbach, U. (1992), 'Social networks, institutionalization, and mortality among elderly people in the United States', *Journal of Gerontology*, 47, pp. 183–90.

Steiner, A., K. Raube, A. E. Stuck *et al.* (1996), 'Measuring psychosocial aspects of well-being in older community residents: Performance of four short scales', *Gerontologist*, 36(1), pp. 54–62.

Steinmetz, S. K. (1998), *Duty Bound Elder Abuse and Family Care*, Newbury Park: Sage Publications.

Stepnowski, C. J. Jr. and S. Ancoli-Israel (2008), 'Sleep and its disorders in seniors', *Sleep Medicine in Clinical Practice*, 3(2), pp. 281–93.

Steptoe, A. and M. Marmot (2002), 'The role of psychobiological pathways in socio-economic inequalities in cardiovascular disease', *European Heart Journal*, 23, pp. 13–25.

Stuck, A. E., J. M. Walthert, T. Nikolaus, C. J. Būla, C. Hohmann and J. C. Beck (1999), 'Risk factors for functional status decline in community-living elderly people: A systematic literature review', *Social Science & Medicine*, 48, pp. 445–69.

Subramanian, S. V. (2003), 'Multilevel methods for public health research' in I. Kawachi and L. F. Berkman (eds), *Neighborhoods and Health*, New York: Oxford University Press, pp. 65–111.

Subramanian, S. V., I. Kawachi and B. P. Kennedy (2001), 'Does the state you live in make a difference? Multilevel analysis of self-rated health in the U.S.', *Social Science & Medicine*, 53(1), pp. 9–19.

Subramanian, S. V., K. A. Lochner and I. Kawachi (2003), 'Neighborhood differences in social capital: A compositional artifact or a contextual construct?', *Health & Place*, 9(1), pp. 33–44.

Sugihara, Y. (2004), 'Chiiki ni okeru tentō tojikomori no risk yōin to kainyū kenkyū (Risk factor and intervention study of falls and housebound behavior)', *Rōnen seishin igaku zasshi* (Japanese journal of geriatric psychiatry), 5, pp. 26–35.

Sugisawa, Atsuko and Hidehiro Sugisawa (1998), 'Kenkōdo jiko hyōka ni kansuru kenkyū no tenkai: Beikoku no kenkyū jirei o chūshin ni (The development of self-assessments of health: The situation in America)', in Kyōichi Sonoda and Chieko Kawada (eds) *Kenkōkan no tenkan: Atarashii kenkō riron no tenkai* (The health revolution: New developments in the theories of health), Tokyo: Tokyo Daigaku Shuppan Kai, pp. 73–83.

Sugisawa, Atsuko *et al.* (1997), 'Rōnenki ni okeru shokugyō karano intai ga seishinteki kenkō to shakaiteki kenkō ni oyobosu eikyō (The impacts of retirement in later life on mental health and social health)', *Nippon kōshū eisei zasshi* (Japanese journal of public health), 44(2), pp. 123–30.

Sugisawa, H. (1994), 'Kōreisha ni okeru shakai-teki tōgō to seimei yogo to no kankei (Social integration and mortality in Japanese elderly)', *Nippon kōshū eisei zasshi* (Japanese journal of public health), 41, pp. 131–9.

Sugisawa, H. and H. Shibata (2000), 'Zenki oyobi kōki kōreisha ni okeru shintaiteki, shinriteki, shakaiteki shigen to seishin kenkō to no kanren (Associations between physical, psychological and social resources and mental health in the early and late elderly)', *Nippon kōshū eisei zasshi* (Japanese journal of public health), 47, pp. 589–601.

Sugisawa, H., J. Liang and X. Liu (1994), 'Social networks, social support, and mortality among older people in Japan', *Journal of Gerontology*, 49, pp. S3–13.

Sugisawa, H., Y. Nakatani, D. Maeda *et al.* (1994), 'Kōreisha ni okeru shakai-teki tōgō to nichijō seikatsu dōsa nōryoku no yogo to no kankei (Social integration and change in activities of daily living in Japanese elderly)', *Nippon kōshū eisei zasshi* (Japanese journal of public health), 41, pp. 975–86.

Sugisawa, Hidehiro and Atsuko Sugisawa (1995), 'Kenkōdo jiko hyōka ni kansuru kenkyū no tenkai' (Development of research on self-rated health in the United States), *Nippon kōshū eisei zasshi* (Japanese journal of public health), 42(6), pp. 366–78.

Sugiyama, M., A. Nishimura, K. Takamoto (2000), 'Tei eiyō jōtai yobō no tame no asesumento – jiko chekku hyō – no katsuyōhō: Herusu asesumento manyuaru (Assessment for preventing poor nutritional status: Use of self-check list)', *Health Assessment Manual*, Research Institute of Health Science, Inc., pp. 164–179.

Sukegawa, T., M. Itoga, H. Seno, S. Miura, T. Inagaki, W. Saito, J. Uegaki, T. Miyaoka, I. Momose, K. Kasahara, R. Oshiro, Y. Shimizu, R. Yasukawa, T. Mihara, T. Maeda, S. Mizuno, K. Tsubouchi, Y. Inami and J. Horiguchi (2003), 'Sleep disturbances and depression in the elderly in Japan', *Psychiatry and Clinical Neurosciences*, 57(3), pp. 265–70.

Suominen, S., R. Gould, J. Ahvenainen *et al.* (2005), 'Sense of coherence and disability pensions: A nationwide, register based prospective population study of 2196 adult Finns', *Journal of Epidemiology and Community Health*, 59(6), pp. 455–9.

Surtees, P., N. Wainwright, R. Luben *et al.* (2003), 'Sense of coherence and mortality in men and women in the EPIC-Norfolk United Kingdom Prospective cohort study', *American Journal of Epidemiology*, 158(12), pp. 1202–9.

Suzuki, M. (2003), *Tentō yobō: Risuku asesumento to kea puran* (Preventing falls: Risk assessment and care planning), Tokyo: Igaku Shoin.

Suzuki, T. (2001), 'Kōreisha no tento jiko (Accidental falls among older citizens)', *Journal of Clinical Rehabilitation*, 10, pp. 955–66.

Szreter, S. and M. Woolcock (2004), 'Health by association? Social capital, social theory, and the political economy of public health', *International Journal of Epidemiology*, 33, pp. 650–67.

Takahashi, M., S. Shibazaki and M. Nagai (2003), 'Rōjin kurabu kaiin no shakai katsudō reberu no genjō (Characteristics of social activities of the elderly who belong to senior citizens' clubs)', *Nippon kōshū eisei zasshi* (Japanese journal of public health), 50, pp. 970–9.

Takasaki, K. *et al.* (1999), 'Rōjin gyakutai no yobō to shien ni kansuru kenkyū (3): Jittai chōsa to denwa sōdan katsudō o chūshin ni (Research on the prevention of elder abuse and support (3): Focus on fact-finding research and telephone counselling)', *Rōjin gyakutai to shien ni kansuru kenkyū: Rōjin gyakutai kenkyū purojekuto hōkokusho* (Research on elder abuse and support: Elder abuse research project report). Nursing of the elderly workshop, Health Department, Medical Faculty, Tokyo Medical and Dental University.

Takasaki, K., Y. Taniguchi, A. Sasaki *et al.* (1998), *'Rōjin gyakutai' no yobō to shien kōreisha / kazoku / sasaete o musubu* (Elder abuse prevention and support: Linking up the elderly, their families and supports), Tokyo, Japanese Nursing Association Publishing Company.

Takayama, N. (1994) 'Household asset and wealth holdings in Japan', in Y. Noguchi and D.A. Wise (eds) *Aging in the United States and Japan: Economic Trends*, Chicago: Chicago University Press.

Takayama, T., Y. Asano, Y. Yamazaki *et al.* (1999), 'Sutoresufuru na seikatsu dekigoto ga shubi ikkan kankaku (Sense of coherence: SOC) to seishin kenkō ni oyobosu eikyō (Effects of stressful life events on sense of coherence (SOC) and mental health)', *Nippon kōshū eisei zasshi* (Japanese journal of public health), 46, pp. 965–76.

Takeda, Tokunori and Katsunori Kondō (2006), 'Chiiki kyojū kōreisha no rippōtai mosha to shinri-shakaimen no tokuchō: Ninchi kinō shōgai no sukuriininguhō toshiteno kanōsei (A cube copy in elderly people and a characteristics of psycho-social life: The possibility of screening for cognitive dysfunction)', *Sōgō rihabiriteishon* (Comprehensive rehabilitation), 34, pp. 377–8.

Takeda, Tokunori, Katsunori Kondō, Kiyoko Yoshii, *et al.* (2005), 'Kyotaku kōreisha no shumi Ikigai: Sagyō ryōhō niyoru kaigo yobō e no tegakari to shite (Leisure activities and IKIGAI in elderly people: A clue to the preventive approaches of occupational therapists)', *Sōgō rihabiriteshon*, (Comprehensive rehabilitation), 33, pp. 469–76.

Takeda, Tokunori, Katsunori Kondō, Hiroshi Hirai, *et al.* (2007), 'Chiiki zaijū kōreisha no ninchishō hasshō to shinri-shakaiteki sokumen to no kanren (Psychosocial factors as predictors for dementia among community-dwelling older people)', *Sagyō ryōhō* (Occupational therapy), 26, pp. 55–65.

Takeda, Tokunori, Katsunori Kondō and Hiroshi Hirai (2009), 'Shinri shakaiteki inshi ni chūmokushita ninchishō yobō no tame no kainyū kenkyū: Popyurēshon senryaku ni motozuku kainyū puroguramu riron to chūkan autokamu hyōka (A study on interventions for dementia prevention focusing on psychosocial factors: Intervention program theory based on population strategy and interim outcome evaluation)', *Sagyō ryōhō* (Occupational therapy), 28 (2), pp. 178–86.

Takeda, Tokunori, Katsunori Kondō, Hiroshi Hirai, and Chiyoe Murata (2008), 'Chiiki zaijū kōreisha no ninchishō hasshō to shinri-shakaiteki sokumen to no kanren (Socio-psychological factors and the incidence of officially recognized ailments among the aged living in regional Japan), *Sagyō ryōhō* (Occupational therapy)', 26(1), pp. 55–65, with some revisions in 27(2), p. 212.

Takekuma, S. and S. Shono (2006) 'Kateinai kōreisha gyakutai ni kansuru chukōnensha no ishiki (Middle-aged and elderly people's perceptions of domestic elder abuse)', Proceedings from the 3rd Osaka Conference of the Japan Academy for the Prevention of Elder Abuse, Tokyo, Japan Academy for the Prevention of Elder Abuse.

Takeo, Y. (2004), 'Kōreisha kaigo yobō kenkōzukuri jigyō eno sanka ikiiki salon to chair exercise (Participation in care prevention and health promotion programs: "Ikiiki Salon" and chair exercise)', *Sportsmedicine*, 6, pp. 22–4.

Takeuchi, T. (1984), 'Netakiri rōjin no seiin tojikomori shōkōgun ni tsuite (Genesis of bedridden elderly: Housebound syndrome)', *Rōjin hoken no kihon to tenkai* (Basis and expansion of Elderly Health Care), pp. 48–52.

Takkinen, S., and I. Ruoppila (2001), 'Meaning in life as an important component of functioning in old age', *International Journal of Aging and Human Development*, 53(3), pp. 211–31.

Tamakoshi, A., R. Aoki, Y. Ōno *et al.* (1995), 'Kōreisha ni okeru shakai katsudō no jittai (Social activities in the elderly)', *Nippon kōshū eisei zasshi* (Japanese journal of public health), 42, pp. 888–96.

Tanaka, H. and S. Shirakawa (2004), 'Sleep health, lifestyle and mental health in the Japanese elderly: Ensuring sleep to promote a healthy brain and mind', *Journal of Psychosomatic Research*, 56, pp. 465–77.

Tanaka, Kō, Hirotaka Mori and Katsumi Shigemura *et al.* (2002), 'Gifu ken ni okeru jisatsu shibō no tokuchō (Distinguishing features of suicide in Gifu prefecture)', *Kosei no shihyo* (Journal of health and welfare statistics), 49(13), pp. 14–20.

Tang Z., H. Wang, C. Meng *et al.* (1999), 'The prevalence of functional disability in activities of daily living and instrumental activities of daily living among elderly Beijing Chinese', *Archives of Gerontology and Geriatrics*, 29, pp. 115–25.

Tatara, K. and E. Okamoto (2009), 'Japan: Health system review', *Health Systems in Transition*, 11(5), pp. 1–164.

Tatara, T. (1999), 'Kōreisha gyakutai no hassei bōshi oyobi enjo hōhō ni kansuru gakutaiteki kenkyū (Academic research on the prevention of elder abuse and ways of helping)', *Heisei 10 nendo kenkyū hōkokusho* (FY1998 Research Report), Tatara Research Lab, Faculty of Sociology, Shukutoku University.

Tatara, T. (2000), 'Kōreisha gyakutai no hassei bōshi oyobi enjo hōhō ni kansuru gakutaiteki kenkyū (Academic research on the prevention of elder abuse and ways of helping)', *Heisei 11 nendo kenkyū hōkokusho* (FY1999 Research Report), Tatara Research Lab, Faculty of Sociology, Shukutoku University.

Taylor, S. E. and T. E. Seeman (1999), 'Psychosocial Resources and the SES-Heath Relationship', *Annals of the New York Academy of Sciences*, 896, pp. 210–26.

Togari, T. and Y. Yamazaki (2005), '13 kōmoku 5 ken hō ban Sense of Coherence Scale no shinrai sei to inshi teki datō sei no kentō (An analysis of the reliability and factorial validity of the 13-item, 5-point version of Sense of Coherence Scale)', *Minzoku eisei* (Journal of health and human ecology), 71(4), pp. 168–82.

Tokyo-fuu Gakukumu-bu Shakai-kaa (Social Affairs Section, Division for Educational Affairs, Tokyo Metropolitan Government) (1928), *Honfu ni okeru jidōo hogo jigyō* (The administration of care for children in Metropolitan Tokyo), see Part 2 on children who were long-term absentees.

Torigoe, T. (1994), *Chiiki jichikai no kenkyū, burakukai, chōnaikai, jichikai no tenkai katei* (A study of local residents' associations: Development process of community, neighborhood and residents' associations), Kyoto: Minerva Shobō.

Torii, J., S. Miyauchi, T. Sawada (2005), 'Ehime ken no kōreisha no gaishutsu hindo no jittai to sono kanren yōin (Frequency of going out of elderly people in Ehime Prefecture and related factors)', *Shikoku kōshū eisei gakkai zasshi* (Shikoku journal of public health), 50, pp. 126–32.

Tornstam, L. (1989), 'Abuse of the elderly in Denmark and Sweden: Results from a population study', *Journal of Elder Abuse and Neglect* 1(1), pp. 35–44.

Tsunoda, Y. (2006), *Kōreisha gyakutai o fusegu chiiki no nettowaaku: Yokosuka kōreisha gyakutai bōshi jigyō kara* (Community network to prevent elder abuse: From the Yokosuka elder abuse prevention project), Tokyo: Gyosei Corporation.

Tsutsui, Takuma (1998), 'Oiru: Kōreisha mondai to josei mondai (Aging: Old age issues and women's issues)' in Kimio Itō and Kazue Muta (eds), *Jendā de manabu shakaigaku* (Sociology from the perspective of gender), Tokyo: Sekai Shisōsha, pp. 206–23.

Turrell, G., A. Kavanagh and S. V. Subramanian (2006), 'Area variation in mortality in Tasmania (Australia): The contributions of socioeconomic disadvantage, social capital and geographic remoteness', *Health & Place*, 12(3), pp. 291–305.

Uryū, N. (2008), *Shitte okitai wagaya no shūkyō* (All you would like to know about your family's religion), Tokyo: Kadokawa Gakugei Shuppan.

Van Doorslaer, E. and A. M. Jones (2003), 'Inequalities in self-reported health: Validation of a new approach to measurement', *Journal of Health Economics*, 22, pp. 61–87.

Varo, J. J., M. A. Martínez-González, J. de Irala-Estévez *et al.* (2003), 'Distribution and determinants of sedentary lifestyles in the European Union', *International Journal of Epidemiology*, 32, pp. 138–46.

Vaz Fragoso, C. A., and T. M. Gill (2007), 'Sleep complaints in community-living older persons: A multifactorial geriatric syndrome', *Journal of the American Geriatrics Society*, 55, pp. 1853–66.

Veenstra, G. (2002), 'Social capital and health (plus wealth, income inequality and regional health governance)', *Social Science & Medicine*, 54(6), pp. 849–68.

Verbrugge, L. (1979), 'Marital status and health', *Journal of Marriage and the Family*, 41, pp. 267–85.

Verghese. J., R. B. Lipton, M. J. Katz *et al.* (2003), 'Leisure activities and the risk of dementia in the elderly', *New England Journal of Medicine*, 48, pp. 2508–16.

Verheji, R. A. (1996), 'Explaining urban-rural variations in health: A review of interactions between individuals and environment', *Social Science & Medicine*, 42(6), pp. 923–35.

Visvanathan R., C. Macintosh, M. Callary *et al.* (2003), 'The nutritional status of 250 older Australian recipients of domiciliary care services and its association with outcomes at 2 months', *Journal of the American Geriatrics Society*, 51(7), pp. 1007–11.

von dem Knesebeck, O., G. Lüschen, W. C. Cockerham, *et al.* (2003), 'Socioeconomic status and health among the aged in the United States and Germany: A comparative cross-sectional study', *Social Science & Medicine*, 57(9), pp. 1643–52.

Vysniauskaite S., N. Kammona, M. M. Vehkalahti *et al.* (2005), 'Number of teeth in relation to oral health behaviour in dentate elderly patients in Lithuania', *Gerodontology*, 22(1), pp. 44–51.

Wagstaff, A. (2002), 'Poverty and health sector inequalities', *Bulletin of the World Health Organization*, 80, pp. 97–105.

Wang, H. X., A. Karp, B. Winblad *et al.* (2002), 'Late-life engagement in social and leisure activities is associated with a decreased risk of dementia: A longitudinal study from the Kungsholmen Project', *American Journal of Epidemiology*, 155, pp. 1081–7.

Wardle, J., M. Farrell, M. Hillsdon *et al.* (1999), 'Smoking, drinking, physical activity and screening uptake and health inequalities', in D. Gordon, D. Shaw, D. Dorling *et al.* (eds.), *Inequalities in health: The evidence*, Bristol: The Policy Press, pp. 213–39.

Watanabe, M., T. Watanabe, T. Matsuura *et al.* (2003), 'Kihonteki nichijō dōsa no jiritsu shiteiru chiiki kōreisha no tojikomori jōtaizō to sono kanren yōin (Housebound state of community dwelling elderly people who were independent of instrumental activities of daily living and related factors)', *Osaka Ika Daigaku zasshi* (Journal of Osaka Medical College), 62, pp. 24–32.

Watanabe, Y. (2005), '(Tokushū) Kōreisha gyakutai bōshi no chiiki shisutemu zukuri, kuni no torikumi: Kōreisha gyakutai no genjō to kongo no kadai ((Special Issue) National initiative to create a community system for the prevention of elder abuse: The current state of elder abuse and future issues)', *Community Care*, 7(2), pp. 10–37.

West, J., J. Hippisley-Cox, C. A. Coupland *et al.* (2004), 'Do rates of hospital admission for falls and hip fracture in elderly people vary by socio-economic status?', *Public Health*, 118, pp. 576–81.

White, J. M. (1992), 'Marital status and well-being in Canada', *Journal of Family Issues*, 13(3), pp. 390–409.

WHO (2003), 'The World Oral Health Report 2003: Continuous improvement of oral health in the 21st century: The approach of the WHO Global Oral Health Program', *Community Dentistry and Oral Epidemiology* (Supplement 1), pp. 3–24.

WHO (2004), *Life Tables for WHO Member States*, http://www.who.int/whr/2004/annex/topic/en/annex_4_en.pdf (accessed on 30 June 2009).

Wildman, J. (2003), 'Income related inequalities in mental health in Great Britain: Analyzing the causes of health inequality over time', *Journal of Health Economics*, 22, pp. 295–312.

Wilkinson, R. G. (2000), *Unhealthy societies: The afflictions of inequality*, London: Routledge.

Williams, D. R., D. T. Takeuchi *et al.* (1992), 'Marital status and psychiatric disorders among blacks and whites', *Journal of Health and Social Behavior*, 33, pp. 140–58.

Wilson, R. S., C. F. Mendes De Leon, L. L. Barnes *et al.* (2002), 'Participation in cognitively stimulating activities and risk of incident Alzheimer's disease', *Journal of the American Medical Association*, 287(6), pp. 742–8.

Winkelmann, L. and R. Winkelmann (1998), 'Why are the unemployed so unhappy? Evidence from panel data', *Economica*, 65, pp. 1–15.

Wynne, R. J. and D. L. Groves (1995), 'Life span approach to understanding coping styles of elderly', *Education*, 115, pp. 448–55.

Yamazaki, Y. (1999), 'Kenkō e no atarashii mikata o rironka shita kenkō seisei-ron to kenkō hoji nōryoku gainen SOC (Theory of a new view on health: Salutogenesis and SOC, a concept of health maintaining ability), *Quality Nursing*, 5(10), pp. 825–32.

Yamazaki, Y. (2003), 'Sutoresu no shinkō to bōshi no katei tettei bunseki (A thorough analysis of the process of progress and prevention of stress)', in Nihonjin no Sutoresu Jittai Chōsa Iinkai (Committee for Survey of Stress Conditions in Japanese People) (ed.), *NHK gendai Nihonjin no sutoresu* (NHK: Stress in modern Japanese people), Tokyo: Nihon Hōsō Shuppan Kyōkai, pp. 177–200.

Yasumura, S. (2006), *Tojikomori yobō shien koukatekina kaigo yobō no tenkai ni mukete* (Housebound prevention: Effective care prevention), Tokyo: Chūō Hōki Shuppan.

Yesavage, J. A., T. L. Brink, T. L. Rose *et al.* (1983), 'Development and validation of a geriatric depression screening scale: A preliminary report', *Journal of Psychiatric Research*, 17(1), pp. 37–49.

Yokoseki, Manami, Katsunori Kondō and Hiroaki Sugimoto (2006), 'Tokubetsu yōgo rōjin hōmu nyūsho taikisha no jittai ni kansuru chōsa (Survey of the situaion of those awaiting admittance to a home with special aged care)', *Shakai fukushigaku* (Study of social welfare), 47, pp. 59–69.

Yokoyama, H., H. Haga, S. Yasumura *et al.* (2005), 'Gishutsu hindo no hikui kōreisha no tokuchō ni kansuru kenkyū jiritsudo no sa ni chakumoku shite (Study on characteristics of house-bound elderly with fewer outings: From the difference in the level of ADL)', *Rōnen shakai kagaku* (Japanese journal of gerontology), 26, pp. 424–37.

Yoshida M., T. Nakamoto, Y. Satō *et al.* (1997), 'Ha no sōshitsu to seikatsu no manzoku-kan (The influence of the extent of missing teeth on the satisfaction of daily living for elderly people)', *Japanese Journal of Gerontology*, 11(3), pp. 174–80.

Yoshihiko, K. (1987), *Rōjin gyakutai* (Elder abuse), Tokyo: Seiwa Shoten.

Yoshii, Kiyoko (2004), 'Socioeconomic inequality in health among the elderly in Japan: A cohort study (Part 1)', World Federation of Public Health Associations 10th International Congress on Public Health, Abstract p. 95.

Yoshii, Kiyoko, Katsunori Kondō, Junko Kuze, *et al.* (2005), 'Chiiki zaijū kōreisha no shakai kankei no tokuchō to sonogo 2-nenkan no yōkaigo jōtai hassei to no kanrensei (Social relationship factors and risk of care requirement in Japanese elderly),' *Nippon kōshū eisei zasshi* (Japanese journal of public health), 52, pp. 456–67.

Yoshii, Kiyoko, Katsunori Kondō, Hiroshi Hirai *et al.* (2005), 'Kōreisha no shinshin kenkō no shakai keizai kakusa to chiiki kakusa no jittai (Self-rated health status and depression)', *Kōshū eisei* (Public health), 69(2), pp. 145–8 (reproduced as Chapter 2 of this book).

Yoshii, Kiyoko, Katsunori Kondō, Junko Kuze and Kyoko Higuchi (2005), 'Chiiki zaijū kōreisha no shakai kankei no tokuchō to sonogo 2 nenkan no yōkaigo jōtai hassei to no kanrensei (Social relationship factors and risk of care requirement in Japanese elderly)', *Nippon kōshū eisei zasshi* (Japanese journal of public health), 52(6), pp. 456–67.

Yukawa, H. (2004), 'Longitudinal study on dietary intake by the elderly in an urban community', *Japanese Journal of Nutrition and Dietetics*, 62(2), pp. 73–81.

Ziersch, A. M. and F. E. Baum (2004), 'Involvement in civil society groups: Is it good for your health?', *Journal of Epidemiology and Community Health*, 58, pp. 493–500.

Index